D0907037

New Comprehensive Biochemistry

Volume 13

General Editors

A. NEUBERGER
London

L.L.M. van DEENEN
Utrecht

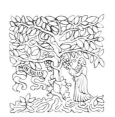

ELSEVIER
AMSTERDAM · NEW YORK · OXFORD

Blood Coagulation

Editors

R.F.A. ZWAAL and H.C. HEMKER

*Biochemistry Department, State University Limburg, Beeldsnijdersdreef 101,
6216 EA   Maastricht (The Netherlands)*

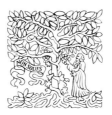

1986
ELSEVIER
Amsterdam · New York · Oxford

ISBN for the series: 0-444-80303-3
ISBN for the volume: 0-444-80794-2

Published by:

Elsevier Science Publishers B.V. (Biomedical Division)
P.O. Box 211
1000 AE Amsterdam
(The Netherlands)

Sole distributors for the U.S.A. and Canada:
Elsevier Science Publishing Company, Inc.
52 Vanderbilt Avenue
New York, NY 10017
(U.S.A.)

Library of Congress Cataloging-in-Publication Data
Main entry under title:
Blood coagulation.

   (New comprehensive biochemistry; v. 13)
   Includes bibliographies and index.
   1. Blood--Coagulation. I. Zwaal, R. F. A. II. Hemker, H. C. III. Series. [DNLM: 1. Blood Coagulation.
W1 NE372F v.13 / WH 310 B6547]
QD415.N48 vol.13 [QP93.5] 574.1'92 s   86-24173
ISBN 0-444-80794-2 (U.S.) [612'.115]

Printed in The Netherlands

Preface

There is no doubt about it; blood coagulation has come of age as a biochemical subject. If you were not aware of this, we hope that this book will convince you. If you knew it already, even though working in a different field, you may feel that biochemical information was too fragmentary and welcome this book for that reason. It is quite remarkable that, despite the flourishing development in the last 10–15 years, the biochemistry of blood coagulation has still remained a rather exotic field. Nevertheless, it has proven to be a very rewarding field for the biochemist to study. Fundamental problems in lipid–protein interaction, in heterogeneous biocatalysis, or in oxidative carboxylation, were recognized and solved in coagulation biochemistry, while many biochemists did not encounter these problems or did not experience situations that made it possible to tackle them. We feel that the solutions found are of interest to every biochemist, particularly to those interested in membranes and in enzymes. Perhaps also the fact that coagulation is a very important chapter of medicine is partly responsible for the reluctance of many biochemists to study it. Indeed two out of three middle aged man in the western world will die from thrombotic disorders, or to put it in simple terms from an excess of thrombin production. This may make the subject so loaded with medical connotations that many biochemists shy off. They should not, if only for scientific reasons.

We have enjoyed editing this book. As most of the workers in the field still know each other it was not too difficult to assemble a list of the best possible authors. We were happy to see that most of them accepted to contribute to this monograph. We were less happy to see that in a single instance we did not receive a manuscript, not even for a considerable time after the deadline. Fortunately, others were quite willing to take their place and on the whole we feel that we have brought together an international set of specialists that cover the subject in a comprehensive and authoritative way. We thought that the editors task should not go as far as to impose much uniformity in style of presentation. We encouraged the authors to present not only the latest news in the field, but also to express — where appropriate — their personal views. We ourselves were quite amused to find well balanced overviews (the majority), besides articles that are clearly written with the intention to stand out the authors' own work; to find strictly scientific reports of what can be considered as established knowledge (again the majority), besides more venturesome articles. Despite — or may be because of — these different approaches we feel that the reader who has finished this book will have obtained a pretty good insight in the biochemistry of blood coagulation as we know it at this moment.

Maastricht
November 1986

R.F.A. Zwaal
H.C. Hemker

R.F.A. Zwaal and H.C. Hemker (Eds.), *Blood Coagulation*
© 1986 Elsevier Science Publishers B.V. (Biomedical Division)

Contents

Chapter 2B
Nonenzymatic cofactors: factor VIII

Chapter 3
Multicomponent enzyme complexes of blood coagulation

Chapter 4
The role of vitamin K in the posttranslational modification of proteins
C. Vermeer (Maastricht)   87

Chapter 5A
Initiation mechanisms: The contact activation system in plasma
Bonno N. Bouma and John H. Griffin (Utrecht and La Jolla)   103

Chapter 5B
Initiation mechanisms: Activation induced by thromboplastin
Bjarne Østerud (Tromsø)   129

Chapter 6
Platelets and coagulation

Chapter 7
Fibrinogen, fibrin and factor XIII

Chapter 8
Fibrinolysis and thrombolysis
D. Collen and H.R. Lijnen (Leuven) 243

R.F.A. Zwaal and H.C. Hemker (Eds.), *Blood Coagulation*
© 1986 Elsevier Science Publishers B.V. (Biomedical Division)

CHAPTER 1

Blood coagulation as a part of the haemostatic system

MARIA C.E. VAN DAM-MIERAS and ANNEMARIE D. MULLER

*Department of Biochemistry, Limburg State University, Beeldsnijdersdreef 101,
6200 MD Maastricht (The Netherlands)*

1. Introduction

Haemostasis is the collective noun for the interrelated processes that cause the cessation of the flow of blood through a damaged vessel wall. The main components of the haemostatic system are: the blood platelets, the humoral coagulation enzymes, the layer of endothelial cells that lines the blood vessels, the subendothelial structures and the smooth muscle cells that support the vessels.

In order to understand the basic mechanisms of haemostasis and the relationships between the different processes involved (see Section 3) it may be useful to start with a short description of the evolution of the haemostatic process.

2. The evolution of the haemostatic system

When in a simple, unicellular organism the plasma membrane is ruptured the flow of cytoplasma is stopped by a 'surface precipitation' reaction. In this surface reaction calcium ions and sulphydryl groups of the membrane are involved [1].

In invertebrates the development of the means for wound closure can be followed [2,3]. In very primitive animals like coelenterates there is no regular circulation of a body fluid and no clotting process is found. When body cavities developed they became populated by amoebocytes; these cells can aggregate at a site of injury. The further evolution of a vascular system was associated with the development of vascular contraction and with the ability of intravascular amoebocytes to extrude long pseudopodia which entrap other cells at the point of vascular injury. Later, amoebocytes evolved which could release a clottable protein to form a coagulum similar to the fibrin meshwork in mammals. This polymerization process is catalysed by a transglutaminase (like factor XIII) [4]. The coagulation process in these invertebrates appears to be a relatively simple process without the cascade system of coagulation enzymes found in mammals. In summary the invertebrate haemostasis consists of an amoebocytic cellular process, a vascoconstrictive process and an extracellular coagulation process. The same three processes can be recognized in vertebrate haemostasis. The fact that human blood platelets contain and secrete fibrinogen, factor V, von Willebrand factor and factor XIII might reflect the evolutionary process [5,6].

Invertebrates are relatively simple organisms in which close connections exist between the defense reactions of the organism, the haemostatic process and the tissue repair mechanisms; the amoebocyte is involved in all these processes. When, for instance, the horseshoe crab (*Limulus polyphemus*) is wounded, the wound is closed by an 'aggregation-like' interaction between the amoebocytes that circulate in the coelomic fluid. When the horseshoe crab is infected by bacteria a 'coagulation-like' defense reaction is seen. The substances involved in this defense reaction are secreted by the amoebocytes [1]. As a result of the reaction the foreign invader is trapped into a meshwork and eliminated by proteolytic, lysosomal enzymes secreted by the amoebocytes. This type of defense mechanism is also found in cells of the monocyte/macrophage series [7,8,9].

In the course of the evolution, organisms became larger and warmblooded. In order to guarantee an efficient blood supply throughout the organism the vertebrates developed a closed vascular system in which the blood flows under a higher pressure. Concomitant with this process specialized haemostatic and immune systems developed; the blood of vertebrates contains different specialized cells that all originate from a pluripotent stem cell [10] (see Table 1).

The nonmammalian vertebrates contain nucleated thrombocytes that activate the clotting process. These cells can be stimulated by thrombin and collagen. The stem cell–thrombocyte system of the nonmammalian vertebrates further evolved to the stem cell–megakaryocyte–thrombocyte system found in mammals and humans [4]. In this system the megakaryocytes in the bone marrow do not divide, but instead the diploid stem cell is transformed into a polyploidic cell by the process of endomitotic polyploidization [11]. The endomitotic polyploidization results in a se-

TABLE 1

The differentiation of human blood cells

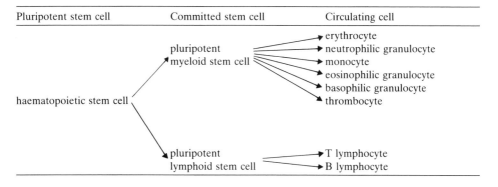

Pluripotent stem cell	Committed stem cell	Circulating cell
	pluripotent myeloid stem cell	erythrocyte
		neutrophilic granulocyte
		monocyte
		eosinophilic granulocyte
		basophilic granulocyte
		thrombocyte
haematopoietic stem cell	pluripotent lymphoid stem cell	T lymphocyte
		B lymphocyte

lective gene amplification, a concomitant increase in the production of functionally important proteins and in an increase in the amount of cytoplasma. This process is stimulated by colony-stimulating factors occurring in plasma. In this way thousands of platelets can be formed from a single megakaryocyte and the efficiency of the haemostatic system increases concomitantly. The degree of polyploidization of the megakaryocytes is not fixed, however, but can be influenced by external factors. Therefore, the stem cell–megakaryocyte–platelet system enables an adaptation of the haemostatic potential to the demand of the organism.

The appearance of a closed vascular system in which the blood circulates under pressure was also accompanied by the development of the highly efficient clotting system found in mammals [3,12,13]. This system consists of a number of coagulation enzymes which circulate in the blood in an inactive zymogen form. These zymogens can be activated into the active proteolytic enzymes by the cleavage of specific peptide bonds. The clotting enzymes have the amino acid serine at their active centre [12,14] and therefore can be classified as serine proteases. Damage to the vascular system not only causes the aggregation of blood platelets at the site of injury but simultaneously induces the activation of the first enzyme of the coagulation cascade. The activated enzyme activates a second enzyme and so forth. The successive reactions take place at the surface of the activated blood platelets [15]. The final result of this process is the conversion of soluble fibrinogen into a fibrin meshwork. It will be evident that the sequential steps in the coagulation cascade yield a large amplification, ensuring a rapid fibrin formation in response to a trauma. In this way rapid reinforcement of the fragile platelet plug by a fibrin meshwork is achieved and furthermore the clotting process is localized at the site of injury. The free circulation of activated clotting factors in the blood would of course create a very dangerous situation and therefore a number of naturally occurring inhibitors of these proteolytic enzymes is present in the blood (cf. Ch. 9A and B). These inhibitors neutralize the activated clotting factors that 'escape' from the site of injury almost immediately [13].

In vertebrates the processes of haemostasis, immune defense and tissue repair are no longer carried out by a single multifunctional type of cell but by a set specialized cells. In spite of the differentiation of the individual cells, close functional relationships between the different types of blood cells are recognized in the processes of tissue repair and immune defense [2,16,17].

3. The human haemostatic system

When damage to a blood vessel occurs the defect must be sealed through the coordinated action of platelets, clotting factors, endothelial cells and the vessel musculature. The relative contribution of these different components to the haemostatic process depends on the extent of the damage and the localization of the process.

(a) The role of vasoconstriction

The vascular contraction during the haemostatic process can be brought about by neurogenic vasospasm, precapillary sphincter constriction and humoral vasospastic phenomena [2]. Neurogenic phenomena occur when during injury of the arterial or the venous wall, pain stimuli from the injured area lead to vasoconstriction by reflex mechanisms through sympathetic fibres. The capillaries do not possess smooth muscle layers but closure of the capillary bed after local haemorrhage can be effected by the precapillary sphincter. Finally, humoral vasoconstrictive agents like serotonin, kinins and thromboxane A_2 are generated during the haemostatic response to injury.

Vasoconstriction may be an effective process to stop a bleeding in the capillary bed, but is not sufficient for a successful achievement of haemostatis in arterioles and venules. In these vessels the critical step is the immediate reaction of the blood platelets with subendothelial structures which become exposed when damage to the vessel occurs [18]. At the same time the coagulation system is also activated [19]. Constriction of the wall of the injured vessel will assist in closing the defect but is not sufficient. Haemostasis in arteries and veins, in which the blood pressure is higher, generally requires outside intervention.

(b) The role of platelets

When platelets are exposed to subendothelial structures they rapidly adhere to these structures and are involved in a further sequence of reactions [20]. Mostly the adhering platelets undergo release reactions. In the primary release the contents of the cytoplasmic dense bodies, which include adenine nucleotides and serotonin, are released into the surrounding medium. The release of ADP from adherent platelets stimulates new platelets to aggregate and serotonin is a mediator of vasoconstriction. Usually a second release reaction occurs during which the contents of the α-granules are freed into the surrounding medium. Stimulated platelets also produce thromboxane A_2, a very potent platelet-aggregating agent.

It has been known for a long time that upon activation of the platelets the platelet surface becomes procoagulant and that the coagulation reactions which ultimately lead to fibrin formation proceed with increased velocity on this surface (cf. Ch. 6). During the last decade it has been shown that platelets contain a number of plasma coagulation factors (von Willebrand factor, fibrinogen, factor V and high molecular weight kininogen), as well as plasma protease inhibitors (α_2-macroglobulin, α_1-antitrypsin and C1 inhibitor). The presence of these factors in platelets suggests a close interaction between platelets and coagulation factors.

Von Willebrand factor is important for the adherence of platelets to damaged endothelium (cf. Ch. 2B). The factor has been identified in plasma [21], endothelial cells, megakaryocytes and platelets [22]. In platelets von Willebrand factor is localized in the α-granules [23,24] and is secreted upon stimulation of the platelets by ADP, collagen and thrombin [24,25]. The platelets contain 10–25% of the von Willebrand factor present in blood. Under normal physiological conditions von Willebrand factor does not readily interact with human platelets. However, interaction between von Willebrand factor and subendothelium is thought to produce a conformational change in this protein which enables recognition of von Willebrand factor receptors on the platelet surface in this way causing platelet adhesion. The secretion of von Willebrand factor upon the stimulation of platelets with thrombin may enhance the formation of the platelet plug. Thus, von Willebrand factor is important for the adherence of platelets to the site of injury. Platelet adhesion results in platelet stimulation and this leads, among others, to the production of metabolites of arachidonic acid, particularly thromboxane A_2 [27]. This potent platelet agonist stimulates further platelet aggregation and secretion of granule contents. The secreted compounds support platelet aggregation and prothrombin activation.

The platelet α-granules also contain fibrinogen [28] and factor V [29]. The potential platelet contributions to the total plasma levels are only 1.5% and 12% respectively [30,31], but during the release reaction a high local concentration of these factors at the platelet surface can be reached. Fibrinogen is an essential cofactor for platelet aggregation [32,33]; platelet stimulation can result in a rapid reversible binding of fibrinogen to receptors on the platelet surface. Factor V and thrombin-activated factor V (= factor V_a) bind to the platelet membrane and serve as a membrane receptor for coagulation factor X ([34,35] and Ch. 2A). This close cooperation between platelets and clotting factors results in the production of a fibrin-reinforced platelet plug localized at the site of the vascular defect.

The presence of high molecular kininogen in blood platelets also points to an involvement of platelets in the contact phase of coagulation but the mechanism of this interaction is still less clear (see also Ch. 5A). The same is true for the function of the protease inhibitors present in platelets although a modulation of the coagulation enzyme–platelet interaction can be supposed.

(c) The role of coagulation factors

It has been described above that the clotting cascade reactions leading to fibrin formation proceed with increased velocity at the surface of stimulated platelets. Platelets are not the first trigger for the activation of the coagulation cascade, however. The activation of the plasma-clotting factors starts when tissue factor exposed in the damaged area activates factor VII (cf. Ch. 5B); the collagen-induced activation of factor XII seems less important for the cessation of traumatic bleeding. The coagulation enzymes will be described in greater detail below.

(d) Tissue repair and fibrinolysis

As soon as the bleeding is stopped the tissue repair process starts. The fibrin meshwork, and the cellular debris are removed by fibrinolytic and phagocytic processes and at the same time the healthy adjacent cells are stimulated to undergo

6

division. Neutrophils and with the progression of time also macrophages are attracted towards the damaged area by chemotactic factors released during the haemostatic process [36–38]. The phagocyting cells release lytic enzymes and take up cellular debris by phagocytosis.

The fibrinolytic system is activated by tissue-type plasminogen activator released from the endothelium (cf. Ch. 8). This proteolytic enzyme activates plasminogen, the zymogen of the fibrinolytic enzyme plasmin, bound to the fibrin–platelet plug thereby confining the fibrinolytic process to the site of injury [39–41]. The physiological role of the factor XII- and kallikrein-dependent plasminogen activation is less clear. The fibrinolytic enzymes that enter the circulation after resolution of the fibrin meshwork are rapidly inactivated by the fibrinolytic inhibitors present in the blood [42–46].

(e) The involvement of endothelial cells

The layer of endothelial cells that constitutes the inner surface of the blood vessels must not be considered as an 'inert container' but as an active participant in both the haemostatic and the fibrinolytic process. This active role of endothelial cells appears from the following:
- When endothelial cells are stimulated by among others thrombin and (activated) platelets the cells synthesize thromboplastin and expose this activator of the coagulation cascade on their surface [47,48].
- Endothelial cells synthesize the clotting cofactors V and VIII [49–51] and can support the activation of factor X and prothrombin [52].
- Endothelial cells synthesize prostacyclin [53].
- A cofactor for antithrombin III is present on the endothelial cells (heparan sulphate?) and this factor catalyses the inhibition of active clotting factors by antithrombin III in vivo (cf. [54–57] and Ch. 9A). Because of the large volume/surface ratio this process is probably not very important in larger vessels. However, it can be important in the microcirculation where the volume/surface ratio is much smaller.
- Thrombomodulin, another cofactor present on the surface of the endothelial cell, binds thrombin, thereby increasing the velocity of protein C activation by thrombin (cf. [58,59] and Ch. 9B). The activated protein C inactivates the coagulation cofactors V_a and VIII_a [60–62] thereby slowing down the thrombin generation. Protein C stimulates the fibrinolytic process, probably by decreasing the activity of the inhibitor of the plasminogen-activating enzyme [63,64].
- The presence of an intravascular thrombus stimulates the endothelial cell to secrete a plasminogen activator [65].

Thus it can be concluded that the physiological state of the blood is determined by a closely regulated interplay of platelets, humoral coagulation factors, fibrinolytic factors, and endothelial cells.

4. The coagulation cascade

The blood coagulation enzymes occur in plasma as inactive zymogens that can be activated in a series of consecutive reactions. The reactions in which the so-called vitamin K-dependent coagulation factors (VII, IX, X and II) are involved proceed at lipid/water interfaces (cf. Ch. 3) and the 'quality of the interface' is one of the parameters that determine the reaction velocity of this process. The affinity of the vitamin K-dependent clotting factors for lipid/water interfaces is caused by the presence of carboxylated glutamic acid residues in the protein molecule; vitamin K is a cofactor in the carboxylation process (cf. [66] and Ch. 4).

In the coagulation cascade the product of the first reaction functions as an enzyme in the second reaction, the product of the second reaction functions as an enzyme in the third reaction, and so on. A description of this cascade process is given in Fig. 1. In this scheme the bold lines represent the 'classical' division of the coagulation cascade in an intrinsic and an extrinsic pathway and the connecting lines show points of interaction between both pathways (see below).

The ordered and controlled interplay of the coagulation cascade reactions is accomplished by the high degree of specificity of the coagulation enzymes and by a

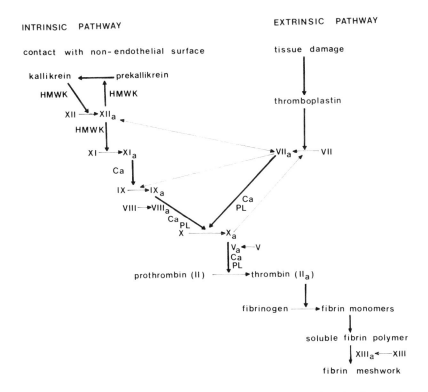

Fig. 1. The coagulation cascade. PL, phospholipid; HMWK, high molecular weight kininogen.

system of positive and negative feedback mechanisms. The majority of the coagulation factors are serine proteases. Factors V_a and VIII_a do not possess intrinsic enzymatic activity, but they form complexes with factors X_a and IX_a respectively. This markedly stimulates the activities of the latter enzymes (cf. Ch. 2 and 3).

The ultimate visible effect of coagulation is the conversion of soluble fibrinogen into insoluble fibrin by thrombin. However, this is not the only function of this enzyme; other functions of thrombin in the haemostatic process are:

- the activation of blood platelets: thrombin causes platelets to aggregate, and – in conjunction with collagen – to make available the phospholipids necessary for the coagulation process (the procoagulant lipid/water interface);
- the activation of (co)factors V and VIII;
- the activation of protein C, a vitamin K-dependent proteinase that inactivates factors V_a and VIII_a;
- the activation of factor XIII; factor XIII_a is a transglutaminase that stabilizes the polymeric fibrin meshwork by covalent cross-linkage of the polymers;

It has been described recently that thrombin, especially in the presence of platelets, increases the thromboplastin exposure on cultured endothelial cells [67]. The physiological significance of this in vitro finding remains to be determined.

Present evidence suggests that the coagulation process is autocatalytic and self-limiting and that thrombin plays a central role. As the generation of active coagulation factors is explosive and is initiated by a local injury of the vessel wall, whilst the inhibitors of these proteolytic enzymes are present in the whole vascular system, the active coagulation enzymes can only exist at the site of injury for a short period of time (during which their formation proceeds much faster than their inactivation).

(a) The serine proteases of blood coagulation

The blood coagulation enzymes are serine proteases with a trypsin-like specificity for arginyl bonds. The clotting enzymes are structurally and mechanistically homologous to trypsin and chymotrypsin but they have a much higher degree of specificity than the digestive enzymes.

The mechanism of action of the digestive serine proteases chymotrypsin, trypsin and elastase has been studied extensively by a combination of kinetics, chemical modifications and crystallographic studies [68–70]. An imporant feature of the serine proteases is the charge relay system in the active site of the enzyme. According to the system described by Blow et al. [68] for chymotrypsin, Ser-195, His-57 and Asp-102 are linked by a hydrogen bond network and the oxygen atom of Ser-195 participates as a strong nucleophile during catalysis (the numbers refer to the numbering system in chymotrypsin).

The different steps of a proteolytic reaction catalysed by a serine protease are given in Fig. 2. In the first step of the reaction sequence the enzyme forms a noncovalent complex, the so-called Michaelis complex, with the substrate (in the reaction scheme the noncovalent bonds are represented by a dot (.)). In the second

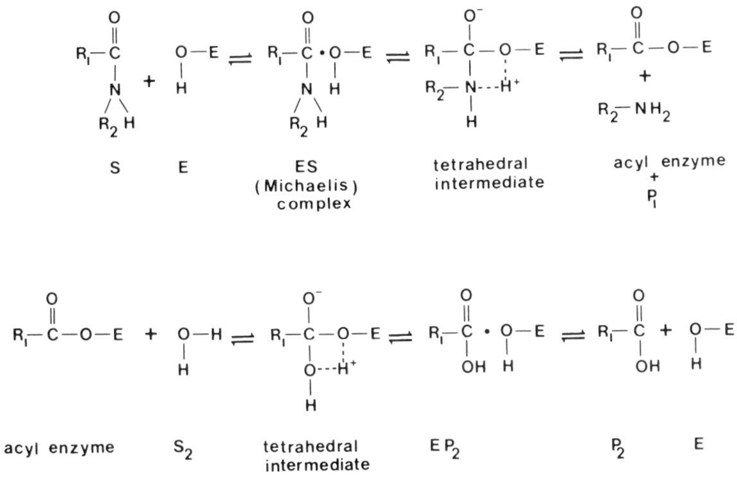

Fig. 2. Schematic representation of the subsequent steps in a reaction catalysed by a serine esterase. S, substrate; E, enzyme; ES, noncovalent enzyme–substrate complex; P, product; EP, noncovalent enzyme–product complex.

step a tetrahedral intermediate between the enzyme and the substrate is formed as a result of a nucleophilic attack of the hydroxyl group of Ser-195 on the substrate. In the third step of the reaction, the destabilized carbon–nitrogen bond is broken; this gives rise to an acyl enzyme intermediate and an amine product that diffuses away. In the next reaction steps the acyl enzyme is split by the reverse of the three steps described above. The acyl enzyme reacts with a water molecule to form a tetrahedral complex and subsequently internal bond shifts lead via a noncovalent complex to the free enzyme and the second product.

The serine residue in the active site of the enzyme derives its nucleophilic reactivity from the fact that it is in the optimum position to attack a tetrahedrally distorted carbonyl carbon atom in the substrate. The distortion in the substrate molecule is induced by the binding to the enzyme and the His–Asp couple functions to facilitate a transfer of a proton either from the attacking serine residue to the leaving group in the acylation step or from an attacking nucleophile (water in the reaction scheme above) to the serine residue during deacylation [69]. All of the serine proteases for which the X-ray structural studies have been carried out have the following features in common (69) (see also Fig. 3):

– the extended polypeptide-binding site on the acyl group side of the susceptible peptide bond;
– a number of sites for binding, with greater or lesser specificity, the side chains of a polypeptide substrate; the side chain specificity is suitably modified from one member of the family to another;
– a site for binding the substrate on its leaving group side;
– a site for binding the carbonyl oxygen atom of the susceptible peptide bond when the carbonyl group is in a tetrahedral configuration;

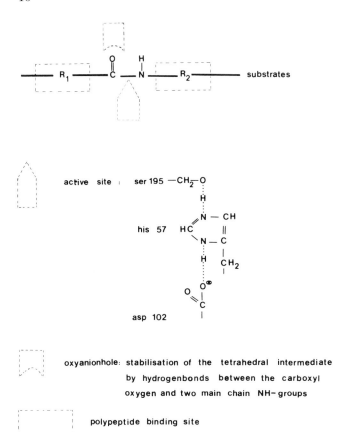

Fig. 3. Schematic representation of the functional domains in a serine esterase (chymotrypsin).

– the reactive serine side chain, which forms a covalent bond with the carbonyl carbon atom of the susceptible peptide bond and the charge relay system in which Ser-195, Asp-102 and His-57 participate [68].

As far as we know, no X-ray diffraction studies of the blood coagulation enzymes have been published until now. Recently Furie et al. [71] have developed three-dimensional computer models of the trypsin-like domains of bovine factor IX_a, factor X_a and thrombin based upon the known tertiary structure of bovine chymotrypsin and trypsin and the sequence homology between the coagulation enzymes and the digestive proteases. It was suggested from this study that the cores of the proteins are highly conserved but that in contrast the surface structures are defined by amino acids that vary from those of trypsin. As a general rule, the charge distribution, topography and hydrophobic grooves on the surfaces of the different coagulation enzymes are highly individualized. This presumably explains the very high substrate specificity that characterizes each of these enzymes.

(b) The physiological course of the coagulation process

As was mentioned above the coagulation process can be triggered either by the contact between blood and subendothelial structures or by the release of thromboplastin from damaged vessels. At present, much is known about the individual reactions of the intrinsic and the extrinsic pathways, especially because during the last years highly purified coagulation factors have become available. A 'confrontation' between theoretical studies of the individual reactions of the coagulation cascade and clinical observations has shown that the familiar picture of an intrinsic and an extrinsic pathway of coagulation joining at the factor X activation step is far too simple and that close connections must exist between both pathways.

How must we explain the clinical observations that patients lacking factor VIII or factor IX (haemophilia patients) show severe bleeding problems, patients having factor VII levels as low as 2% may show only a mild bleeding tendency and patients lacking factor XI, factor XII, prekallikrein or high molecular weight kininogen have no abnormal bleeding tendency? Already in 1961 Biggs and Nossel [72] showed that the amount of thrombin generated by diluted thromboplastin is lower in factor VIII- and factor IX-deficient plasmas and in 1965 Josso and Prou-Wartelle [73] postulated that factor VII can activate factor IX. This means that factor X can be activated either directly by factor VII and tissue thromboplastin or indirectly by factor IX_a (together with factor VIII_a), which in turn has been activated by factor VII. The activation of factor IX by the factor VII–thromboplastin complex has been firmly establish by later studies [74–77]. These studies appear to support a vital role for a thromboplastin-triggered pathway.

The current view on the starting mechanism of coagulation is based on the observation that the zymogen factor VII has a non-negligible enzymatic activity [78,79]. Once it becomes absorbed onto tissue thromboplastin, the activity of factor VII is enhanced enough to start the coagulation process (see also Ch. 5B). However, it has been observed that a more active two-chain factor VII_a can be formed from the single-chain factor VII. This activation of factor VII can be accomplished by contact factors, factor IX_a and factor X_a [80–86]. Once factor VII_a is formed the coagulation reactions proceed with an increasing velocity due to the 'reinforcement loops' in the cascade pathways.

References

1 Belamarich, F.A. (1975) Progr. Haemostas. Thromb. 3, 191–209.
2 Mason, R.G. and Saba, H.I. (1978) Am. J. Pathol. 92, 774–811.
3 Archer, R.K. (1981) in: Recent Advances in Blood Coagulation (Poller, L., Ed.) pp. 211–226, Churchill, London.
4 Schneider, W., Scharf, R.E., Hagen-Aukamp, Ch. and Winkelmann, M. (1983) Arzneim.-Forsch. (Drug Res.) 33 (II), 1351–1354.
5 Walsh, P.N. (1982) in: Hemostasis and Thrombosis: Basic Principles and Clinical Practice (Colman, R.W., Hirsh, J., Marder, V.Z. and Salzman, E.W., Eds.) pp. 404–420, Lippincott, Philadelphia, PA.

12

6 Niewiarowski, S. and Varma, K.G. (1982) in: Hemostasis and Thrombosis: Basic Principles and Clinical Practice (Colman, R.W., Hirsh, J., Marder, V.J. and Salzman, E.W., Eds.) pp. 421–430, Lippincott, Philadelphia, PA.

7 Jókay, I. and Karczag, E. (1973) Experientia 29, 334–335.

8 Edgington, T.S. (1983) Nouv. Rf. Hématol. 25, 1–6.

9 Geczy, C.L. and Hopper, K.E. (1981) J. Immunol. 126, 1059–1065.

10 Begeman, H. and Rastetter, J. (1979) Atlas of Clinical Hematology, pp. 28–29, Springer, Berlin.

11 Williams, N. and Levine, R.F. (1982) Br. J. Haematol. 52, 173–180.

12 Davie, E.W., Fujikawa, K., Kurachi, K. and Kisiel, W. (1979) Adv. Enzymol. 48, 227–318.

13 Rao, A.K., Schmaier, A.H. and Colman, R.W. (1982) Pathobiol. Ann. 12, 35–64.

14 Nemerson, Y. and Zur, M. (1979) in: The Chemistry and Physiology of the Human Plasma Proteins (Bing, D.H., Ed.) p. 145, Pergamon, New York.

15 Zwaal, R.F.A. and Hemker, H.C. (1982) Haemostasis 11, 12–39.

16 Weksler, B.B. (1983) Clin. Lab. M. 3, 667–676.

17 Roit, I. (1982) Essential Immunology, Blackwell, Oxford.

18 Jaffe, R.H. (1976) in: Platelets in Biology and Pathology (Gordon, J.L., Ed.) pp. 261–292, Elsevier/North-Holland, Amsterdam.

19 Østerud, B. (1984) Scand. J. Haematol. 23, 337–345.

20 Zucker, M.B. and Nachmias, V.T. (1985) Arteriosclerosis 5, 2–18.

21 Sixma, J.J., Kater, L., Bouma, B.N., Schmitzl, F., de Graaf, S. and Trit, C. (1976) J. Lab. Clin. Med. 87, 112–119.

22 Piovella, F., Nalli, G., Malamani, G.D., Majolino, I., Frassonis, F., Sitar, G.M., Ruggeri, A., Delloboro, C. and Scari, E. (1978) Br. J. Haematol. 39, 209–213.

23 Nachman, R.L. and Jaffe, E.A. (1975) J. Exp. Med. 141, 1101–1112.

24 Zucker, M.B., Broekman, M.J. and Kaplan, K.L. (1979) J. Lab. Clin. Med. 94, 675–682.

25 Koutts, J., Walsh, P.N., Plow, E.F., Fenton, J.W., Bouma, B.N. and Zimmerman, J.S. (1978) J. Clin. Invest. 62, 1255–1263.

26 Hawiger, J., Fujimoto, T. and Ohara, S. (1981) Thromb. Haemostas. 46, 24.

27 Haluschka, P.V., Dollery, C.T. and MacDermot, J. (1983) Q.J. Med. 52, 461–470.

28 Kaplan, K.L., Broekman, J., Chernoff, A., Lesnik, G.R. and Drillings, M. (1979) Blood 53, 604–618.

29 Chesney, C.M., Pifer, D. and Colman, R.W.L. (1981) Proc. Natl. Acad. Sci. (U.S.A.) 78, 5180–5184.

30 Keenan, J.P. and Solum, N.O. (1972) Br. J. Haematol. 23, 461–466.

31 Tracy, P.B., Peterson, J.M., Nesheim, M.E. and Katzman, J.A. (1981) Thromb. Haemostas. 46, 89.

32 Mustard, J.F. and Packham, M.A. (1970) Pharmacol. Rev. 22, 97–187.

33 Bang, N.U., Heidenreich, R.O. and Trygstad, C.W. (1972) Ann. N.Y. Acad. Sci. 201, 280–299.

34 Kane, W.H., Lindhout, M.J., Jackson, C.M. and Majerus, P.W. (1980) J. Biol. Chem. 255, 1170–1184.

35 Tracy, P.B., Neshheim, M.E. and Mann, K.G. (1981) J. Biol. Chem. 256, 743–751.

36 Ryan, G.B. and Majno, G. (1977) Am. J. Pathol. 86, 185–276.

37 Carr, I. (1973) The Macrophage. A Review of Ultrastructure and Function, Academic Press, London.

38 Bar-Shavit, R., Kahn, A., Fenton, J.W. and Wilner, G.D. (1983) J. Cell. Biol. 96, 282–285.

39 Collen, D. (1980) Thromb. Haemostas. 43, 77–89.

40 Mullertz, S. (1984) Sem. Thromb. 10, 1–5.

41 Miles, L.A. and Plow, E.F. (1985) J. Biol. Chem. 260, 4303–4311.

42 Aoki, N. and Harpel, P.C. (1984) Sem. Thromb. 10, 24–41.

43 Wiman, B. and Collen, D. (1977) Eur. J. Biochem. 78, 19–26.

44 Kruithof, E.K.O., Ransijn, A. and Bachman, F. (1983) Progr. Fibrinolys, 6, 362–366.

45 Chmielewska, J., Rånby, M. and Wiman, B. (1983) Thromb. Res. 31, 427–436.

46 Erickson, L.A., Ginsberg, M.H. and Loskutoff, D.J. (1984) J. Clin. Invest. 74, 1465–1472.

47 Cazenave, J.P., Klein-Soyer, C. and Peretz, A. (1982) Nouv. R.J. Hématol. 24, 167–171.

48 Johnsen, U.L.H., Lyberg, T., Galdal, K.S. and Prydz, H. (1983) Thromb. Haemostas. 49, 69–72.

49 Cerveney, T.J., Fass, D.N. and Mann, K.G. (1984) Blood 63, 1467–1474.
50 Jaffe, E.A. (1982) Ann. N.Y. Acad. Sci. 401, 163–170.
51 Reinders, J.H., de Groot, P.G., Dawes, J., Hunter, N.R., van Heugten, H.A.A., Zandbergen, J., Gonsalves, M.D. and van Mourik, J.A. (1985) Biochim. Biophys. Acta 844, 306–313.
52 Stern, D.M., Nawroth, P.P., Kisiel, W., Handley, D., Drilling, M. and Bartos, J. (1984) J. Clin. Invest. 74, 1910–1921.
53 Willems, C.H., van Aken, W.G., Peuscher-Prakke, F.M., van Mourik, J.A., Dutilh, C. and ten Hoor, F. (1978) J. Mol. Med. 3, 195–201.
54 Bounassisi, V. (1973) Exp. Cell. Res. 76, 363–368.
55 Busch, C. and Owen, W.G. (1982) J. Clin. Invest. 69, 726–729.
56 Owen, W.G. (1982) Arch. Pathol. Lab. Med. 106, 209–213.
57 Lollar, P. and Owen, W.G. (1980) J. Clin. Invest. 66, 1222–1230.
58 Esmon, C.T. and Owen, W.G. (1981) Proc. Natl. Acad. Sci. (U.S.A.) 78, 2249–2252.
59 Owen, W.G. and Esmon, C.T.J. (1981) J. Biol. Chem. 256, 5532–5535.
60 Kisiel, W., Canfield, W.M., Ericsson, L.H. and Davie, E.W. (1977) Biochemistry 16, 5824–5831.
61 Walker, F.J., Sexton, P.W. and Esmon, C.T. (1979) Biochim. Biophys. Acta 571, 333–342.
62 Vehar, G.A. and Daine, F.W. (1980) Biochemistry 19, 401–410.
63 van Hinsberg, V.W.M., Bertina, R.M. van Wijngaarden, A., van Tilburg, N.H., Emeis, J.J. and Haverkate, F. (1985) Blood 65, 444–451.
64 Sakata, Y., Curriden, S., Lawrence, D., Griffin, J.H. and Loskutoff, D.J. (1985) Proc. Natl. Acad. Sci. (U.S.A.) 82, 1121–1125.
65 Kwaan, H.X. (1984) Sem. Thromb. Haem. 10, 71–79.
66 Stenflo, J., Fernlund, P., Egan, W. and Roepstorff, P. (1974) Proc. Natl. Acad. Sci. (U.S.A.) 71, 2730–2733.
67 Brox, J.H., Østerud, B., Bjørklid, E. and Fenton, J.W. (1984) Br. J. Haematol. 57, 239–246.
69 Blow, D.M., Birktoft, J.J. and Hartley, B.S. (1969) Nature (London) 221, 337–340.
69 Kraut, J. (1977) Annu. Rev. Biochem. 46, 331–358.
70 Stryer, L. (1981) Biochemistry, pp. 157–183, Freeman, San Francisco, CA.
71 Furie, B., Bing, D.H., Feldman, R.J., Robinson, D.J., Burnier, J.P. and Furie, B.C. (1982) J. Biol. Chem. 257, 3875–3882.
72 Biggs, R. and Nossel, H.L. (1961) Thromb. Diath. Haemorrh. 6, 1–14.
73 Josso, F. and Prou-Wartelle, O. (1965) Thromb. Diath. Haemorr. Suppl. 17, 35–44.
74 Østerud, B. and Rapaport, S.I. (1977) Proc. Natl. Acad. Sci. (U.S.A.) 74, 5260–5264.
75 Zur, M. and Nemerson, Y. (1980) J. Biol. Chem. 25, 5703–5707.
76 Jesty, J. and Silverberg, S.A. (1979) J. Biol. Chem. 25, 12337–12345.
77 Marlar, R.A. and Griffin, J.H. (1981) Ann. N.Y. Acad. Sci. 370, 325–335.
78 Jesty, J. and Nemerson, Y. (1974) J. Biol. Chem. 249, 509–515.
79 Nemerson, Y. (1983) Haemostasis 13, 150–155.
80 Altman, R. and Hemker, H.C. (1967) Thromb. Diath. Haemorrh. 18, 525–531.
81 Kisiel, W., Fujikawa, K. and Davie, E.W. (1977) Biochemistry 16, 4189–4149.
82 Radcliffe, R., Bagdassarian, A., Colman, R. and Nemerson, Y. (1977) Blood 50, 611–617.
83 Radcliffe, R. and Nemerson, Y. (1975) J. Biol. Chem. 250, 388–395.
84 Selgihsohn, U., Kasper, C.K., Østerud, B. and Rapaport, S.I. (1979) Blood 53, 828–837.
85 Nemerson, Y. (1976) Thromb. Haemostas. 35, 96–100.
86 Muller, A.D., van Deijk, W.A., Dévilée, P.P., van Dam-Mieras, M.C.E. and Hemker, H.C. Br. J. Haematol. 62, 367–377.

R.F.A. Zwaal and H.C. Hemker (Eds.), *Blood Coagulation*
© 1986 Elsevier Science Publishers B.V. (Biomedical Division)

Nonenzymatic cofactors: factor V*

KENNETH G. MANN[1], MICHAEL E. NESHEIM[2] and PAULA B. TRACY[3]

[1]*Department of Biochemistry, University of Vermont College of Medicine, Burlington,
VT 05405 (U.S.A.),*[2]*Department of Biology and Medicine, Queens University, Kingston,
Ont. (Canada), and* [3]*Department of Medicine and Biology, University of Vermont College
of Medicine, Burlington, VT 05405 (U.S.A.)*

1. Early history

The existence of factor V was deduced by Owren in Norway in 1943 when he studied a patient that had a bleeding diathesis which could not be accounted for by virtue of the known coagulation factor deficiencies [1,2]. Owren correctly deduced that the missing factor enhanced the rate of thrombin formation, and that it appeared to circulate in plasma as a less active species which could be converted to a more active form by the action of thrombin. Owren named the absent factor, factor V, and was perhaps prescient to adopt the roman numeral identification system for this coagulation factor. As a consequence, factor V is one of the few factors for whom the nomenclature has endured from discovery to the present.

The pioneering work of Seegers and coworkers [3] identified that factor V (accelerator globulin) was an essential cofactor in the conversion of prothrombin to thrombin. The work of Papahadjopoulos and Hanahan [4] and Cole and coworkers [5] showed that the physiologically significant activator of prothrombin was a complex of two proteins, factor X_a, factor V (factor V_a), phospholipids and calcium ions.

A number of investigators have provided useful purification procedures which provided functionally active factor V, however the isolation of homogenous preparations of factor V eluded investigators for nearly 40 years following Owren's discovery [6]. During this interval, factor V earned the nickname, 'labile factor' because of its notorious property of losing activity during storage under virtually all conditions. In retrospect, attempts at the isolation of homogenous factor V were plagued by the fact that factor V itself is an inactive or barely active cofactor that requires activation by thrombin or factor X_a before activity is expressed. In ad-

---

* Supported by HL-17430 and HL-34575.

dition, the product of activation, factor V_a, is immensely susceptible to proteolytic inactivation by a regulatory biochemical mechanism involving activated protein C and protein S [7–9]. Thus, in many early investigations, the activity difference between factor V and factor V_a was not addressed. In retrospect, studies of the isolated proteins have shown that factor V_a is (at least) 400 times more active than factor V, hence, an activity assay has the potential of giving enormously misleading results. For example, let us suppose one conducted a step of purification of factor V from 1 ml of plasma (1 unit) and the isolation step on one hand resulted in the activation of factor V to factor V_a, but on the other hand resulted in a 99.8% loss in total factor V. The investigator, using a non-discriminate activity assay, would conclude an 80% yield of activity based upon a one-stage factor V assay.

The isolation procedure developed in my laboratory for factor V was based upon the operational hypothesis that factor V was a *pro*cofactor, and would require activation by thrombin in order to express activity [10,11]. Consequently, steps of isolation were followed by measurements of factor V_a activity, both before and after treatment with thrombin. The various steps of purification were optimized with respect to total yield of factor V_a (after thrombin activation) and to the activation quotient, the ratio of factor V_a activity before and after treatment with thrombin.

Homogenous preparations of bovine factor V have been reported by this laboratory, Esmon [12] and by Dahlbäck [13]. Other investigators have reported essentially minor modifications to these isolation techniques. Human factor V has proven to be more difficult to isolate as a homogenous, single-chain form, than bovine factor V. We have had our best results for isolation of human factor V using a monoclonal antibody technique [14,15]. Kane and Majerus [16] have reported a human factor V isolation technique using conventional chromatographic procedures. Factor V has also been isolated from baboon, canine and porcine plasmas by our laboratory.

2. Factor V biosynthesis

In human blood, factor V is divided among two principal compartments: the blood plasma and the platelet [17,18]. A small fraction of factor V is also contained within the white cell populations in human blood [19]. Surveys of plasma factor V, based upon both radioimmunoassay and bioassay techniques indicate a mean of about 7 μg of factor V/ml of plasma after correction for hematocrit. In addition, the platelet compartment contains on the average approximately 2–3 μg/ml of whole blood after correction for hematocrit. In the bovine species, however, the factor V appears to be almost totally contained within the plasma compartment. 2–3% of bovine factor V is found within platelets while the remaining factor V is in plasma. In addition, bovine plasma contains between 4 and 5 times the amount of factor V found in human plasma [20]. When isolated, both bovine and human factor V have approximately the same specific activity (1500 units/mg) [17]. One should exercise great caution when comparing results for bovine and human factor V, with respect to the plasma standard used in the assay. A human factor V-deficient plasma standard, standardized with human plasma, will result in a quite different factor V activity value than a human deficient plasma assay standardized with bovine plasma. One unit (factor V/1ml) of bovine factor V in a human plasma deficient assay will equal approximately 5 human units.

Two sources have been identified as the potential sites of synthesis of the plasma factor V pool. Our laboratory has shown that bovine aortic endothelial cells grown in culture synthesize and secrete factor V [21]. In contrast, human umbilical vein endothelium synthesizes but does not secrete factor V [22,23]. Thus, all blood vessels are not equivalent with respect to factor V synthesis and secretion. Factor V synthesis has also been demonstrated in human hepatocellular carcinoma cell line (HepG2) [23]. However, it is not known whether normal (nonmalignant) liver cells are also capable of synthesizing factor V.

The other major site of factor V synthesis appears to be within the bone marrow stem cell pool. Human platelets, as pointed out previously, contain approximately 20% of the total factor V in blood. This factor V appears to be located in the α-granules [24]. Immunohistochemistry, as well as synthesis studies, indicate the major stem cell product containing factor V is the differentiated megakaryocyte [25,26]. Both human platelet and plasma factor V cross-react equivalently with antisera that we have produced in burros immunized with plasma factor V [17]. However, recent data from our laboratory indicate that our collection of monoclonal antibodies produced against human plasma factor V react differently with platelet factor V. Thus, it is not clear at the present time that platelet factor V and plasma factor V are completely identical with respect to molecular detail. It is also not clear that the functions of platelet factor V and plasma factor V are indeed identical. A family with defective platelet factor V, but normal plasma factor V, has been observed to express a significant bleeding diathesis [27], suggesting a special role for platelet-secreted factor V in the hemostatic process, at least under the circumstances of certain hemostatic challenge. We have also observed an individual with high-titer autoantibody to factor V, who appeared to be protected from bleeding by the factor V present in the platelet compartment alone [28]. Hence, a great deal more work is required to elucidate the relative function of the various synthetic routes for factor V and the presentation of factor V from both platelets and plasma in the expression of hemostatic competence.

3. Factor V structure

Factor V is a relatively unusual plasma protein. It is a large, single-chain molecule, with a molecular weight of 330 000 [10,29]. Our initial observation that factor V had such a large molecular weight led to intensive investigations of its molecular architecture using hydrodynamic procedures. Extensive sedimentation equilibrium and sedimentation velocity studies, carried out under native, and reduced–denatured conditions, confirm the fact that the 330 000-dalton molecule represents the covalent unit of factor V. The sedimentation coefficient of a molecule (9.2 S) suggests that the molecule is highly asymmetric. Gel filtration studies indicate that the Stokes radius of the factor V molecule is in the range of 91–95 Å [12,29]. These data are also consistent with a highly asymmetric molecule; a globular protein with a Stokes radius of 90 Å, would be expected to have a molecular weight between 7×10^5 and 1×10^6. Recently electron micrographic studies from two laboratories have indicated that the factor V molecule is a multi-lobed irregular structure, containing 3–4 globular domains [30,31]. The study from Mosseson's laboratory made use of scanning-transmission electron microscopy of unstained preparations of factor V. These techniques also made possible mass analysis of the imaged particles. These image data are consistent with a molecular weight of 330 000.

4. Proteolytic cleavages of the factor V molecule

At least 3 proteases associated with blood clotting can cleave the factor V peptide chain. The sites of these peptide cleavages are identified for bovine factor V in Fig. 1. Both thrombin [32] and factor X_a [33] are capable of activating factor V to factor V_a. The activation of bovine and human factor V to factor V_a has been extensively studied by our laboratory and by Suzuki and colleagues [34]. The sites of cleavage identified in Fig. 1 for thrombin cleavage of factor V are consistent with the data by all laboratories mentioned for both the human and the bovine molecule. There are, however, differences in reports with respect to the order of bond cleavage during human and bovine factor V activation. It is not known at the present time whether the various differences observed reflect species differences, differences in the preparations or differences in activation conditions used by the various laboratories which have studied these phenomena.

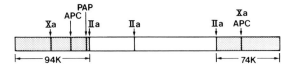

CLEAVAGE PATTERN OF BOVINE FACTOR V

Fig. 1. Schematic representation of the cleavage sites of bovine factor V by 4 proteases. The thrombin (IIa) cleavages yield activated factor V composed of 2 subunits, one of $M_r = 94\,000$ from the amino terminus of factor V, and one of $M_r = 74\,000$ from the carboxyl terminus. Factor X_a cleaves factor V_a at one position in each subunit, as does activated protein C (APC). Both cleave the light chain at the same position, while each attacks at a different position in the heavy chain. The APC cleavage in the heavy chain is associated with the inactivation of factor V_a by APC. Factor V_a bound to the surface of platelets exhibits a cleavage of the heavy chain by a platelet-associated protease (PAP).

(a) Factor X$_a$ and activated protein C cleavage of factor V

Since uncleaved factor V possesses little or no cofactor activity in the prothrombinase complex prior to its activation by thrombin [33,35], it becomes relevant to ask the question of how the initial factor V$_a$ becomes available to serve in the activation of prothrombin to thrombin. We have used monoclonal antibodies specific for factor V$_a$ [36] and dansylarginine N-(3-ethyl-1,5-pentanedyl) amide, a potent inhibitor of thrombin [37] to show conclusively that factor V can also be proteolytically activated to a fully active species by factor X$_a$. The rate of this reaction is small compared to the rate of activation of factor V by thrombin; however, it is potentially quite significant since the initial level of active prothrombinase enzyme (V$_a$:X$_a$) would be explicitly related to the level of factor X$_a$ available. The sites of factor X$_a$ cleavage of factor V have not been specifically identified. However, studies conducted with factor V$_a$ indicate that factor X$_a$ cleaves both the NH$_2$-terminal-derived D chain (heavy chain), and the C-terminal-derived E chain (light chain) of bovine factor V$_a$ [38]. These two peptide chains of factor V$_a$ are also cleaved by activated protein C (cf. [38–40] and Ch. 9B). In the case of the light chain, or E chain of factor V$_a$, activated protein C and factor X$_a$ give rise to identical products. However, activated protein C cleaves the heavy chain of factor V$_a$ to give rise to a 70 000 and 24 000 molecular weight peptide while factor X$_a$ cleaves the 94 000-dalton chain NH$_2$-terminal peptide of factor V$_a$ (heavy chain) to give rise to 45 000 and 56 000 molecular weight products. In the case of factor X$_a$ cleavage, the rate of cleavage of the E chain is fast while, for activated protein C the rate of cleavage of the D chain is fast. Inactivation of factor V$_a$ by activated protein C appears to correspond to cleavage of the NH$_2$-terminal D chain, and can be blocked by prior complex formation of factor V$_a$ with factor X$_a$ [38,41].

(b) Platelet protease cleavage of factor V

Two platelet-related cleavages of factor V/factor V$_a$ have been reported. Kane and coworkers [42] have reported that high concentrations of a platelet lysate, when incubated with factor V gave rise to numerous polypeptide chains, and an increase in factor V$_a$ activity. Subsequent treatment of the extract-treated factor V$_a$ with thrombin gave rise to full factor V$_a$-like activity.

Our laboratory has identified a protease associated with the intact bovine platelet which is capable of inducing significant cleavages in platelet-bound factor V [43] and factor V$_a$ [38]. This platelet-related cleavage is restricted to the heavy chain of factor V$_a$ and gives rise to a 90 000-dalton product. The cleavage appears to occur at the carboxyl terminus of the 94 000 chain. This cleavage does not appear to influence the expression of proteolytic activity of prothrombinase with respect to prothrombin as a substrate. The surface-bound protease cleaves factor V to yield peptides indistinguishable from the 94 000-dalton heavy chain of factor V$_a$ with additional proteolysis giving rise to the 90 000-dalton peptide. The platelet-associated protease cleavage of factor V and V$_a$ is blocked by EDTA, pepstatin and leupeptin. In addition, if platelets are pretreated with prostaglandin E_1 to block platelet activation, the platelet membrane protease activity is not expressed. Present data also indicate that the substrate for this platelet protease is membrane-bound factor V or V_a and not the proteins in solution. The significance of this platelet reaction, which appears to be quite specific, has not yet been elaborated.

5. Homologies of factor V and factor VIII

Our laboratory was fortunate to develop a murine monoclonal antibody to human factor V which binds to factor V with high affinity but which can be displaced at high ionic strength [14]. Human factor V in our laboratory is routinely isolated using this monoclonal antibody for immunoaffinity isolation. Dr. David Fass, my associate at the Mayo Clinic, utilized similar techniques to prepare monoclonal antibodies against the partially purified porcine factor VIII coagulant protein, which could be used for the isolation of active factor VIII:C [44].

Factor V and factor VIII:C appear to be homologous in terms of their function as cofactors in reactions involving vitamin K-dependent enzymes and vitamin K-dependent substrates (see Ch. 2B). As isolated from plasma, porcine factor VIII:C appears to be represented as a two-chain protein with molecular weights of 166 000 and 76 000 which remain associated in the presence of a divalent cation [44,45]. From the gene sequence of factor VIII:C, it is clear that a high molecular weight precursor gives rise to these plasma fragments [46,47]. Treatment of the isolated porcine factor VIII:C with thrombin gives rise to an 82 000 molecular weight chain obtained from the NH$_2$-terminus of the 166 000 peptide and the 69 000 chain de-

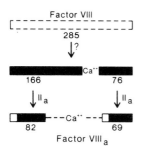

Fig. 2. A schematic representation of the process of factor VIII activation. The present physical data obtained on porcine factor VIII indicate that the isolated molecule is composed of 2 chains of apparent molecular weights 166 000 and 76 000 with Ca^{2+} involved in the noncovalent association of these chains. A hypothetical precursor is shown by a dotted line with an apparent molecular weight of 285 000. The products obtained from the two chains of the isolated factor VIII molecule upon thrombin treatment are illustrated at M_r values of 82 000 and 69 000, and are associated in the presence of calcium ion. The open segments at the NH$_2$-termini of each of these chains represent regions of the peptides that are homologous to factor V_a (from Mann, K.G. (1984) Membrane-bound enzyme complexes in blood coagulation, in: Progress in Hemostasis and Thrombosis (Spaet, T.H., Ed.) Vol. 7, pp. 1–23, reprinted by permission of the publisher, Copyright 1984 by Grune and Stratton, Inc., New York).

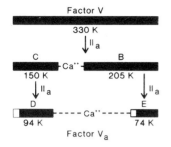

Fig. 3. The activation of factor V represented schematically. Procofactor factor V is cleaved by throm-bin first to give rise to 2 intermediate peptide chains that are noncovalently associated in the presence of calcium ion. These chains are subsequently cleaved to give rise to 2 polypeptide chains, D and E, that are obtained from the NH_2- and COOH-terminal of the parent molecule, respectively. These two chains are noncovalently associated with the process involving calcium ion. The open areas indicated at the NH_2-termini of the D and E chain represent areas that have been shown to be homologous to similar areas of the factor VIII_a peptide chains (from Mann, K.G. (1984) Membrane-bound enzyme complexes in blood coagulation, in: Progress in Hemostasis and Thrombosis (Spaet, T.H., Ed.) Vol. 7, pp. 1–23, reprinted by permission of the publisher, Copyright 1984 by Grune and Stratton, Inc., New York).

rived from the carboxyl terminus of the 76 000 molecular weight chain. This scheme of activation is represented in Fig. 2.

The scheme of thrombin activation of bovine factor V that we have observed is represented in Fig. 3. Under the conditions that we have employed, thrombin first cleaves the 330 000 molecular weight factor V procofactor giving rise to 2 peptide chains, C and D, with apparent molecular weights of 150 000 and 205 000 based upon gel electrophoresis in SDS. These two chains remain noncovalently associated [48]. Cleavage of the 150 000 molecular weight chain gives rise to a 94 000 molecular weight peptide from the NH_2-terminus, and at this point factor V_a activity is expressed. Subsequent cleavage of the 205 000-dalton chain gives rise to a COOH-terminal fragment of molecular weight 74 000 (component E) and these two chains remain noncovalently associated in the presence of divalent cations. Suzuki and coworkers [34] have reported that in the activation of human factor V the cleavage which gives rise to component D occurs first, while Esmon [49] has reported that activation of bovine factor V by the Russell's viper venom coagulant protein gives rise to the cleavage which would give rise to component E as the first product.

Sequence studies of the NH_2-terminals of peptides liberated from factor V upon activation with thrombin and the peptides derived from factor VIII:C activation by thrombin, indicated that these two proteins were remarkably homologous with respect to amino acid sequence. The NH_2-terminal sequences of the bovine factor V_a heavy and light chains and the respective porcine factor VIII homologues rep-resented in Fig. 4 are indeed homologous to one another, even though the factor V and factor VIII of two different species are represented. In addition, sequences within the respective chains show significant internal homology, giving evidence of internal duplication in the structure of factor V and factor VIII [50,51]. When

22

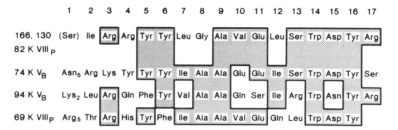

RELATIVE RESIDUE POSITION

Fig. 4. The 4 amino acid sequences given are aligned to the sequence occurring in the 166-, 130-, and 82-kDa polypeptides of the porcine factor VIII with serine (parentheses denote tentative assignment) as the initial residue. The 74-kDa chain of bovine factor V has, as the first relative residue in this alignment, the asparagine found in position 5 of the polypeptide. The 94-kDa bovine factor V chain and the 69-kDa porcine factor VIII chain have been similarly juxtaposed as indicated in the figure (reprinted with permission of Fass, D.N. et al. (1985) Internal duplication and sequence homology in factors V and VIII, in: Proc. Natl. Acad. Sci. (U.S.A.) 82, 1688–1691).

computer searches were performed on the sequences in factor V and factor VIII, it was observed that the two molecules share homology with another plasma protein, ceruloplasmin (cf. [52] and Ch. 2B). Ceruloplasmin is a blue, copper-containing protein in blood that has a molecular weight of about 150 000. This unexpected observation with respect to homology prompted a search for copper in factor V. Atomic absorption and atomic emission analyses of the factor V isolated either by conventional techniques for the bovine species, or by monoclonal antibody techniques for the human factor V, gave evidence of 1 g atom of copper ion/mole of factor V [53]. Ceruloplasmin exhibits amine oxidase activity, however, initial studies have indicated that factor V does not possess this activity, at least when challenged with sample substrates. Ceruloplasmin does not possess cofactor activity in the prothrombinase complex. However, it is interesting to speculate that the presence of copper ion in the factor V/factor V_a molecule, indicates a potential oxidase-related enzymatic role for factor V in addition to its cofactor role in prothrombinase.

6. Factor V/factor V_a metal and lipid interactions

The dependence of factor V_a activity on metal ions was observed well prior to the isolation of the molecule [54]. Equilibrium binding studies of calcium ion interaction with factor V conducted by our laboratory, indicate that factor V contains two relatively simple calcium-binding sites which do not interact and which have an association constant of 5×10^{-5} M. In addition, factor V contains one very tightly bound calcium ion with a K_d of less than 10^{-8} M [55]. As pointed out previously, copper has also been implicated in factor V structure however the relative participation of copper ion and calcium ion for the maintenance of the overall structure of the molecule has not been elaborated. Guinto and Esmon have reported calcium-binding data for bovine factor V_a [56]. These investigators found one calcium-binding site for the two peptides in factor V_a with an association constant of 2.4×10^{-5} M. This site was not displayed by either of the isolated peptide chains.

Treatment of factor V_a with EDTA is accompanied by a time-dependent loss in factor V procofactor activity which can be restored after reincorporation of metal ion [12,55]. Addition of a variety of metal ions can result in restoration of factor V_a activity. These include manganese, calcium, cobalt, chromium and cadmium. In the presence of added metal ion, dissociated light and heavy chains of factor V_a reassemble to form the active factor V_a molecule. The exact nature of the metal ion interaction associated with chain–chain association, has not been deduced; nor does there appear to be a significant spectral or fluorescence change associated with peptide chain interactions. However, monoclonal antibodies have been produced which will recognize the apo-factor V but not the metal ion-containing form [36]. This observation suggests that a limited conformational change may occur upon removal of the metal ion. Recently, we have performed high-resolution protein NMR experiments on factor V and factor V_a after treatment with EDTA (Woodworth and Church, unpublished observations). These studies indicate significant chemical shifts, particularly associated with histidine and tyrosine residues which may be related to the metal ion-binding 'pocket' of the molecule.

The early work of Papahadjopoulos and Hanahan [4] indicated a factor V interaction with phospholipids. Quantitative interpretation, however, of the association of factor V and factor V_a with phospholipids, has been rather controversial. Three laboratories have reported factor V- and factor V_a-binding data with each laboratory using different physical techniques for measurement [57–61]. Qualitatively, the data appeared to be similar, however the quantitative data are not. We have used light-scattering techniques to show that both factor V and factor V_a bind to acidic phospholipids [57,58]. The binding we have observed is independent of added metal ion, and has a significantly higher affinity than that observed for the vitamin K-dependent proteins ($\sim 10^{-8}$ M). Further, from conventional and quasi-elastic light-scattering data we have observed binding which is independent of ionic strength up to 1 M salt. Further our studies have shown that the association of factor V_a with phospholipids is quantitatively dependent upon the 74 000-dalton E chain of factor V_a [58,59]. Data from our laboratory have also shown that this same chain corresponds to the platelet-binding site of factor V_a [62].

Data reported by Nelsestuen's laboratory [60] indicate a significantly lower dissociation constant for factor V_a binding to phospholipids ($\sim 10^{-10}$ M). In this instance, the investigators used kinetics of association and dissociation of factor V_a with phospholipids to estimate the dissociation constant. Studies by van de Waart and coworkers [61] have used a non-equilibrium technique of sedimentation of large vesicles from suspension, followed by activity measurements of the fraction of factor V_a bound and free. These investigators reported a K_d in agreement with our laboratory. Their data also are consistent with the lipid-binding component of factor V_a residing in the 74 000-dalton carboxyl terminal-derived E chain; however their data suggest that the binding is ionic strength dependent.

Overall then, there is qualitative agreement with respect to factor V and factor V_a binding requiring acidic phospholipids and with the binding site residing in the 74 000-dalton (light) chain. However, the quantitative details of the binding interaction remain controversial.

7. Factor V_a binding to factor X_a, prothrombin and activated protein C

The study of the protein interactions in the prothrombinase complex has been elaborated by a variety of techniques. Papahadjopoulos and Hanahan [4] and Cole and coworkers [5] used sedimentation techniques to establish qualitatively the interactions amongst the proteins in prothrombinase. The availability of the pure proteins in more recent years has made it possible to quantitatively estimate dissociation constants, stoichiometry and peptide chain specificities of the protein–protein interactions associated with factor V and factor V_a. Most of the measurements currently available are kinetic in origin, and depend upon the expression of prothrombinase activity toward prothrombin or a synthetic peptide substrate [11,18,35,61,63–65]. Thus many of the reports give rise to only 'apparent' K_d and n data. Equilibrium binding studies of peptide association have been performed using light-scattering techniques [57,58] as well as fluorescence polarization utilizing active site [65–67] modified factor X_a and active site modified activated protein C [68]. Affinity chromotography utilizing immobilized protein has also been used to assess protein–protein interactions [69]. Direct platelet-binding studies have also been performed under equilibrium conditions using radiolabeled proteins and an oil centrifugation technique [20,70,71].

For studies in which evaluation of stoichiometry is possible, all data are consistent with the molar stoichiometry of 1 mole of factor V_a bound per 1 mole of factor X_a. In addition, all studies are consistent with this complex being described by a dissociation constant of approximately 10^{-10} M indicating a very high affinity between factor V_a and factor X_a and a lipid or platelet receptor. Published kinetic data suggest that the interaction between factor X_a and factor V_a in the absence of lipid is of the order of 10^{-8} M [72]. Light-scattering experiments performed in our laboratory suggest the dissociation constant between factor V_a and factor X_a in the absence of lipid is $\sim 10^{-7}$ M.

Two studies from our laboratory implicate the 74 000-dalton E chain of factor V_a in the factor X_a-binding process. We have made use of a covalently modified fluorescent factor X_a derivative to study interactions of factor X_a with factor V_a. Factor X_a has been modified at the active site histidine with 1,5-dansyl-glutamyl, glycyl, arginyl-chloromethyl ketone (dansyl-EGR-X_a) and the interactions of this inactivated enzyme with factor V_a/phospholipid have been evaluated. Monoclonal antibodies, directed against the light chain of factor V_a but not antibodies toward the heavy chain of factor V_a, have the property of blocking the binding of dansyl-

EGR-X_a to lipid-bound factor V_a [66]. In studies with platelets, we were able to show that platelet-bound factor V_a, treated with EDTA to remove the heavy chain, results in platelet-bound light chain. This product is still capable of binding factor X_a from solution in the presence of calcium ion [62]. In both of these studies, the 74 000-dalton E chain of factor V_a is implicated as both the lipid-binding chain of factor V_a and also as a significant contributor to factor X_a binding. These studies, however, do not exclude contributions of the 94 000-dalton D (heavy) chain to factor X_a binding. In this regard, van de Waart and coworkers [61] and Esmon [69] have not been able to show binding of the light chain of factor V_a to factor X_a bound to agarose.

The heavy chain of factor V_a has been implicated in the binding of prothrombin [69]. Binding of the factor V_a 94 000-dalton heavy chain to prothrombin immobilized on agarose was shown to be calcium independent. Factor V did not bind to this column, and the binding of the heavy chain of factor V_a to the immobilized prothrombin was not influenced by EDTA.

We have recently developed a fluorescent chloromethyl ketone reagent which can be used to study the binding of activated protein C to factor V_a bound to a membrane. This reagent, 2,5-dansyl-EGRCK, labels the active site histidine in activated protein C and gives an excellent polarization signal when activated protein C binds the lipid or to lipid-containing factor V_a [68]. In contrast to the binding of factor X_a to factor V_a, but consistent with the binding of prothrombin to factor V_a, the binding of activated protein C to factor V_a is independent of calcium ion. The studies of the isolated chains of factor V_a indicated that the binding interaction is quantitatively associated with the light chain of factor V_a, and that the interaction of activated protein C with either factor V_a or factor V_a light chain occurs with a 1:1 stoichiometry. 2,5-dansyl-EGR-activated protein C has also been studied with respect to its binding to factor V. In contrast to prothrombin, the labeled activated protein C also binds to a nonactivated factor V.

8. Factor V_a-related complex interaction on natural membrane surfaces

Membranes composed of synthetic phospholipids provide convenient models for the study of complex assembly related to prothrombin activation, however the most likely natural surfaces for assembly of these complexes are peripheral blood cell membranes. We have studied the interaction of factor V_a, factor X_a and prothrombin with platelets, monocytes and lymphocytes [18–20,70]. In addition, Rogers and Schuman have reported prothrombinase complex assembly on vascular endothelial cells in culture [73]. Equilibrium binding measurements have been performed for bovine and human factor V and factor V_a with platelets [20,71]. For the bovine system, binding is saturable with respect to both factor V and factor V_a, and totally reversible. Thus, binding data for bovine platelets can be treated quantitatively.

Bovine platelets, either collected in inhibitors such as prostaglandin E_1 or intentionally activated by thrombin, express the same number of binding sites for factor V and factor V_a. A single class of sites is seen for factor V with approximately 1000 sites. For factor V_a, 2 classes of sites are seen; a high-affinity class, which numbers approximately 1000, and a lower-affinity class, with approximately 4000 sites.

For human platelets, the equilibrium binding studies are made complex by the fact that human platelets are not saturable with respect to factor V or factor V_a. When saturable binding is not observed in equilibrium binding measurements, quantitative interpretation of the equilibrium binding data is not feasible.

We have used kinetic studies to estimate the number of human platelet-binding sites for the prothrombinase complex. For the activation of prothrombin to occur at physiologically relevant concentrations of prothrombin and factor X_a ($\sim 10^{-6}$ M and $\sim 10^{-9}$ M, respectively), factor V_a and a membrane receptor are obligate for expression of activity. Because of this, we deduced the functional level of the factor V_a/factor X_a interaction with the platelet surface, using the titration of the rate of activation of prothrombin as a mechanism of interpretation of the binding sites and binding site interactions. Using bovine platelets, a functional assessment of factor V_a-binding sites indicated that only the high-affinity sites determined from equilibrium binding experiments were related to the functional expression of prothrombinase activity. Equilibrium binding measurements which made use of labeled factor X_a and labeled factor V_a indicated an interaction stoichiometry of 1:1. Thus, the kinetic data could be interpreted in terms of the number of receptor sites on the platelet for factor X_a–factor V_a binding [70].

As pointed out previously, true equilibrium binding studies for factor V_a binding to human platelets have been made impossible because of the nonsaturable nature of this binding. In addition, the high content of factor V present in human platelets and secreted to a variable extent during platelet experiments complicates estimates of platelet factor V binding. Semi-quantitative estimates from binding measurements by Kane and Majerus indicate 2000–3000 factor V_a-binding sites for human platelets. Quantitative assessment of functional binding sites using a kinetic approach indicate approximately 3000 factor V_a–factor X_a-binding sites which participate in prothrombin activation. The number of sites expressed in a functional prothrombinase titration of factor V_a binding to human platelets, was not influenced by platelet activation by thrombin or thrombin plus collagen (with mixing but without continuous stirring). However, the ultimate specific activity obtained per site was influenced by prior activation of platelets with thrombin. Thus, one could conclude that: (a) the formation of factor V_a–factor X_a-binding sites on the platelet, was not influenced by the state of platelet activation, however (b) the ultimate expression of activity by that site did depend upon platelet activation. Human monocytes express approximately 16 000 factor V_a–factorX_a-binding sites of high affinity based upon kinetic-functional titration assays, and these cells may provide a significant role in fibrin deposition during inflammation.

Recently, we have had the opportunity to study both factor V_a and factor X_a

binding, using the kinetic method, in an individual who is factor V antigen deficient, both in plasma and in platelets [18]. In these experiments, the functional stoichiometry of the human platelet factor V_a–X_a interaction could be confirmed as 1:1.

Data from our laboratory, and from that of Majerus indicate that the factor V_a–factor X_a complex assembles on the surface of unactivated platelets. The binding interaction of these complexes with platelets is not altered by platelet activation, however, the maximum activity per site appears to require platelet activation and inhibitors of the latter do result in a lower overall turnover number per complex. Recent data from Hemker's laboratory have concluded that platelet activation with agents such as thrombin and collagen separately, result in similar numbers of binding sites as those reported by our laboratory [74]. However, this group also reports that with multiple stimuli and vigorous stirring, platelets will express additional factor V_a–factor X_a receptors (see Ch. 6 for recent summary on this topic). We have reproduced the experiments reported by these investigators, and find that the time course of expression of the additional receptor sites, does not coincide with the time course normally associated with the 'standard' events associated with platelet activation i.e., pseudopod formation, release of dense granules, and aggregation. Rather, the increase in sites reported by these coworkers, occurs at a significant interval following the afore-mentioned events of platelet activation and thus represents further activation and shear-related prothrombinase sites on platelets. The exact relevance of the various prothrombinase receptors on platelets awaits further studies.

9. The prothrombinase complex

Based upon binding interactions produced from both kinetics and equilibrium measurements of binding a hypothetical working model of the prothrombinase complex in cartoon form was developed in 1979 and is shown in Fig. 5 [75]. Although this model is presently 'long in the tooth' it still represents a reasonable, if incomplete representation of prothrombinase. The factor V_a molecule is shown bound to phospholipid forming the receptor on the membrane surface for the factor X_a protease. The requirement for activation of factor V for binding is implied by the fissures in the model, and factor X_a is represented by a two-domain protein bound both to factor X_a and to the phospholipid surface. The substrate, prothrombin, is represented as a three-domain molecule composed of prothrombin fragment 1, prothrombin fragment 2, and prethrombin 2. The prothrombin is represented as binding to phospholipids through the γ-carboxyglutamic acid-containing region (fragment 1). This interaction somehow involves calcium ions and these are represented schematically as attachment sites for the phospholipid surface. It should be pointed out, however, that the exact nature of vitamin K-dependent protein interaction with acidic phospholipids involving calcium ions is not well understood, and may or may not involve ion bridging. The prothrombin fragment 2 domain has

28

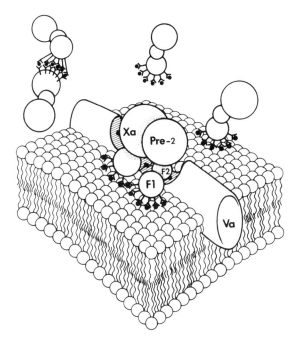

Fig. 5. The hypothetical model of the prothrombinase complex. Factor V_a is shown as a relatively hydrophobic protein binding to the phospholipid bilayer and forming the receptor for 1 molecule of factor X_a. Factor X_a is shown represented to interact both with factor V_a, and through its γ-carboxyglutamic acid-containing region, with the phospolipid surface itself. A molecule of prothrombin with its 3 domains, prothrombin fragment 1, fragment 2, and prethrombin 2, is shown associated with factor V_a, factor X_a, and the phospholipid surface, the latter occurring through the Gla-containing fragment 1 region. The interaction between prothrombin and factor V_a is represented through the fragment 2 region. Calcium ions, represented by small black dots, are shown associated with factor X_a·factor V_a, prothrombin·factor V_a, and factor V_a D and E chain interactions. Calcium ions are shown represented also in the interaction at Gla of the fragment 1 region of prothrombin and the NH_2-terminal segment of factor X_a with the phospholipid membrane. Prothrombin molecules are represented also, in solution both as dimers and monomers. Prothrombin molecules are represented also binding directly to the phospholipid membrane (from Nesheim, M.E., Hibbard, L.S., Tracy, P.B. et al. (1980) Participation of factor V_a in prothrombinase, in: The Regulation of Coagulation (Mann, K.G. and Taylor Jr., F.B., Eds.) p. 145, Elsevier/North-Holland, New York, reprinted by permission of the publisher, Copyright 1980 by Elsevier Science Publishing Co. Inc., New York).

been implicated by a number of kinetic studies as that through which factor V_a participates in prothrombin activation. It is therefore shown in close proximity to the factor V_a molecule. As represented, factor X_a is bound to membranes by a tight interaction ($K_d = 10^{-10}$ M) while prothrombin is interacting both with the assembled enzyme cofactor complex and with the lipid membrane directly.

A number of key features of this model are apparent. First of all, the model implies that at factor X_a concentrations potentially present in a clotting situation

($\sim 10^{-8}$–10^{-9} M) all factor X_a would be bound as long as sufficient receptors (membrane and factor V_a) were available. Thus, the enzyme would be fixed at a cellular site. Secondly, both prothrombin and the factor V_a–factor X_a complex in the cartoon are binding to acidic phospholipid. Thus, there is a potential for competition of prothrombin and enzyme (factor V_a–factor X_a) at fixed membrane composition and concentration since both enzyme and substrate can compete for the same surface. Thirdly, as represented, the binding site is represented by a pure phospholipid membrane without receptor proteins. While this is without question, and by design the situation which occurs with synthetic phospholipid vesicles, it remains uncertain whether additional receptor proteins in the platelet membrane are involved in the formation of a similar complex on cell surfaces.

10. Prothrombinase activity

If one assumes physiologic concentrations of factor V and prothrombin, and estimates that in coagulation between 1 and 10% of the coagulation factor X may be activated, one could compare the rate of prothrombin activation in the presence of a complete catalyst (X_a–V_a lipid complex) to that for factor X_a alone with all reagents at 'physiologic concentrations'. In this illustration, phospholipids are used, platelets substitute equivalently, and the assumption here is that sufficient membrane-binding sites are available in the system and are not limiting. Under this set of conditions, the turnover rate for prothrombin, per mole of factor X_a, in the presence of saturating V_a, receptor sites and calcium ion, would be approximately 1200 moles of thrombin/min/mole of factor X_a. If one were to delete any constituent from this reaction mixture, the reaction rate would fall dramatically. This is illustrated in Table 1, which represents the measured rate under the conditions discussed in the preceding section. Table 1 illustrates why Owren's patient bled in 1943 because of a lack of factor V. In the absence of factor V, 10^{-9} M factor X_a, converts prothrombin to thrombin at a rate which is approximately

TABLE 1

Relative rates of prothrombin activation in the presence of various combinations of the components of the 'prothrombinase' complex

Components present[a]	Relative rate[b]
X_a	1
X_a, Ca^{2+}	2
X_a, Ca^{2+}, phospholipid	22
X_a, Ca^{2+}, V_a	356
X_a, Ca^{2+}, phospholipid, V_a	278 000

[a] Proteins are present at potential physiological concentration; prothrombin $\sim 10^{-6}$ M, factor V_a $\sim 10^{-8}$ M, factor X_a $\sim 10^{-9}$ M. Phospholipid is present at a concentration adequate to saturate the reaction.
[b] Relative rates are expressed in comparison to factor X_a by itself.

1/10 000 rate that would occur in the presence of saturating levels of factor V_a. Deletion of a membrane receptor (lipid) results in a 1000-fold change in rate while deletion of both would decrease the rate by approximately 5 orders of magnitude. Under the set of conditions described in Table 1, virtually all the factor X_a and factor V_a will be bound to the membrane receptor and only a fraction of the prothrombin would occupy phospholipid-binding sites. However, owing to the tremendous relative preponderance of prothrombin in the system ($\sim 10^{-6}$ M), approximately half the surface of each phospholipid vesicle would be covered by substrate molecules while only 10% would be covered by enzyme (factor V_a–factor X_a complexes).

An attractive rationalization for the dramatic increase in rate (3×10^5) of a complete prothrombinase complex over an equivalent concentration of factor X_a alone at potential plasma concentrations of constituents relates to the changes in specific activity and co-concentration of enzyme and substrate. Since both enzyme and substrate are condensed in a relatively small element of the total volume of solution, the relevant 'K_m' relates to local concentration [63,76,77] (see also Ch. 3 for an extensive discussion). Work from our laboratory using prothrombin, with no lipid-binding capacity, obtained from warfarinized animals indicates that the intrinsic K_m of prothrombin, without lipid-binding capacity for factor X_a–factor V_a bound to a membrane surface is approximately 12 μM [78]. Since in the experiments described, the nominal concentration of prothrombin is approximately 1 μM, it is approximately 10% of K_m. However, in the region of bound enzyme, the concentration of prothrombin, owing to lipid binding, is quite in excess of the apparent K_m, and the membrane-bound enzyme is saturated by the local environmental concentration of prothrombin. The second major feature of catalyst formation involves intrinsic alterations in the enzyme factor X_a, the substrate prothrombin, or both, and brings about a significant alteration in the catalytic rate constant; in other words, a 'k_{cat}' effect.

Work from Rosing and coworkers suggests that the principal effect of lipid on prothrombinase is to reduce the 'apparent K_m' for the reaction while the effect of factor V_a is to stimulate the k_{cat} for the reaction [76]. A more complete discussion of the influence of lipid binding on the apparent K_m and k_{cat} of this reaction can be found in ref. 77 and in Ch. 3.

One unique feature alluded to earlier, for reactions in which membrane-bound enzyme acts upon membrane-bound substrate, deals with competition of enzyme and substrate for membrane-binding sites. We have constructed a computer model to evaluate the influence of binding factors X_a, V_a, and prothrombin and lipid concentration on the observed rate and/or K_m observed for a given set of reaction conditions [77]. As suggested by the prothrombinase model in Fig. 4, both the factor V_a–X_a complex and prothrombin should compete for the same lipid site and thus, one should see for this reaction, characteristic competition and inhibition by excess enzyme or excess substrate as one or the other displaces the membrane-bound counterpart from the surface. This model has also been tested in terms of lipid concentrations since one would predict that increasing the concentration of surface could in fact inhibit the reaction by dispersing enzyme and substrate. This is indeed observed for normal (10 Gla) prothrombin and not observed for Gla-deficient prothrombin [78].

Two peptide bonds are cleaved in prothrombin to give rise to thrombin and hence, there are two potential mechanisms in terms of order of bond cleavage which could give rise to active thrombin. In factor V-free systems, the predominant reaction appears to go through prothrombin fragment 1·2, prethrombin 2 as a first cleavage i.e., cleavage at Arg_{273}–Thr_{274} followed by cleavage of prethrombin 2 at Arg_{322}–Ile_{323} to give rise to thrombin [79]. Current data obtained for a fully saturated factor X_a–factor V_a complex indicate that the predominant intermediate seen for the prothrombinase catalyst corresponds to meizo-thrombin with the first cleavage occurring at Arg_{322}–Ile_{323}, and the subsequent cleavage giving rise to α-thrombin and fragment 1·2 by virtue of cleavage at Arg_{273}–Thr_{274}. This change in reaction order may relate to an altered mechanism of the reaction and this may give rise to the observed change in k_{cat} for thrombin production [80].

11. The cell membrane receptor for factor V_a

Although phospholipids provide a convenient source upon which to construct synthetic models of prothrombinase, a growing body of data suggest that the platelet receptor for the factor V_a–factor X_a complex may involve something more than phospholipids per se. Studies of one of Dr. Harvey Weiss' patients have suggested that this individual had a platelet prothrombinase defect even in the presence of a surplus of factor V_a and factor X_a, thus implicating the lack of expression of a receptor on the surface of the platelets for the factor V_a–X_a complex (cf. [81] and Ch. 6). This observation suggests that some protein may be absent which is required to assemble the entire receptor. Secondly, we have prepared monoclonal antibodies to factor V_a which have no effect on binding of factor V_a to phospholipid vesicles, but inhibit factor V_a binding to platelets. In addition, data (at least from our laboratory) suggest a gross difference in the capacity and affinity with which lipids bind to factor V_a as compared to the affinity of the receptor of bovine platelets for factor V_a. All of these studies are circumstantial; they can be explained by a variety of phenomena besides the existence of a specific protein receptor, which either participates in or organizes a lipid receptor for the factor V_a–factor X_a complex (see Ch. 6 for a balanced discussion). Recently, we have conducted experiments which suggest that there is another explicit difference between the factor V_a–factor X_a complex on platelets as a prothrombinase catalyst, and the factor V_a–factor X_a complex on phospholipids. Since factor X_a, factor V_a and prothrombin compete for the same phospholipids, one can show substrate-competitive inhibition for prothrombinase formed on a synthetic phospholipid vesicle. However, this same competition is not shown for prothrombinase formed on the surface of the cell. These data strongly suggest that in contrast to prothrombinase assembly on phospholipids where both prothrombin and the factor V_a–factor X_a complex bind to the same 'receptors' (phospholipids), enzyme (factor V_a–factor X_a) and substrate (prothrombin) bind to different receptors on the cell surface.

32

12. Concluding remarks

Factor V_a was the first cofactor isolated to homogeneity. This isolation has led to a rapid growth of physical data related to the activation of factor V, to factor V_a, the regulation of factor V_a activity by activated protein C and protein S, the binding of factor V_a to a variety of cell types, and the participation of factor V_a in the prothrombinase complex. Many of the observations that have been made for factor V_a and factor V_a–factor X_a interactions have their equivalent in factor IX_a–factor VIII_a interactions, including isolation of factor VIII:C, activation of factor VIII:C, function of factor VIII:C and sequence homology with factor VIII:C. Whether similar homologies can be expected with respect to the complexes in which thrombomodulin and tissue factor participate remains for further study.

References

1 Owren, P.A. (1947) Acta Med. Scand. Suppl. 194, 1–327.
2 Owren, P.A. (1947) Lancet 1, 446–448.
3 Seegers, W.H. (1962) Prothrombin, Harvard University Press, Cambridge, MA.
4 Papahadjopoulos, D. and Hanahan, D.J. (1964) Biochim. Biophys. Acta 90, 436–439.
5 Cole, E.R., Koppel, J.L. and Olwin, J.H. (1965) Thromb. Diath. Haemorrh. 14, 431–444.
6 Colman, R.W. and Weinberg, R.M. (1976) in: Methods in Enzymology (Lorand, L., Ed.) Vol. 45, pp. 107–122, Academic Press, New York.
7 Kisiel, W., Canfield, W.M., Ericsson, L.H. and Davie, E.W. (1977) Biochemistry 16, 5824–5831.
8 Marlar, R.A. and Griffin, J.H. (1980) J. Clin. Invest. 66, 1186–1189.
9 Walker, F.J. (1981) J. Biol. Chem. 256, 11128–11131.
10 Nesheim, M.E., Myrmel, K., Hibbard, L. and Mann, K.G. (1979) J. Biol. Chem. 254, 508–517.
11 Nesheim, M.E., Katzmann, J.A., Tracy, P.B. and Mann, K.G. (1981) in: Methods in Enzymology (Lorand, L., Ed.) Vol. 80, pp. 249–274, Academic Press, New York.
12 Esmon, C.T. (1979) J. Biol. Chem. 254, 964–973.
13 Dahlbäck, B. (1980) J. Clin. Invest. 66, 583–591.
14 Katzmann, J.A., Nesheim, M.E., Hibbard, L.S. and Mann, K.G. (1981) Proc. Natl. Acad. Sci. (U.S.A.) 78, 162–166.
15 Foster, W.B., Tucker, M.M., Katzmann, J.A., Miller, R.S. and Mann, K.G. (1983) Blood 61, 1060–1067.
16 Kane, W.H. and Majerus, P.W. (1981) J. Biol. Chem. 256, 1002–1007.
17 Tracy, P.B., Eide, L.L., Bowie, E.J.W. and Mann, K.G. (1982) Blood 60, 59–63.
18 Tracy, P.B., Eide, L.L. and Mann, K.G. (1985) J. Biol. Chem. 260, 2119–2124.
19 Tracy, P.B., Rohrbach, M.S. and Mann, K.G. (1983) J. Biol. Chem. 258, 7264–7267.
20 Tracy, P.B., Peterson, J.M., Nesheim, M.E., McDuffie, F.C. and Mann, K.G. (1980) in: The Regulation of Coagulation (Mann, K.G. and Taylor, F.B., Eds.) pp. 237–243, Elsevier, New York.
21 Cerveny, T.J., Fass, D.N. and Mann, K.G. (1984) Blood 63, 1467–1474.
22 Cerveny, T.J. (1984) Doctoral Dissertation, University of Minnesota.
23 Wilson, D.B., Salem, H.H., Mruk, J.S., Maruyama, I. and Majerus, P.W. (1984) J. Clin. Invest. 73, 654–658.
24 Chesney, C.McI., Pifer, D.D. and Colman, R.W. (1983) Thromb. Res. 29, 75–84.
25 Nichols, W.L., Gastineau, D.A., Solberg, L.A. and Mann, K.G. (1985) Blood 65, 1396–1406.
26 Chiu, H.C., Schick, P. and Colman, R.W. (1983) Fed. Proc. 42, 1994 (abstr.).
27 Tracy, P.B., Giles, A.R., Mann, K.G., Eide, L.L., Hoogendoorn, H. and Rivard, G.E. (1984) J. Clin. Invest. 1221–1228.

28 Nesheim, M.E., Nichols, W.L., Cole, T.L., Houston, J.G., Schenk, R.B., Mann, K.G. and Bowie, E.J.W. (1986) J. Clin. Invest., 77, 405–415.
29 Mann, K.G., Nesheim, M.E. and Tracy, P.B. (1981) Biochemistry 20, 28–33.
30 Mosseson, M.W., Nesheim, M.E., DiOrio, J., Hainfield, J.F., Wall, J.S. and Mann, K.G. (1985) Blood 65, 1158–1162.
31 Dahlbäck, B. (1985) J. Biol. Chem. 260, 1347–1349.
32 Nesheim, M.E. and Mann, K.G. (1979) J. Biol. Chem. 254, 1326–1334.
33 Foster, W.B., Nesheim, M.E. and Mann, K.G. (1983) J. Biol. Chem. 258, 13970–13977.
34 Suzuki, K., Dahlbäck, B. and Stenflo, J. (1982) J. Biol. Chem. 257, 6556–6564.
35 Nesheim, M.E., Taswell, J.B. and Mann, K.G. (1979) J. Biol. Chem. 254, 10952–10962.
36 Foster, W.B., Katzmann, J.A., Miller, R.S., Nesheim, M.E. and Mann, K.G. (1982) Thromb. Res. 28, 649–661.
37 Nesheim, M.E., Prendergast, F.G. and Mann, K.G. (1979) Biochemistry 18, 996–1003.
38 Tracy, P.B., Nesheim, M.E. and Mann, K.G. (1983) J. Biol. Chem. 258, 662–669.
39 Canfield, W., Nesheim, M., Kisiel, W. and Mann, K.G. (1978) Circulation 57–58(II), 210 (abstr.).
40 Walker, F.J., Sexton, P.W. and Esmon, C.T. (1979) Biochim. Biophys. Acta 571, 333–342.
41 Nesheim, M.E., Canfield, W., Kisiel, W. and Mann, K.G. (1981) J. Biol. Chem. 257(3), 1443–1447.
42 Kane, W.H., Mruk, J.S. and Majerus, P.W. (1982) J. Clin. Invest. 70, 1092–1100.
43 Tracy, P.B. and Mann, K.G. (1983) Fed. Proc. 42, 31 (abstr.).
44 Fass, D.N., Knutson, G.J. and Katzmann, J.A. (1982) Blood 59, 594–600.
45 Fass, D.N., Knutson, G.J. and Hewick, R. (1983) Thromb. Haemost. 50, 255 (abstr.).
46 Toole, J.J., Knopf, J.L., Wozney, J.M., Sultzman, L.A., Buecker, J.L., Pittman, D.D., Kaufman, R.J., Brown, E., Shoemaker, C., Orr, E.C., Amphlett, G.W., Foster, W.B., Coe, M.L., Knutson, G.J., Fass, D.N. and Hewick, R.M. (1984) Nature (London) 312, 342–347.
47 Gitschier, J., Wood, W.I., Goralka, T.M., Wion, K.L., Chen, E.Y., Eaton, D.H., Vehar, G.A., Capon, D.J. and Lawn, R.M. (1984) Nature (London) 312, 326–330.
48 Nesheim, M.E., Foster, W.B., Hewick, R. and Mann, K.G. (1984) J. Biol. Chem. 259, 3187–3196.
49 Esmon, C.T. (1980) in: The Regulation of Coagulation (Mann, K.G. and Taylor, F.B., Eds.) pp. 137–144, Elsevier, New York.
50 Fass, D.N., Hewick, R., Knutson, G., Nesheim, M.E. and Mann, K.G. (1983) Thromb. Haemostas. 50, 255 (abstr.).
51 Fass, D.N., Hewick, R.M., Knutson, G.J., Nesheim, M.E. and Mann, K.G. (1985) Proc. Natl. Acad. Sci. (U.S.A.) 82, 1688–1691.
52 Church, W.R., Jernigan, R.L., Toole, J., Hewick, R.M., Knopf, J., Knutson, G.J., Nesheim, M.E., Mann, K.G. and Fass, D.N. (1984) Proc. Natl. Acad. Sci. (U.S.A.) 81, 6934–6937.
53 Mann, K.G., Lawler, C.M., Vehar, G.A. and Church, W.R. (1984) J. Biol. Chem. 259, 12949–12951.
54 Day, W.C. and Barton, P.G. (1972) Biochim. Biophys. Acta 261, 457–468.
55 Hibbard, L.S. and Mann, K.G. (1980) J. Biol. Chem. 255, 638–645.
56 Guinto, E.R. and Esmon, C.T. (1982) J. Biol. Chem. 257, 10038–10043.
57 Bloom, J.W., Nesheim, M.E. and Mann, K.G. (1979) Biochemistry 18, 4419–4425.
58 Higgins, D.L. and Mann, K.G. (1983) J. Biol. Chem. 258, 6503–6508.
59 Higgins, D.L., Prendergast, F.G., Nesheim, M.E. and Mann, K.G. (1982) Circulation 65–66(II), 172 (abstr.).
60 Pusey, M.L., Mayer, L.D., Wei, G.J. et al. (1982) Biochemistry 21, 5262–5269.
61 van de Waart, P., Bruls, H., Hemker, H.C. and Lindhout, T. (1983) Biochemistry 22, 2427–2432.
62 Tracy, P.B. and Mann, K.G. (1983) Proc. Natl. Acad. Sci. (U.S.A.) 80, 2380–2384.
63 Nesheim, M.E., Eid, S. and Mann, K.G. (1981) J. Biol. Chem. 256, 9874–9882.
64 Rosing, J., Tans, G., Govers-Riemslag, J.W.P., Zwaal, R.F.A. and Hemker, H.C. (1980) J. Biol. Chem. 255, 274–283.
65 Nesheim, M.E., Kettner, C., Shaw, E. and Mann, K.G. (1981) J. Biol. Chem. 256, 6537–6540.
66 Tucker, M.M., Foster, W.B., Katzmann, J.A. and Mann, K.G. (1983) J. Biol. Chem. 258, 1210–1214.
67 Tucker, M.M., Nesheim, M.E. and Mann, K.G. (1983) Biochemistry 22, 4540–4546.

34

68 Krishnaswamy, S., Tucker, M., Williams, B. and Mann, K.G. (1985) Thromb. Haemostas. 54, 242 (abstr.).
69 Guinto, E.R. and Esmon, C.T. (1984) J. Biol. Chem. 259(22), 13986–13992.
70 Tracy, P.B., Nesheim, M.E. and Mann, K.G. (1981) J. Biol. Chem. 256, 743–751.
71 Kane, W.H. and Majerus, P.W. (1982) J. Biol. Chem. 257, 3963–3969.
72 Skogen, W.F., Esmon, C.T. and Cox, A.C. (1984) J. Biol. Chem. 259, 2306–2310.
73 Rogers, G.M. and Schuman, M.A. (1983) Proc. Natl. Acad. Sci. (U.S.A.) 80, 7001–7005.
74 Hemker, H.C., van Rijn, J.L.M.L., Rosing, J., Van Dieijen, G., Bevers, E.M. and Zwaal, R.F.A. (1983) Blood Cells 9, 303–317.
75 Nesheim, M.E., Hibbard, L.S., Tracy, P.B., Bloom, J.W., Myrmel, K.H. and Mann, K.G. (1980) in: The Regulation of Coagulation (Mann, K.G. and Taylor, F.B., Eds.) pp. 145–160, Elsevier, New York.
76 Rosing, J., Tans, G., Govers–Riemslag, J.W.P., Zwaal, R.F.A. and Hemker, H.C. (1980) J. Biol. Chem. 255, 274–283.
77 Nesheim, M.E., Tracy, R.P. and Mann, K.G. (1984) J. Biol. Chem. 259, 1447–1453.
78 Malhotra, O.P., Nesheim, M.E. and Mann, K.G. (1985) J. Biol. Chem. 260, 279–287.
79 Nesheim, M.E. and Mann, K.G. (1983) J. Biol. Chem. 258, 5386–5391.
80 Krishnaswamy, S., Mann, K.G. and Nesheim, M.E. (1986) J. Biol. Chem. 261 (19), 8977–8984.
81 Miletich, J.P., Kane, W.H., Hofmann, S.L., Stanford, N. and Majerus, P.W. (1979) Blood 54, 1015–1022.

R.F.A. Zwaal and H.C. Hemker (Eds.), *Blood Coagulation*
© 1986 Elsevier Science Publishers B.V. (Biomedical Division)

Nonenzymatic cofactors: factor VIII

PHILIP J. FAY, STEPHEN I. CHAVIN, DOMINIQUE MEYER[1] and
VICTOR J. MARDER

*Hematology Unit, Department of Medicine, University of Rochester School of Medicine
and Dentistry, Rochester, New York (U.S.A.), and [1]Institut de Pathologie Cellulaire,
INSERM, U 143, Hôpital de Bicêtre , Paris (France)*

1. Introduction

The critical role of factor VIII in hemostasis is vividly illustrated by the severe hemorrhagic disorder of classic hemophilia that results from its deficiency, whether congenital or acquired. Interest in the structure, function and metabolism of this coagulation protein has been commensurate with its biochemical and clinical importance, although progress has been painstakingly slow because of the unavailability of pure protein. This limitation is the result primarily of its very low plasma concentration of less than 100 ng/ml and its apparent high sensitivity to protease degradation. Recently, progress has occurred in two directions that has allowed for a significant increase in experimental observation. First, relatively pure preparations have been obtained from blood, especially by use of highly specific antibodies to factor VIII. Second, recombinant DNA technology has been successfully applied, and new insights are now provided for the structure of factor VIII as well as for its gene. As a result of these advances, our understanding of factor VIII will certainly accelerate in the next several years. This chapter will summarize our current appreciation of the biochemistry, immunology, function and metabolism of newly synthesized and circulating forms of factor VIII, and will also consider its striking similarity to factor V and its unique characteristic of binding to von Willebrand factor (vWF). Since factor VIII has until recently been purified mostly in its complexed form with vWF, some ambiguity in terminology exists in the literature, especially in the outmoded designation of vWF as 'factor VIII-related antigen'. In this chapter, we define factor VIII as an entity entirely distinct from vWF, which has its own unique molecular structure, biologic function, genetic control and, in its absence or malfunction, disease states.

Reference	Source			Gel filtration / Gel elution and su-		
Fay et al. [7,8]	Purified human	1 400 000	20 000	230 000	155 000 146 000 120 000 90 000 / 82 000 80 000	90 000 (51 000; 38 000) / 75 000 73 000
Hoyer and Trabold [13]	Partially purified	–	–	285 000		116 000 (70 000)

38

2. Biochemistry

(a) Purification and molecular weight of polypeptide chains

Until the report by Vehar and Davie in 1980 [1], preparation of active factor VIII contained mostly fibrinogen and von Willebrand protein with relatively little factor VIII protein. Vehar and Davie utilized bulk quantities of bovine plasma as starting material and conventional fractionation and chromatographic techniques to achieve a preparation with specific activity about 300 000-fold higher than plasma. SDS–urea–polyacrylamide gel electrophoresis (SDS–PAGE) of the final preparation showed only 3 polypeptides of equal staining intensity, with M_r of 93 000, 88 000 and 85 000 (Table 1). Although these chains apparently were not disulfide-linked, one of the purification steps involved disulfide bond reduction and therefore the polypeptides originally may have been disulfide bonded. Fass et al. [2,3] and Lollar et al. [4] reported a similar degree of purification for porcine factor VIII. By use of an immunoadsorbant column of anti-factor VIII monoclonal antibody coupled to agarose, they obtained a preparation consisting of 4 polypeptides, of which the smallest (M_r 76 000) had the greatest staining intensity. Amino acid sequence analysis indicated that the 3 largest polypeptides derived from the same amino terminal portion of the protein, and that the polypeptides of M_r 130 000 and 82 000 were proteolytic products of the M_r 166 000 polypeptide [5]. The smallest chain (M_r 76 000) had a distinctly different amino terminal sequence, suggesting its origin from a different portion of the molecule. The data were considered to be compatible with a two-chain molecule, in which 1 of the 3 larger polypeptides was bound to the smallest, presumably by a non-covalent bond.

Fulcher and Zimmerman [6] purified human factor VIII by application of therapeutic concentrates to an anti-von Willebrand protein monoclonal immunosorbant column and elution of column-bound factor VIII with a 0.25 M calcium chloride-containing buffer to dissociate it from the antibody-bound protein. Electrophoresis of this preparation identified at least 6 faintly staining bands of M_r 90 000–188 000, and a major doublet of M_r 79 000, 80 000. Fay et al. [7] purified human factor VIII to a specific activity of 20 000 U/mg (about 1.4×10^6-fold higher than plasma) by means of chemical fractionation, filtration and anion exchange chromatography, and have identified polypeptides of M_r 155 000, 146 000, 120 000 and an 82 000/80 000 doublet. A polypeptide of M_r 100 000 that was present in an earlier preparation [8,9] could be separated in the last purification step from the factor VIII coagulant activity.

Rotblat et al. [10] described a human factor VIII preparation produced by a combination of chemical and immunological techniques, in which cryoprecipitate was adsorbed to a specially modified insoluble polymer (polyelectrolyte E5), then eluted and applied to an anti-vW protein monoclonal antibody immunosorbant column. Factor VIII was eluted with calcium, then directly adsorbed on an anti-factor VIII monoclonal antibody column; eluted factor VIII had a specific activity of about 4000 U/mg and some preparations showed a very high molecular weight

TABLE 1

polypeptide of about 365 000. This preparation was analyzed by Vehar et al. [11] by two-dimensional thin-layer chromatography, and polypeptides of M_r 210 000, 170 000, 150 000, 120 000, and 90 000 all had remarkably similar fingerprint patterns, in distinction to polypeptides of M_r 82 000 and 80 000. The same conclusion as reached by Fass et al. was drawn, namely that the polypeptides greater than 80 000 were all derived from the amino terminal portion of the molecule by progressive cleavages at the C-terminal part of the peptide, and each was bound to a small polypeptide chain of 80 000. The occasional presence of a very high molecular weight polypeptide by Rotblat et al. [10] suggests that a single high molecular weight precursor factor VIII polypeptide may exist which undergoes proteolysis during purification. Separation of the putative two-chain protein by calcium-chelating agents into large plus small polypeptide chains suggests that a calcium bridge holds the two chains together as a complex [12].

(b) Total molecular weight

Molecular weight estimates or measurements of undissociated factor VIII preparation have indicated a large molecule of 250 000 or greater. Hoyer and Trabold [13] used a partially purified preparation of human factor VIII and calculated the molecular weight of the active moiety by measurement of the Stokes radius after gel filtration and the sedimentation coefficient by sucrose density gradient centrifugation. The calculated value was 285 000 (Table 1), but the preparation was not pure enough or sufficiently concentrated to detect subunit polypeptide chains of the factor VIII protein. Vehar and Davie [1] estimated the size of bovine factor VIII at 250 000–300 000 using gel permeation chromatography, and this value was in reasonable agreement with the sum of the 3 individual polypeptides (266 000) that they identified in the preparation. Fass and colleagues [3] surmised that the molecular size of a 2-chain molecule would be approximately 242 000, representing the largest of the peptides (M_r 166 000) plus the small peptide (M_r 76 000). Fay and colleagues [8] used HPLC gel filtration and found that the activity eluted at the position of approximately 230 000, compatible with the 2-chain polypeptide model of Fass et al. [3]. Weinstein et al. [14,15] used a method of electrophoretic analysis of a complex of human factor VIII with radiolabeled anti-factor VIII Fab, using non-reducing conditions in the presence of SDS. On the assumption that no more than one Fab fragment binds to each factor VIII molecule, the molecular weight of factor VIII was estimated to be 240 000 in both plasma and factor VIII concentrates. They also noted single-chain molecular weight species of M_r 180 000, 120 000 and 100 000. The highest single polypeptide chain observed under conditions of SDS–PAGE was that of Rotblat et al. [10] (M_r 365 000), but this single-chain moiety was not a predominant species and was probably easily degraded to smaller derivatives by protease digestion during preparation.

An accurate determination of the amino acid content of the intact factor VIII species was obtained from cloned human factor VIII, as reported by Vehar et al. [11,16] and Toole et al. [17] in November 1984. The dramatic success of cloning technology (discussed below) allowed for a molecular weight determination based upon amino acid sequence analysis alone, with virtual agreement between the two studies of 265 000 and 267 000. The molecular size of the cloned factor VIII does not include a contribution by carbohydrate, since this portion of the protein has not yet been determined. Nevertheless, this value agrees with most of the determinations by physico-chemical analysis of purified plasma factor VIII. Although the intact factor VIII molecule probably is significantly larger than 265 000, the predominant circulating form of factor VIII in plasma appears to be a 2-chained molecule of approximately 250 000. All of the preparations reported to date possess the required properties of being potentiated by both thrombin and factor X_a, and of being inactivated by both activated protein C and human acquired antibodies to factor VIII.

(c) Carbohydrate content

Most of the carbohydrate in the factor VIII–von Willebrand protein complex is part of the von Willebrand protein rather that the factor VIII since the latter comprises less than 1% of the total protein [18–20]. Nevertheless, there is evidence that factor VIII also is a glycoprotein. Purified bovine factor VIII binds to concanavalin agarose and can be eluted with α-methylglucopyranoside [1] and furthermore, the polypeptides in a purified preparation of human factor VIII react with periodic acid-Schiff stain after electrophoresis in denaturing polyacrylamide gels [21]. The carbohydrate of factor VIII probably does not influence coagulant activity, since Sodetz et al. [22] showed that neuraminidase and β-galactosidase had no effect on the factor VIII clotting activity. More recently, Fay et al. [9] depleted carbohydrate with a mixture of endoglycosidases and exoglycosidases without significant change in clotting activity. Furthermore, activity of sugar-depleted factor VIII could still be potentiated by thrombin and the decay rate of activity after such activation was the same as untreated factor VIII.

(d) Disulfide and calcium bridges

Thus far, evidence in support of the 2-chain structure of factor VIII has been indirect, with no clear-cut demonstration of disulfide or calcium bridges holding the two polypeptide chains together. However, the role of calcium in the integrity of factor VIII structure is strongly implied by the sensitivity of coagulant activity to storage in citrated plasma in contrast to its stabilization in heparinized plasma [23] or in buffer containing physiological levels of calcium ions [24]. The presence of homologies in factor VIII with ceruloplasmin (see below) suggests that copper or other divalent metal ion-binding sites may be present in factor VIII although not necessarily as a bridge between the two polypeptide chains.

Agents which react with free sulfhydryl groups have little or no effect on factor VIII activity [25–27] and even reduction of some disulfide bonds with low concentrations of dithiothreitol followed by alkylation does not affect factor VIII activity

[26,27]. With higher concentrations of reducing agents (2.3–3.9 mM) followed by alkylation, factor VIII levels are reduced by up to 73%, coincident with a reduction in size of the molecule, as measured by changes in gel filtration behavior [26]. These results suggest that disulfide bonds play an as yet uncertain role in maintenance of the structure of factor VIII, perhaps more with regard to intrachain bonds than with bridges between the two polypeptide chains. The best evidence yet available for the non-covalent nature of bridges between two chains of factor VIII is that of Fass and colleagues [12], based upon the differential elution of polypeptide chains from immunoabsorbant anti-factor VIII columns in the presence or absence of calcium-chelating agents.

(e) Protease (thrombin) cleavage

Changes in polypeptide size and overall molecular weight of factor VIII have been noted after thrombin exposure (Table 1), such experiments usually performed in association with measurements of factor VIII activity, its potentiation or loss. The considerable controversy regarding the association of such activity changes with structural changes (considered below) is to some degree a reflection of the differences and heterogeneity of factor VIII preparations and the complex changes that follow thrombin exposure. Hoyer and Trabold [13] showed a conversion from an M_r 285000 molecule to a species of M_r 116000 in association with thrombin activation of activity, followed by a decrease in molecular size to M_r 70000 in association with thrombin inactivation of factor VIII. McKee et al. [28,29] showed similar changes in gel filtration behavior followed by the exposure of partially purified factor VIII to thrombin. Weinstein and Chute [15] demonstrated thrombin-induced conversion of a single polypeptide chain of M_r 240000 to an M_r 100000 species and subsequent one of M_r 80000, also in association with initial potentiation and ultimate inactivation of factor VIII function. Gel electrophoretic analyses of highly purified bovine factor VIII [1] showed conversion of 3 polypeptide chains of 93000, 88000 and 85000 to a doublet of about 75000 and a small polypeptide of 38000, but the relationship between the resultant polypeptides and the parent chains is not certain. Lollar et al. [4] showed that the larger polypeptides of porcine factor VIII were cleaved to chains of 69000, 44000 and 35000, but that the initial polypeptide of 76000 was unchanged. Fulcher et al. [6,21] indicated that polypeptides of 100000 or greater were all converted to a chain of 92000 which was subsequently split approximately in half (54000 and 44000), and that the doublet of 79000/80000 was converted to a smaller doublet of 71000/72000. Data by Fay et al. [7] most closely approximate that of Fulcher and Zimmerman, with a polypeptide of 90000 deriving from the larger chains and conversion of the doublet moiety to a smaller doublet after loss of mass of approximately 10000.

Thus, there does appear to be some general agreement that the larger of the two polypeptides that constitute factor VIII is progressively converted to a moiety of M_r slightly under 100000, which is then clipped approximately in half, while the smaller polypeptide chain is retained after thrombin treatment as a moiety only slightly reduced from the untreated form. The corresponding changes in undissociated factor VIII molecules after thrombin treatment will require further correlative studies.

3. Gene cloning

Recently, two groups have successfully cloned the human factor VIII gene. Both Genentech [11,16,30], in collaboration with Tuddenham and Genetics Institute [17], with Fass, used similar methods for the DNA cloning and expression of active factor VIII and report similar results. Using information obtained from the amino acid sequence of portions of purified, plasma-derived factor VIII, specific oligonucleotide probes were constructed and used to probe a genomic library containing DNA derived from an individual with 4 X-chromosomes. The factor VIII gene was very long, consisting of about 186 kb, equivalent to about 0.1% of the X-chromosome. DNA sequence analysis of the cloned gene revealed 26 exons (coding sequences) ranging in size from 69 to 3106 base pairs and introns (intervening DNA sequences) which range in size from 207 to 32 400 base pairs. The complete gene sequence consists of about 9 kb of exon and 177 kb of intron sequences.

Genomic clones of exon sequences provided a probe with which to identify a tissue source for factor VIII mRNA. Analysis of human liver mRNA demonstrated the presence of a single mRNA of about 9 kb specific for the factor VIII probe. An mRNA of this size could encode for a single-chain factor VIII precursor of about M_r 300 000. The isolated mRNA in turn was used to construct a cDNA library. Selected cDNA and genomic exon DNA fragments were assembled and ultimately gave rise to a full-length factor VIII cDNA clone. This sequence subsequently was inserted into a plasmid capable of transcribing heterologous sequences upon transfection into mammalian cell cultures. Monkey kidney cells served as the host for the Genetic Institute clone whereas hamster kidney cells were used by Genentech.

A predominant 9-kb RNA from transfected, but not from control untransfected cells, hybridized to an oligonucleotide probe specific for factor VIII, thus indicating the transcription of the factor VIII DNA sequences. Monoclonal antibodies directed against both N- and C-terminal sequences of plasma-derived factor VIII showed a 300-fold increase in factor VIII cross-reactivity in the recombinant cells, indicating translation of the factor VIII mRNA into protein. To determine if the recombinant factor VIII was functionally active, protein secreted into the medium by the transfected cells was partially purified using an anti-factor VIII monoclonal antibody immunosorbant column, similar to that employed for the purification of plasma-derived factor VIII. The immunoaffinity-purified protein shortened the clotting time of plasma from a hemophilia A patient. The levels of secreted factor VIII were about 0.01 and 0.07 units/ml for the Genetics Institute and Genentech preparations, respectively. The recombinant factor VIII activity was neutralized by anti-factor VIII monoclonal antibodies as well as by antibody from a patient

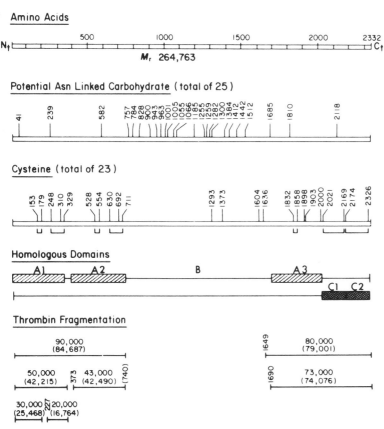

Fig. 1. Line diagram illustrating the salient features of the recombinant factor VIII precursor protein. Asparagine-linked glycosylation sites and cysteine residues are potential, not proven sites of carbohydrate additions and disulfide bridges, respectively. Domain structures show boxes indicating the triplicated domains ('A') homologous to ceruloplasmin as well as a different duplicated domain ('C') and a unique 'B' domain. The molecular weights of the thrombin-derived fragments were determined by SDS–polyacrylamide gel electrophoresis. The M_r value is calculated from the actual amino acid composition shown in parentheses. The position of cleavage of the M_r 90 000 polypeptide has not been determined. (Reproduced with permission from Nature; Vehar et al. (1984) [11]).

with factor VIII inhibitor, and was potentiated by thrombin and inactivated by activated protein C. Genentech also showed that the recombinant protein bound to immobilized von Willebrand protein, a high molecular weight plasma protein presumed to serve in vivo as a carrier for factor VIII. The bound factor VIII could be eluted with high concentrations of calcium ions, as is the case with the plasma factor VIII. These functional results confirm that the factor VIII cDNA codes for an active factor VIII protein which possesses many of the characteristics described for plasma factor VIII.

The sequence of the cDNA clone indicates that the mature protein contains 2351 amino acids from the initiator methionine to the terminating tyrosine residues and begins with a hydrophobic, secretory leader peptide sequence of 19 amino acids (Fig. 1). This corresponds to a molecular weight of 264 763 [11] or 267 039 [17] (Table 1). Searches for internal homologies in the amino acid sequence, derived from the DNA sequence, revealed 3 types of domain structures: a triplicated 'A' unit of about 350 amino acids located at positions 1–329, 380–711 and 1649–2019; a unique 'B' unit of about 926 amino acids at position 712–1648; and a duplicated 'C' unit of about 160 amino acids located at the carboxy terminus of the molecule. The A domain has remarkable sequence homology with sequences of ceruloplasmin [11,17,31], a plasma protein that functions in copper transport, and amino acid sequence analysis identified a structure consisting of 3 contiguous domains sharing about 30% homology [32,33]. While no copper has been identified in the structure of factor VIII, the sensitivity of factor VIII to chelating reagents and the stabilization of factor VIII activity by calcium ions suggest that metal ions are important for the maintenance of factor VIII structure. Most of the 23 cysteine residues of the mature factor VIII polypeptide are contained in the A and C domains. The determination of disulfide bridging in ceruloplasmin predicts two types of arrangements for the A domain of factor VIII. The disulfide structures depicted in the C domains are based on the assumption that linkages form between the two cysteine residues within each domain. The B domain is extremely rich in potential asparagine-linked glycosylation sites (19 of 25) thus suggesting that this region may contain a large amount of carbohydrate side chains (Fig. 1).

Exposure of plasma-derived factor VIII to thrombin results in activation of factor VIII clotting activity and the appearance of new polypeptides. Information made available by the cDNA sequence has allowed for the analysis of the cleavage sequences and mapping of fragments. The most consistent sequences found at thrombin sites are arginine–serine or arginine–alanine. Only some of these potential sites are cleaved, suggesting the involvement of secondary structure in thrombin specificity. The cleavage which liberates the M_r 80 000 polypeptide occurs at an arginine–glutamic acid sequence, and is probably not a thrombin-generated fragment. The precursor factor VIII protein therefore may be cleaved to the free M_r 80 000 by a protease other than thrombin. This is consistent with the purification of plasma-derived factor VIII containing 2 polypeptide chains, a heavy chain of approximately M_r 200 000 (or a fragment derived from this chain) and a light chain of M_r 80 000. Thrombin activation of factor results in the appearance of an M_r 90 000 polypeptide (residues 1–740) resulting from the removal of the B domain or its fragments. Thrombin subsequently cleaves the M_r 90 000 polypeptide to products of M_r 50 000 and M_r 43 000; this site is located at the junction of the A1 and A2 domains. Thrombin further cleaves the M_r 50 000 polypeptide to products of M_r 30 000 and 20 000. The M_r 80 000 polypeptide is cleaved after residue 1689 to an M_r 73 000 fragment thereby releasing an M_r 4500 peptide. This peptide contains a single glycosylation site and is highly acidic, containing 15 acidic residues and only 4 basic residues out of 41 amino acids.

Thus, the abundant information provided by the gene-cloning success has not only helped to explain the polypeptide chain structure of purified plasma factor

VIII and its thrombin cleavage products, but it has highlighted dramatic new observations, such as the ceruloplasmin homology, and extends the potential for understanding function and especially for producing therapeutic material in quantity.

4. Immunological aspects

The availability of purified factor VIII has provided the means for producing large quantities of heterologous antibodies, both polyclonal [6] and monoclonal [21,34–39], all of which have been applied effectively for purification and assay of factor VIII. Even without these relatively new tools, the use of human anti-factor VIII antibodies obtained from hemophiliacs or previously normal individuals with factor VIII inhibitors have been used to develop sensitive in vitro assays for measuring small quantities of factor VIII. The techniques have involved neutralization of function by antibody [40] or very sensitive radiometric assays [39–42] that use radiolabeled and immunopurified antibody either in solid phase [39,41] or liquid phase by precipitation of immune complexes [41,42]. The sensitivity of these immunoradiometric assays is 0.01–0.03 U/ml, considering normal plasma to contain 1 U/ml. The assays have been utilized to study factor VIII content of normal and hemophilic samples and especially to compare protein concentration with coagulant activity.

Factor VIII antigen is present in serum but at a level only approximately 70% of that present in plasma [39,40,43]. The antigen retains reactivity in the immunologic assays at 37 or 4°C but is destroyed at a temperature of 56°C or at a pH of 4 or less. The concentration of factor VIII antigen is increased in the presence of EDTA [44] and decreased in the presence of phospholipid [45,46]. There is excellent correlation in most plasma samples between the concentration of factor VIII antigen and functional coagulant activity, in normals as well as in plasma from most patients with classical hemophilia or von Willebrand's disease [41]. About 70–90% of patients with severe hemophilia A and less than 1% of coagulant activity have undetectable levels of plasma factor VIII antigen. About 10–30% of severe hemophiliacs have less than 1% activity but higher levels of factor VIII antigen (1–10%) and 1 patient with undetectable activity has been reported with normal amounts of factor VIII antigen [47]. Patients with mild to moderate hemophilia usually have slightly more immunoreactive material than clotting activity. Those hemophilic patients who have greater amounts of antigenic material than relative clotting activity have been designated as A+ or CRM+ [38,41,48].

Factor VIII antigen assays have made it possible to measure this antigen in fetal blood [49], thereby allowing for prenatal diagnosis of classical hemophilia. Since amniotic fluid has no detectable factor VIII antigen, small amounts of fetal blood obtained at 18–20 weeks of gestation, even when mixed with small amounts of amniotic fluid, can be used to determine the plasma factor VIII level [49,50].

5. Function

(a) Coagulation

The majority of the plasma-clotting proteins are serine proteases, with two major exceptions being factors V and VIII. These coagulation cofactors seem to lack enzymatic activity and are thought to be non-catalytic components involved respectively in the formation of factor X_a and thrombin [51]. Regarding factor VIII, Østerud and Rapaport [52] used antisera that specifically inhibited either factor VIII or IX and showed that factor IX_a and factor VIII formed a bimolecular complex, both components of which were needed in order to achieve optimal activation of factor X.

Purified factor IX_a, in the absence of factor VIII, converts factor X to factor X_a; however, the addition of factor VIII increases the maximum velocity (V_{max}) of the reaction [53–56]. The major effect of phospholipid in this reaction is to lower the K_m for factor X from 299 μM to 0.057 μM [57]. In the absence of phospholipid, the K_m for factor X is 1000 times higher than the plasma concentration of factor X, and the reaction would proceed very slowly or not at all; in the presence of the optimal amount of phospholipid, the K_m is low enough for the reaction to proceed

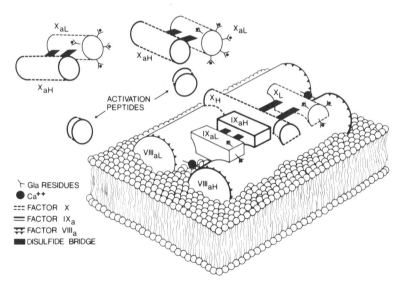

Fig. 2. Schematic representation of the factor X activating system ('tenase') consisting of factors IX_a, VIII_a, calcium and phospholipid. The phospholipid is shown as a typical membrane bilayer, with the polar head groups of each leaf oriented outward, and the aliphatic fatty acid chains directed internally. The factor VIII_a is represented as two polypeptides held together by two divalent calcium bridges, although the exact number of such bridges has yet to be determined. The binding of factors IX_a and X to factor VIII has yet to be demonstrated directly, although there is indirect evidence of interactions between factor IX_a and factor VIII_a. Once the activation peptide is cleaved from factor X_a, the active protease presumably is released and goes on to form a prothrombinase complex.

efficiently at the physiological concentration of factor X, provided that factor VIII is present as well (see Ch. 3). This effect of phospholipid probably is due largely to binding of factors VIII (or VIII$_a$), IX$_a$ and X to the lipid surface, thereby increasing their effective concentrations (Fig. 2). These results and conclusions are analogous to those presented for the prothrombinase complex [58,59], although the mechanism(s) by which factors VIII$_a$ and V$_a$ can increase markedly the maximum velocity of generation of factor X$_a$ and thrombin, respectively, are not known.

The possibility that factor VIII has enzymatic activity was suggested by Vehar and Davie [60], who showed that prior treatment of partially purified factor VIII with diisopropyl fluorophosphate (DFP) affected its level and stability. The known inhibitory effects of DFP on factors IX$_a$, X$_a$ and thrombin did not explain the loss of activity and it was proposed that this might have been the result of acylation of a reactive serine in factor VIII molecule, i.e. that factor VIII may be a serine protease. Attempts in other laboratories to reproduce this observation have not been successful [28] and, therefore, supportive evidence for the proposal that factor VIII is a serine protease is not yet available. Nevertheless, if one assumes that factor VIII has an M_r 200 000, and a plasma concentration of approximately 100 ng/ml [1,8], then the molar concentration is approximately 0.5 nM, about 200-fold lower than that of factors IX or X. The low molar ratio of factor VIII relative to factor X is compatible with the hypothesis [60] that one molecule of factor VIII interacts with many of factor IX and/or factor X, that is, that the mechanism has catalytic as well as stoichiometric features.

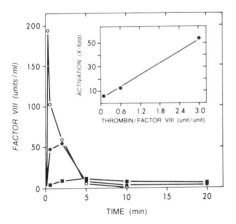

Fig. 3. Potentiation and inactivation of factor VIII coagulant activity by thrombin. Purified human factor VIII (4 U/ml) was incubated with 12.5 (○), 2.5 (●) or 0.25 (■) U/ml of human thrombin (kindly provided by Dr. John Fenton, Albany Medical Center) and the changes in factor VIII activity were monitored using a one-stage assay. The inset shows the linear relationship of the extent of coagulant activity potentiation to the unit ratio of thrombin:factor VIII. The values of 'activation' indicate the ratio of coagulant activity at peak potentiation relative to activity prior to thrombin interaction, plotted against the unit ratio of thrombin to factor VIII.

48

(b) Modulation of coagulant activity by thrombin

Factor VIII coagulant activity is potentiated by thrombin, then diminished to a level below that existing before thrombin exposure and finally eliminated. Although this effect occurs with an enzyme:substrate ratio as low as 1:50 [1,6,14], the data suggest that activation more closely resembles a stoichiometric rather than a catalytic reaction [3,8,28,61]. For example, a ratio of thrombin:factor VIII of 0.07 (unit:unit) results in a 5-fold potentiation, higher ratios produce a 50-fold potentiation (Fig. 3) and also result in a more rapid rate of inactivation. Thus, the higher the molar ratio of thrombin to factor VIII the greater will be the enhancement of activity. Although most investigators suggest that activation and inactivation each occur by proteolysis of the factor VIII substrate, other evidence suggests that the inactivation step is independent of a proteolytic cleavage. Switzer and McKee [28] showed that dansyl-arginine-4-ethylpiperadine amide (DAPA), a rapid competitive inhibitor of thrombin, has essentially no effect on the loss of thrombin-enhanced factor VIII activity. Additionally, rapid removal of factor VIII_a from continued exposure to a thrombin–agarose resin did not alter the rate of decay of activity from that expected with continued thrombin exposure. Detailed kinetic data reflecting the effect of thrombin inhibitors on potentiation and inactivation of factor VIII were reported by Hultin and Jesty [62]. They noted that thrombin-potentiated factor VIII activity decreased in the presence of either the competitive inhibitor DAPA or either of two irreversible inhibitors, diisopropylfluorophosphate (DFP), or hirudin, and that the initial period of decay was even more rapid than

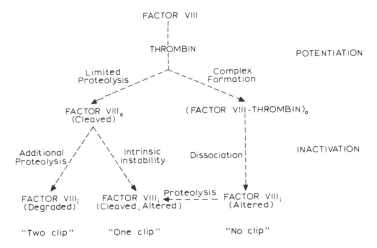

Fig. 4. Hypothetical mechanisms regarding the potentiation and inactivation of factor VIII coagulant activity by thrombin. The terms 'no-clip', 'one-clip', and 'two-clip' indicate proteolytic events that are postulated to occur during potentiation and/or inactivation of factor VIII coagulant activity but do not necessarily indicate the cleavage of single peptide sites at each step. Factor VIII_i (altered), the product of the 'no-clip' pathway, would be cleaved by thrombin to factor VIII_i (cleaved, altered) in an event unrelated to changes in functional activity.

in the absence of the inhibitor. They concluded that only the initial potentiation step depends upon the concentration of thrombin, whereas inactivation was the result of a first-order decay reaction, perhaps because factor VIII_a is intrinsically, or conformationally unstable. More recently, Lollar et al. [4] have succeeded in stabilizing the thrombin-potentiated level of porcine factor VIII in the presence of both factor IX_a and phospholipid. It is postulated that such stabilization of activity prevents the loss of conformational integrity of the potentiated factor VIII molecule by formation of the complex between phospholipid, factor IX_a and factor VIII_a (Fig. 2).

Three molecular mechanisms relating to the thrombin-mediated potentiation and inactivation of factor VIII activity are illustrated schematically in Fig. 4. The most widely accepted mechanism for potentiation is that of limited proteolysis of factor VIII. Subsequent inactivation may proceed by either a second proteolytic event which yields a more highly degraded molecule ('two-clip' model), but this explanation does not explain the failure of thrombin inhibitors to impede the rate of inactivation following the initial potentiation step. If this 'two-clip' pathway were correct, inhibitors would be expected to stabilize the potentiated factor VIII moiety by preventing or slowing down the second cleavage. A more attractive possibility is that potentiated factor VIII is intrinsically unstable and inactivation results from the loss of required confirmation, perhaps that which holds the two polypeptide chains together ('one-clip' model). The 'no-clip' model proposed by Hultin and Jesty [62] suggests that thrombin and factor VIII form a bimolecular complex which possesses enhanced clotting activity, and inactivation results from dissociation of this active complex. While this model was proposed to explain the failure of thrombin inhibitors to stabilize potentiated factor VIII, it also offers an explanation for the stoichiometric ratio of thrombin and factor VIII which seems to be required for maximal potentiation. The evidence to date favors the 'one-clip' model.

The relationship of potentiation and inactivation of factor VIII activity with the observed changes in polypeptide chain structure of purified factor VIII exposed to thrombin (Table 1) is still uncertain. The 'one-clip' model would suggest that thrombin converts the higher molecular weight polypeptides to an intermediate size during the potentiation step, possibly in association with the loss of a small peptide from the light chain, but that further changes in the polypeptide chains do not occur during the inactivation step. The model proposed by Fulcher et al. [21] is that of a 'two-clip' pattern in which potentiation is associated with accumulation of the M_r 92 000 moiety from the heavier chains, and inactivation is associated with cleavage of this moiety to the M_r 54 000 and 44 000 species. Other studies of partially purified factor VIII or factor VIII in plasma suggest a two-step proteolytic process [13,15].

A related question is whether 'native' factor VIII has intrinsic clotting activity or whether proteolysis converts an inactive factor VIII to one with coagulant activity. Experiments by Switzer et al. [63] showed that blood collected directly into protease inhibitors had less intrinsic factor VIII activity but could be potentiated to a greater degree by thrombin than could factor VIII prepared in the absence of inhibitors. The experiments were interpreted to indicate that factor VIII circulates as a relatively inactive precursor and that maximal clotting activity was expressed after limited proteolytic activation by thrombin or another serine protease, compatible with the 'one-clip' or 'two-clip' mechanism shown in Fig. 4.

(c) Interactions with other clotting proteins (Table 2)

The specific thrombin inhibitor, hirudin, partially inhibits factor X activation by a mixture of factors VIII and IX_a, but has no inhibitory effect on factor X activation by factor IX_a when factor VIII is absent [53,55]. One possible explanation for this failure of the thrombin inhibitor to block factor VIII-dependent activation of factor X is that more than one activator exists, only one of which is blocked by hirudin. Further evidence of the multiplicity of catalytic and cofactor pathways involved in factor X activation is indicated by the presence of and duration of a lag phase prior to developing maximum factor X_a generation by factors IX_a and VIII [1,54]. The elimination of the lag phase by preincubation of factors VIII and IX_a prompted the suggestion by Vehar and Davie [1] that the effect of factor IX_a on the lag phase was the result of a different mechanism from that of factor X_a or thrombin. The role of factor VIII in the activation of factor X_a is therefore complex, given the interaction and feedback mechanisms between thrombin and factor X_a as well as other possible physiological activators that may participate in the reaction. Just as feedback potentiation of factor V by thrombin is important for the action of the prothrombinase complex (factor X_a–prothrombin–factor V_a–calcium) [58,64,65], factor X_a may be important in feedback potentiation of factor VIII in the generation of factor X_a by the 'tenase' complex (factor IX_a–factor X–factor VIII_a–calcium). The mechanism of potentiation of factor VIII activity by factor X_a is probably similar to that of thrombin, based upon similar rates of potentiation

TABLE 2

Plasma serine proteases that affect factor VIII coagulant activity

Protein	Action	Probable mechanism
Thrombin	Activation	Limited proteolysis
	Inactivation	Intrinsic instability
Factor X_a	Activation	Limited proteolysis
	Inactivation	Intrinsic instability
Factor IX_a	Activation	Not known
Activated protein C (C_a)	Inactivation	Limited proteolysis
Protein S	Accelerates protein C_a inactivation	Enhances phospholipid binding of protein C_a

and inactivation [1,8] as well as studies of protease inhibitors which failed to stabilize factor X_a-potentiated factor VIII coagulant activity, as has been noted for thrombin [62].

Modulation of enhanced factor VIII procoagulant activity is also achieved by interaction with the activated form of protein C [66]. This plasma protein is an important inhibitor of blood coagulation that is converted from an inactive zymogen by the thrombin:thrombomodulin complex on endothelial surfaces [67,68], and requires calcium and phospholipid for efficient inactivation of factor VIII_a (and factor V_a) coagulant activity (cf. [1,8] and Ch. 9B). Several studies have shown proteolytic cleavages of the factor VIII polypeptide chains, specifically the M_r 93 000 moiety of bovine factor VIII [1] and the M_r 92 000 polypeptide of human factor VIII [69]. A second vitamin K-dependent serine protease, protein S [70], enhances the rate of factor V_a inactivation by activated protein C [71,72], presumably by stoichiometric interaction that enhances the binding of activated protein C to phospholipid vesicles (cf. [72] and Ch. 9B). Presumably, protein S also enhances factor VIII_a inactivation by activated protein C.

6. Biosynthesis and metabolism

Determination of the site of biosynthesis of factor VIII prior to the application of monoclonal antibody and recombinant DNA technology was based primarily upon physiological experiments such as epinephrine stimulation and transplantation experiments in animals, which produced somewhat ambiguous thought-provocative suggestions, reviewed comprehensively by Webster et al. [73] and Bloom [74]. That the liver is the major organ of factor VIII synthesis was further suggested by studies of rat liver perfusion, using normal or von Willebrand protein-deficient plasma, which demonstrated a significant shortening of clotting time in the perfusate that was inhibited by cyclohexamide and/or actinomycin. The result indicated hepatic synthesis, but did not distinguish whether such synthesis occurred in the hepatocyte or other cells of the liver.

Using immunochemical techniques with anti-human factor VIII antibody, Kelly et al. [75] reported the presence of factor VIII protein in liver, spleen and kidney extracts from guinea pigs and suggested that the hepatocyte was the major source of factor VIII. However, Stel et al. [76] and van der Kwast et al. [77] used mouse monoclonal antibodies against human factor VIII to study cryostat sections of intact liver and found factor VIII in the hepatic sinusoidal endothelial cells as well as in non-lymphoid mononuclear cells of lung, spleen and lymph nodes, but not in the hepatic parenchymal cell. Neither of these studies demonstrated factor VIII coagulant activity or distinguished between de novo synthesis and factor VIII storage.

The most definitive information yet available comes from successful molecular cloning of factor VIII [17,30]. By means of in vitro hybridization techniques with factor VIII DNA probes, factor VIII mRNA has been detected in extracts from hepatocyte and non-hepatocyte liver cells as well as from spleen, kidney and placenta, but not in peripheral blood cells. This demonstration of an active factor VIII gene and its mRNA transcription in different tissues suggests but does not prove that factor VIII is translated in several types of cell. Still, the liver appears to be the major organ for factor VIII synthesis. The recent report providing evidence that factor V is definitely synthesized by endothelial cells [78] suggests that new technology or more strenuous study of factor VIII biosynthesis by endothelial cells may also demonstrate that this cell is the source for plasma factor VIII as well.

The concentration of factor VIII in plasma is regulated primarily by genes located on the X-chromosome (see discussion on gene cloning above), but genetic control of von Willebrand protein concentration also influences factor VIII levels, primarily by virtue of its factor VIII transport property (see below). In addition to these genetic controls, a number of pathologic conditions and pharmacologic agents can cause transient changes in the level of factor VIII, including pregnancy, chronic liver disease, physical exertion, hypoxia, adrenergic agents, vasopressin and disseminated intravascular coagulation (DIC) [73,74].

Following intravenous infusion of factor VIII, the increased level of clotting activity shows approximately two phases of decay, an initial decrease during the first several hours which was presumed to be due to equilibration with extravascular pools, followed by a longer linear phase with a half-time of 8–12 h [79]. This half-time occurs in normals and hemophiliacs and is the same with plasma, cryoprecipitate or factor VIII concentrate. Factor VIII protein and factor VIII coagulant activity disappear at the same rates, indicating that disappearance is most likely due to removal of the protein rather than inactivation. The survival of factor VIII may be shortened by the presence of antibodies against factor VIII, although overall consumption in the course of active hemostasis or hypercatabolic states such as after surgery does not significantly change the decay rates [79,80]. Infusion of factor VIII into patients with von Willebrand's disease results in a much longer survival with little or no decrease in concentration at 24–48 h. In addition, a small secondary rise in factor VIII level may occur at 18–24 h after injection. It is not known whether these differences between hemophiliacs and von Willebrand disease patients are due to differences in transport and catabolism of the exogenous factor VIII, to release of stored factor VIII, or to induction of synthesis of factor VIII consequent upon the infusion.

7. Comparison with factor V

Factors V and VIII appear to share structural and functional features (see also Ch. 2A). Both serve cofactor roles in the intrinsic clotting cascade, interacting with an activated vitamin K-dependent protein, phospholipid and calcium to activate a second vitamin K-dependent protein, factor X_a or thrombin for factors VIII and V respectively (see Ch. 3).

Precursor factor V purified from bovine [81,82] or human [83] plasma is a single-chain glycoprotein of M_r 330 000, similar in size to the largest single-chain factor VIII isolated from plasma [10], and is compatible with the precursor deduced from amino acid sequence of the recombinant molecule, to which carbohydrate is probably added [11,17] (Table 1). While the entire sequence of factor VIII is known [11,17], only limited portions of the factor V sequence have been determined and therefore the full extent of sequence similarity of these two proteins has not been determined [84].

Factors V and VIII are cleaved at several sites by thrombin to generate the activated forms. Human factor V_a [83] consists of an M_r 105 000 amino-terminal-derived fragment that is non-covalently bound to an M_r 71 000–74 000 doublet derived from the carboxy terminus. Internal fragments of M_r 150 000 and 71 000 are activation peptides that contain a high proportion of carbohydrate. The amino- and carboxy-terminal fragments are linked by calcium ions and are separable by treatment with EDTA, and the separated fragments, which are individually inactive, can be recombined in the presence of calcium or manganese ions with restoration of functional activity.

These results are remarkably similar to those postulated and observed for factor VIII. Thrombin cleavage of factor VIII generates an amino-terminal-derived heavy chain (M_r 90 000) and a carboxy-terminal-derived light chain (M_r 80 000) [11] with an internal region of factor VIII containing most of the asparagine residues which potentially carry sugar linkages [11,17]. When treated with EDTA, the factor VIII polypeptides are dissociated and activity is lost [3], suggesting a similar calcium bridge, although recombination of the dissociated fragments or regeneration of activity with calcium have not been successful. Factors V and VIII are substrates for activated protein C, which cleaves factor V [85,86] and factor VIII [1,8,69] to yield inactive forms.

Although there exist both structural and functional similarities between factors V and VIII, subtle differences also exist. Thrombin-activated factor V (V_a) is a relatively stable cofactor, whereas the activity of factor VIII_a is labile in the absence of phospholipid and factor IX_a. Factor V is present in human plasma at a much higher concentration, approximately 18 μg/ml or about 55 nM [83] in comparison to estimates of factor VIII plasma concentration of about 50–200 ng/ml or 0.2–1 nM [1,8]. This latter concentration is 50–200-fold lower than that for factor V and may indicate significant functional or regulatory differences between the two clotting proteins.

8. Relationship with von Willebrand factor

Factor VIII probably exists in plasma primarily in a non-covalent complex with von Willebrand factor, representing no more than 1% of the total mass of this complex, with about 10–15% of factor VIII circulating in free form. The evidence for the existence of such a factor VIII/von Willebrand factor complex is mostly indirect, derived from clinical, immunological and biochemical data. Clinically, there is excellent correlation between factor VIII coagulant activity and von Willebrand factor activity in normal individuals as well as in most patients with von Wille-brand's disease, in contrast with a lack of correlation between factor VIII and any of the other coagulation or carrier proteins. Polyclonal or monoclonal antibodies specific for von Willebrand factor bind factor VIII in addition to von Willebrand factor [87–89], presumably by way of the bimolecular interaction between them, and this property has been used for the purification of human factor VIII [6,10]. The non-covalent complex is further indicated by gel filtration experiment in which physiologic ionic strength buffers elute factor VIII together with von Willebrand factor in the void volume fractions after agarose gel filtration. Analysis of normal plasma by SDS–agarose gel electrophoresis indicates that 60–70% of factor VIII is present in complex with the largest molecular weight multimers of von Wille-brand factor [90]. The complex can be separated into component parts by high ionic strength buffers, a high concentration of calcium, detergents or traces of thrombin [91–94], and reassociation of the component parts in vitro may occur with resto-ration of proper ionic strength conditions [95,96] or in vivo following the infusion of von Willebrand factor–free factor VIII fraction into patients with hemophilia A [97]. The non-covalent association of factor VIII and von Willebrand factor is also disrupted by EDTA [24,44] and the resultant inactive factor VIII moieties sub-sequently elute as a smaller protein. Thus, calcium may play a role not only in the non-covalent binding of the presumed 2-chained structure of factor VIII but also in the stabilization of the quaternary structure of factor VIII/von Willebrand fac-tor complexes. Although the major function of von Willebrand factor is to pro-mote the adhesion of platelets to subendothelial matrix or to each other [98], this protein appears to play an important role as a carrier protein for factor VIII and possibly as a mechanism for stabilizing its coagulant activity.

9. Conclusion

Our understanding of factor VIII has finally reached the tangible level of straightforward protein chemistry, now that sufficient quantities of purified ma-terial are available. With the added impetus of cloned material for study and ul-timately treatment, the expectation is for rapid elucidation of fine-point details of immunology, structure–function relationships, binding sites to von Willebrand fac-tor, cell biosynthesis, genetic control and plasma regulation. Previously elusive in-sights to this most important clotting protein are now attainable.

Acknowledgements

We gratefully acknowledge Carol Weed for typing the manuscript and Vince Sullivan for drawing the illustration shown in Fig. 2.

This work was supported in part by Grant No. HL 30616 from the National Heart, Lung and Blood Institute, National Institutes of Health, Bethesda, MD. Dr. Fay is the recipient of a New Investigator Research Award, No. HL 34050 from the National Heart, Lung and Blood Institute.

References

1 Vehar, G.A. and Davie, E.W. (1980) Biochemistry 19, 401.
2 Fass, D.N., Knutson, G.J. and Katzmann, J.A. (1982) Blood 59, 594.
3 Knutson, G.J. and Fass, D.N (1982) Blood 59, 615.
4 Lollar, P., Knutson, G.J. and Fass, D.N. (1984) Blood 63, 1303.
5 Fass, D.N., Hewick, R., Knutson, G.J., Nesheim, M.E. and Mann, K.G. (1983) Thromb. Haemostas. 50, 801.
6 Fulcher, C.A. and Zimmerman, T.S. (1982) Proc. Natl. Acad. Sci. (U.S.A.) 79, 1648.
7 Fay, P.J., Anderson, M.T., Chavin, S.I. and Marder, V.J. (1985) Thromb. Haemostas. 54, 45.
8 Fay, P.J., Chavin, S.I., Schroeder, D., Young, F.E. and Marder, V.J. (1982) Proc. Natl. Acad. Sci. (U.S.A.) 79, 7200.
9 Fay, P.J., Chavin, S.I., Schroeder, D., Young, F.E. and Marder, V.J. (1984) Biochim. Biophys. Acta 800, 152.
10 Rotblat, F., O'Brien, D.P., Middleton, S.M. and Tuddenham, E.G.D. (1983) Thromb. Haemostas. 50, 108.
11 Vehar, G.A., Keyt, B., Eaton, D., Rodriguez, H., O'Brien, D.P., Rotblat, F., Opperman, H., Keck, R., Wood, W.I., Harkins, R.N., Tuddenham, E.G.D., Lawn, R.M. and Capon, D.J. (1984) Nature (London) 312, 337.
12 Fass, D.N., Knutson, G.J. and Hewick, R. (1983) Thromb. Haemostas. 50, 817.
13 Hoyer, L.W. and Trabold, N.C. (1981) J. Lab. Clin. Med. 97, 50.
14 Weinstein, M., Chute, L. and Deykin, D. (1981) Proc. Natl. Acad. Sci. (U.S.A.) 78, 5137.
15 Weinstein, M.J. and Chute, L.E. (1984) J. Clin. Invest. 73, 307.
16 Wood, W.I., Capon, D.J., Simonsen, C.C., Eaton, D.L., Gitschier, J., Keyt, B., Seeburg, P.H., Smith, D.H., Hollingshead, P., Wion, K.L., Delwart, E., Tuddenham, E.G.D., Vehar, G.A. and Lawn, R.M. (1984) Nature (London) 312, 330.
17 Toole, J.J., Knopf, J.L., Wozney, J.M., Sultzman, L.A., Buecker, J.L., Pittman, D.D., Kaufman, R.J., Brown, E., Shoemaker, C., Orr, E.C., Amphlett, G.W., Foster, W.B., Coe, M.L., Knutson, G.J., Fass, D.N. and Hewick, R.M. (1984) Nature (London) 312, 342.
18 Legaz, M.E., Schmer, G., Counts, R.B. and Davie, E.W. (1973) J. Biol. Chem. 248, 3946.
19 Switzer, M.E. and McKee, P.A. (1976) J. Clin. Invest. 57, 925.
20 Switzer, M.E. and McKee, P.A. (1977) J. Clin. Invest. 60, 819.
21 Fulcher, C.A., Roberts, J.R. and Zimmerman, T.S. (1983) Blood 61, 807.
22 Sodetz, J.M., Pizzo, S.V. and McKee, P.A. (1977) J. Biol. Chem. 252, 5538.
23 Krachmalnicoff, A. and Thomas, D.P. (1983) Thromb. Haemostas. 49, 224.
24 Mikaelsson, M.E., Forsman, N. and Oswaldsson, U.M. (1983) Blood 62, 1006.
25 Austin, D.E.G. (1970) Br. J. Haematol. 19, 472.
26 Blomback, B., Hessel, B., Savidge, G., Wikstoom, L. and Blomback, M. (1978) Thromb. Res. 12, 1177.
27 Harris, R.B., Newman, J. and Johnson, A.J. (1981) Biochim. Biophys. Acta 668, 456.
28 Switzer, M.E. and McKee, P.A. (1980) J. Biol. Chem. 255, 10606.
29 McKee, P.A., Andersen, J.C. and Switzer, M.E. (1975) Ann. N.Y. Acad. Sci. 240, 8.
30 Gitschier, J., Wood, W.I., Goralka, T.M., Wion, K.L., Chen, E.Y., Eaton, D.H., Vehar, G.A., Capon, D.J. and Lawn, R.M. (1984) Nature (London) 312, 326.
31 Church, W.R., Jernigan, T.L., Toole, J., Hewick, R.M., Knopf, J., Knutson, G.J., Nesheim, M.E., Mann, K.G. and Fass, D.N. (1984) Proc. Natl. Acad. Sci. (U.S.A.) 81, 6934.

32 Takahashi, N., Ortel, T.L. and Putnam, F.W. (1984) Proc. Natl. Acad. Sci. (U.S.A.) 81, 390.

33 Dwulet, F.E. and Putman, F.W. (1981) Proc. Natl. Acad. Sci. (U.S.A.) 78, 2805.

34 Brown, J.E., Thuy, L.P., Carton, C.L. and Hougie, C. (1983) J. Lab. Clin. Med. 101, 793.

35 Muller, H.P., van Tilburg, N.H., Derks, J., Klein-Breteler, E. and Bertina, R.M. (1981) Blood 58, 1000.

36 Rotblat, F., Goodall, A.H., O'Brien, D.P., Rawlings, E., Middleton, S. and Tuddenham, E.G.D. (1983) J. Lab. Clin. Med. 101, 736.

37 Stel, H.V., Veerman, E.C.I., Huisman, J.F., Janssen, M.C. and van Mourik, J.A. (1983) Thromb. Haemostas. 50, 860.

38 Hoyer, L.W. and Breckenridge, R.T. (1968) Blood 32, 962.

39 Peake, I.R., Bloom, A.L., Giddings, J.C. and Ludlam, C.A. (1979) Br. J. Haematol. 42, 269.

40 Holmberg, L., Borge, L., Ljung, R. and Nilsson, I.M. (1979) Scand. J. Haematol. 23, 17.

41 Lazarchick, J. and Hoyer, L.W. (1978) J. Clin. Invest. 62, 1048.

42 Reisner, H.M., Barrow, E.S. and Graham, J.B. (1979) Thromb. Res. 14, 235.

43 Muller, H.P., van Tilburg, N.H., Bertina, R.M., Terweil, J.P. and Veltkamp, J.J. (1980) Clin. Chim. Acta 107, 11.

44 Tran, T.H. and Duckert, F. (1983) Thromb. Haemostas. 50, 547.

45 Yoshioka, A., Peake, I.R., Furlong, B.L., Furlong, R.A., Giddings, J.C. and Bloom, A.L. (1983) Br. J. Haematol. 55, 27.

46 Broden, K., Brown, J.E., Carton, C. and Andersson, L.O. (1983) Thromb. Res. 30, 651.

47 Rotblat, F. and Tuddenham, E.G.D. (1981) Thromb. Res. 21, 431.

48 Girma, J.P., Lavergne, J.M., Meyer, D. and Larrieu, M.J. (1981) Br. J. Haematol. 47, 269.

49 Firshein, S.I., Hoyer, L.W., Lazarchick, J., Forget, B.G., Hobbins, J.C., Clyne, L.P., Pittlick, F.A., Muir, A., Merkatz, I.R. and Mahoney, M.J. (1979) New Engl. J. Med. 300, 937.

50 Mibashan, R.S. and Thumpston, J.K. (1979) Lancet 8130, 1309.

51 Nemerson, Y. and Furie, B. (1980) CRC Crit. Rev. Biochem. 9, 45.

52 Østerud, B. and Rapaport, S.I. (1970) Biochemistry 9, 1854.

53 Brown, J.E., Baugh, R.F. and Hougie, C. (1978) Thromb. Res. 13, 893.

54 Hultin, M.B. and Nemerson, Y. (1978) Blood 52, 928.

55 Neal, G.G. and Chavin, S.I. (1979) Thromb. Res. 16, 473.

56 Hultin, M.B. (1982) J. Clin. Invest. 69, 950.

57 Van Dieijen, G., Tans, G., Rosing, J. and Hemker, H.C. (1981) J. Biol. Chem. 256, 3433.

58 Jackson, C.M. (1978) Br. J. Haematol. 39, 1.

59 Rosing, J., Tans, G., Govers-Riemsing, J.W.P. and Hemker, H.C. (1980) J. Biol. Chem. 255, 274.

60 Vehar, G.A. and Davie, E.W. (1977) Science 197, 374.

61 Weinstein, M., Fulcher, C.A., Chute, L.E. and Zimmerman, T.S. (1983) Blood 62, 1114.

62 Hultin, M.B. and Jesty, J. (1981) Blood 57, 476.

63 Switzer, M.E., Pizzo, S.V. and McKee, P.A. (1979) Blood 54, 310.

64 Davie, E.W., Fujikawa, K., Kurachi, K. and Kisel, W. (1979) Adv. Enzymol. 48, 277.

65 Jackson, C.M. and Nemerson, Y. (1980) Annu. Rev. Biochem. 49, 765.

66 Stenflo, J. (1976) J. Biol. Chem. 251, 355.

67 Esmon, C.T. and Owen, W.G. (1981) Proc. Natl. Acad. Sci. (U.S.A.) 78, 2249.

68 Esmon, N.L., Owen, W.G. and Esmon, C.T. (1982) J. Biol. Chem. 257, 859.

69 Fulcher, C.A., Gardiner, J.E., Griffin, J. and Zimmerman, T.S. (1984) Blood 63, 486.

70 DiScipio, R.G. and Davie, E.W. (1979) Biochemistry 18, 899.

71 Walker, F.J. (1980) J. Biol. Chem. 255, 5521.

72 Walker, F.J. (1981) J. Biol. Chem. 256, 11128.

73 Webster, W.P., Zukoski, C.F., Hutchen, P., Reddick, R.L., Mandel, S.R. and Penick, G.D. (1971) Am. J. Physiol. 220, 1147.

74 Bloom, A.L. (1979) Clin. Haematol. 8, 53.

75 Kelly, D.A., Summerfield, J.A. and Tuddenham, E.G.D. (1983) Thromb. Haemostas. 50, 17.

76 Stel, H.V., van der Kwast, T.H. and Veerman, E.C.I. (1983) Nature (London) 303, 530.

77 van der Kwast, T.H., Stel, H.V., Veerman, E.C.I. and Bertina, R.M. (1983) Thromb. Haemostas. 50, 17.

78 Cerveny, T.J., Fass, D.N. and Mann, K.G. (1984) Blood 63, 1467.

79 Barrow, E.M. and Graham, J.B. (1974) Physiol. Rev. 54, 23.

80 Hoyer, L.W. (1982) in: Hemostasis and Thrombosis. Basic Principles and Clinical Practice (Colman, R.W., Hirsh, J., Marder, V.J. and Salzman, E.W., Eds.) p. 48, Lippincott, Philadelphia, PA.

81 Nesheim, M.E., Myrmel, K.H., Hibbard, L. and Mann, K.G. (1979) J. Biol. Chem. 254, 508.

82 Mann, K.G., Nesheim, M.E. and Tracy, P.B. (1981) Biochemistry 20, 28.

83 Suzuki, K., Dahlback, B. and Stenflo, J. (1982) J. Biol. Chem. 257, 6556.

84 Church, W.R., Jernigan, R.L., Toole, J., Hewick, R.M., Knopf, J., Knutson, G.J., Nesheim, M.E., Mann, K.G. and Fass, D.N. (1984) Proc. Natl. Acad. Sci. (U.S.A.) 81, 6934.

85 Kisiel, W., Canfield, W., Ericsson, L. and Davie, E.W. (1977) Biochemistry 16, 5824.

86 Walker, F.J., Sexton, P.W. and Esmon, C.T. (1979) Biochim. Biophys. Acta 571, 333.

87 Zimmerman, T.S. and Edgington, T.S. (1973) J. Exp. Med. 138, 1015.

88 Peake, I.R. and Bloom, A.L. (1976) Thromb. Haemostas. 35, 191.

89 Holmberg, L. and Ljung, R. (1978) Thromb. Res. 12, 667.

90 Moake, J.L., Weinstein, M.J., Troll, J.H., Chute, L.E. and Colannino, N.M. (1983) Blood 61, 1163.

91 Owen, W.G. and Wagner, R.H. (1976) Thromb. Diath. Haemorrh. 27, 502.

92 Rick, M.E. and Hoyer, L.W. (1973) Blood 42, 737.

93 Weiss, H.J. and Hoyer, L.W. (1973) Science 182, 1149.

94 Lavergne, J.M., Meyer, D. and Jenkins, C.S.P. (1976) Thromb. Haemostas. 35, 186.

95 Cooper, H.A., Griggs, T.R. and Wagner, R.H. (1973) Proc. Natl. Acad. Sci. (U.S.A.) 70, 2326.

96 Brockway, W.J. and Fass, D.N. (1977) J. Lab. Clin. Med. 89, 1295.

97 Tuddenham, E.G.D., Lane, R.S., Rotblat, F., Johnson, A.J., Snape, T.J., Middleton, S. and Kernoff, P.B.A. (1982) Br. J. Haematol. 52, 259.

98 Hoyer, L.W. (1981) Blood 58, 1.

R.F.A. Zwaal and H.C. Hemker (Eds.), *Blood Coagulation*
© 1986 Elsevier Science Publishers B.V. (Biomedical Division)

CHAPTER 3

Multicomponent enzyme complexes of blood coagulation

G. TANS and J. ROSING

Department of Biochemistry, University of Limburg, Biomedical Centre, Maastricht (The Netherlands)

1. Introduction

A large number of plasma proteins have been discovered to participate in the process of blood coagulation. Upon initiation of blood coagulation various proteins and enzymes interact with each other in a sequential fashion described in a scheme that is known as the blood coagulation cascade [1,2]. This cascade system summarizes the sequence of reactions that eventually leads to the formation of a fibrin clot. All enzymatically active coagulation factors that participate in the blood coagulation cascade belong to the class of serine proteases and show considerable homology with trypsin and chymotrypsin, the proteolytic enzymes of the digestive tract [3,4]. The in vivo activity of blood coagulation factors is controlled by the fact that they circulate in the blood as non-enzymatic precursors (zymogens) of serine proteases. When needed the zymogens of the coagulation factors are converted into an enzymatically active form by limited proteolysis, a process which occurs according to a mechanism basically similar to that described for the activation of the zymogens of the gastrointestinal proteinases.

In one important aspect coagulation factor activations differ from the activations of trypsinogen and chymotrypsinogen. Compared to the rates by which the proteases of the digestive tract activate their corresponding zymogens the serine proteases of the blood coagulation cascade have a remarkably low activity towards their natural zymogen substrates. Therefore, during blood coagulation additional components (protein cofactors, metal ions and so-called procoagulant surfaces) are needed to sufficiently speed up in vivo rates of coagulation factor activation. Thus apart from the enzyme the catalytic units of coagulation-factor-activating complexes consist of more components which together ensure efficient reaction.

In this chapter we will treat the current concepts concerning the assembly and molecular mechanism of the multicomponent enzyme complexes of blood coagulation. Especially the prothrombin-activating complex will be dealt with in detail since this is the best documented example and its molecular mechanism is most likely representative for the other enzyme complexes that participate in the blood coagulation cascade.

2. Mechanism of zymogen activation by serine proteases

Activation of coagulation factors occurs through proteolysis of one or more peptide bonds in the zymogen molecule, a reaction that is catalyzed by another active coagulation factor. Since most enzymatically active coagulation factors belong to the class of serine proteases it is not surprising that their proteolytic action is thought to adhere to that of the well known serine proteases chymotrypsin and trypsin. The molecular mechanism of peptide bond cleavage by serine proteases is depicted in Fig. 1 [3,5–10]. The first step is the formation of a noncovalent complex between enzyme and substrate (the so-called Michaelis complex). In all serine proteases with known three-dimensional structure the active site serine is hydrogen bonded to a histidine residue which in its turn is hydrogen bonded to an aspartate residue. This line-up of Ser-His-Asp, called the catalytic triad or charge–relay system, greatly facilitates the next step in the reaction sequence that is the formation of a covalent intermediate (tetrahedral intermediate) through nucleophilic attack of the active site serine on the carbonyl group of the peptide bond that has to be cleaved. This intermediate has a very short lifetime and rapidly dissociates into the acyl enzyme and the first product (P1). The final step is hydrolysis of the acyl enzyme intermediate which results in the dissociation of the second product (P2).

3. Activation of zymogens of blood coagulation factors

A schematic representation of the zymogens that are activated during blood coagulation is shown in Fig. 2. The carboxy-terminal region of the coagulation factors is highly homologous to trypsin [11–20] and it is thought that the generation

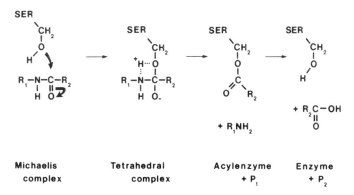

Fig. 1. Mechanism of peptide bond cleavage by serine proteases.

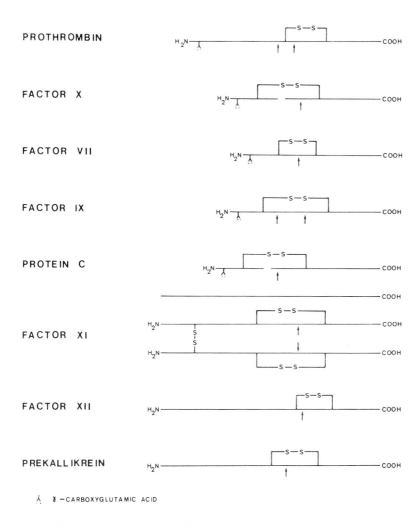

Fig. 2. Zymogens activated during blood coagulation.

of the active site is analogous to the active site formation during trypsinogen activation. Thus the cleavage of a peptide bond in these zymogens generates a new amino terminus at or near the end of the region homologous to trypsin. This new peptide chain changes its conformation and the active site becomes exposed. Thus activated clotting factors are two chain molecules which consist of a trypsin-like chain with molecular weights ranging from 30 000 to 40 000 dalton, that contains the active site and a second domain that appears to contain the structural information for specific interactions with accessory components such as cofactor recognition, metal ion-binding sites and surface-binding sites.

A typical feature of the zymogen activations in the coagulation cascade is that

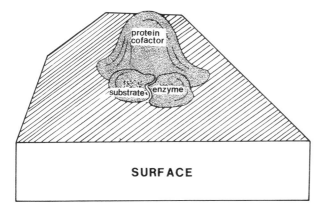

Fig. 3. Schematic model for multicomponent enzyme complexes of blood coagulation.

the enzyme–substrate interactions are very inefficient. On the one hand this prevents undesired activation of the circulating zymogens but on the other hand it is the reason for the fact that accessory components are needed to sufficiently speed up the reaction rates of in vivo coagulation factor activation. Fig. 3 shows a schematic representation of the basic assembly of the enzyme–cofactor–substrate complexes that participate in blood coagulation. Most coagulation reactions are confined to a negatively charged surface and for optimal activation all proteins involved (i.e. enzyme, substrate and protein cofactor) have to bind to the procoagulant surface. For this binding sometimes the divalent metal ion Ca^{2+} is required. Based on the nature of the participating surface the enzyme complexes of blood coagu-

TABLE 1

Multicomponent enzyme complexes in coagulation

Enzyme	Substrate	Cofactors
X_a	II	V_a, Ca^{2+}, phospholipid
IX_a	X	VIII_a, Ca^{2+} phospholipid
VII_a	X, IX	Thromboplastin, Ca^{2+} [a]
Activated protein C	V_a, VIII_a	Protein S, Ca^{2+}, phospholipid
II_a	Protein C	Thrombomodulin, endothelial cell surface[b]
XII_a	Prekallikrein, XI	HMWK, surface[c]
Kallikrein	XII	HMWK, surface[c]

[a] Thromboplastin contains a protein cofactor (tissue factor apoprotein) and phospholipid.

[b] Endothelial cells stimulate this reaction rather poorly in in vitro experiments [28] but it is thought that in the microvascular circulation the stimulation will be much greater since the concentration of endothelial cells in the microvascular bed of the capillaries is much higher than can be reached in in vitro cultures.

[c] A wide variety of substances is known to function as procoagulant surface in contact activation reactions.

lation can be divided into different groups with similar characteristics (Table 1).

The assembly of the enzyme–substrate complex in the activations of vitamin K-dependent clotting factors takes place on phospholipid membranes that contain negatively charged phospholipids (for a review see ref. 21). In vivo this surface is likely provided by activated platelets (cf. [22–25] and Ch. 6). Vitamin K-dependent clotting factors contain the so-called γ-carboxyglutamic acid residues that are formed upon post-ribosomal carboxylation of specific glutamic acid residues present in the amino-terminal region of these proteins (see Ch. 4). The γ-carboxyglutamic acid residues are essential for calcium-dependent binding of these proteins to phospholipid. Except for the activation of factor IX by factor XI_a the activations of the vitamin K-dependent clotting factors have an absolute requirement for a protein cofactor since in the absence of cofactors the reaction rates are too low to be important in vivo. Thus in prothrombin activation, factor V_a is the protein cofactor; in factor X and IX activation by factor VII_a the reaction rate is enhanced by tissue factor apoprotein and factor X activation by factor IX_a is stimulated enormously by activated factor VIII:C. The activities of factors V_a and VIII_a are controlled by activated protein C since this enzyme can proteolytically degrade these cofactors in a reaction stimulated by protein S, Ca^{2+} and phospholipid (cf. [26,27] and Ch. 9B). Finally, the activation of protein C by thrombin is greatly enhanced by the protein cofactor thrombomodulin and the endothelial cell surface [28–30]. Recently, it was reported that factor V_a can also act as a cofactor in the activation of protein C by thrombin [31].

The proteins involved in contact activation require for optimal interaction a surface different from phospholipids. A wide variety of substances such as glass, kaolin, dextran sulfate, bacterial lipopolysaccharides and sulfatides have been shown to stimulate contact activation reactions (for recent reviews see refs. 32–34). Many of these compounds do, however, not occur in the human body. Procoagulant surfaces of potential physiological importance are cerebroside sulfates (sulfatides) [35,36], lipopolysaccharides from bacteria [37–40] and sulfated glycosaminoglycans such as chondroitin sulfate and heparin [41,42]. The presence of a sulfate group seems to be essential for the procoagulant activity of the surface. Only one protein cofactor, high molecular weight kininogen (HMWK), appears to be involved in contact activation (43–48]. The presence of this cofactor stimulates the reciprocal activation of prekallikrein and factor XII and HMWK is also involved in the activation of factor XI by factor XII_a in plasma.

4. Activation of vitamin K-dependent coagulation factors

In this section we will review the current concepts of the molecular mechanism of activation of the vitamin K-dependent coagulation factors by multicomponent enzyme complexes. We will focus on the activation of prothrombin because a large amount of data is available concerning this reaction. Although prothrombin activation is a somewhat more complex reaction than the activations of other vitamin

K-dependent coagulation factors the prothrombinase complex is generally thought to be a useful example for the other multicomponent enzyme complexes.

(a) Prothrombin activation

Prothrombin is the zymogen precursor of thrombin, the serine protease responsible for the conversion of fibrinogen to fibrin. When the activation of purified prothrombin by factor X_a is followed on SDS gels a rather complex pattern of activation products is observed. This is caused by the fact that a number of peptide bonds in the prothrombin molecule are susceptible to proteolytic cleavage (Fig. 4). It was not until 1974 that work of different laboratories [49–61] culminated in the complete description of the peptide bond cleavages that occur during factor X_a-catalyzed prothrombin activation [62–67].

It appears that the cleavage of two peptide bonds in prothrombin is necessary for thrombin formation. These are at the positions Arg_{274}–Thr_{275} (site 1) and Arg_{323}–Ile_{324} (site 2). Both peptide bonds are available for proteolytic cleavage in the native prothrombin molecule. Prothrombin activation by the venom of *Echis carinatus* leads to meizothrombin [68,69] a reaction product in which only the Arg_{323}–Ile_{324} bond has been cleaved. During factor X_a-catalyzed prothrombin activation prethrombin 2 has been observed as an intermediate which indicates that the Arg_{274}–Thr_{275} bond is also accessible to proteolytic cleavage. A complication in the analysis of prothrombin activation is that the reaction product thrombin can act on prothrombin near the amino-terminal region at position Arg_{156}–Ser_{157} (site 3) resulting in fragment 1 (the fragment containing the γ-carboxyglutamic acid residues) and prethrombin 1. In human prothrombin an additional fourth peptide bond in the A chain region of thrombin can be cleaved [70].

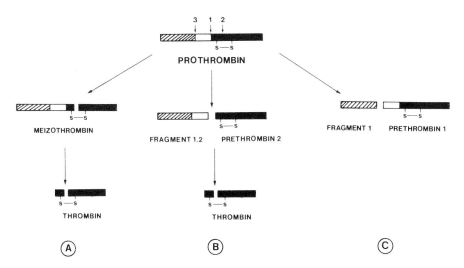

Fig. 4. Peptide bonds in prothrombin susceptible to proteolytic cleavage.

TABLE 2

Effect of accessory components on the rate of prothrombin activation by factor X_a

Activating mixture	Relative rate		
	a	b	c
X_a, Ca^{2+}	1	1	1
X_a, Ca^{2+}, PL	51	50	10
X_a, Ca^{2+}, V_a	318	350	155
X_a, Ca^{2+}, V_a, PL	1 640	19 000	121 000

a, from Jobin and Esnouf [72]; b, from Esmon et al. [66]; c, from Nesheim et al. [73] (compare also ch. 2A).
PL, phospholipid.

The cleavage at site 2 is a prerequisite for the exposure of the active site since prethrombin 2 has no proteolytic or amidolytic activity whereas both meizothrombin and thrombin have. The substrate specificity of the latter two differs, however. Both enzymes are equally active on small oligopeptide substrates such as S 2238 but thrombin is much more active than meizothrombin on the natural substrate fibrinogen [71].

The physiologic pathway by which thrombin is formed from prothrombin is currently still unsure. Thrombin can either be generated via meizothrombin (pathway A) or prethrombin 2 (pathway B). In 1974 Esmon et al. [67] suggested that pathway B describes the most plausible sequence of reactions during factor X_a-catalyzed prothrombin activation either with or without accessory components. This proposal was based on the observation that substantial amounts of prethrombin 2 were generated during prothrombin activation, whereas meizothrombin, the intermediate in pathway A was not detectable. It should be emphasized, however, that the gel electrophoretic techniques employed in this kind of study do not allow the detection of low amounts of intermediates. Steady-state concentrations of intermediate (e.g. meizothrombin) equal to or even below the concentration of enzyme present can be kinetically compatible with a catalytic pathway via such an intermediate. Since such low amounts of meizothrombin would have escaped detection we feel that it is as yet not unequivocally proven whether A or B describes the actual pathway of prothrombin activation*.

Over the past 20 years a lot has been learned concerning the molecular mechanism and assembly of the various constituents of the prothrombinase complex. Jobin and Esnouf [72] were among the first to quantitatively assess the effects of accessory components on the relative rates of prothrombin activation (Table 2). They observed that the addition of each accessory component caused rate enhancements of 1 or 2 orders of magnitude. Their data were later confirmed by the groups of Jackson in 1974 [66] and Mann in 1979 [73]. The magnitude of the effect

* While this Chapter was in print it has been reported that meizothrombin indeed occurs as a transient intermediate during Factor X_a-catalyzed prothrombin activation (J. Rosing, R.F.A. Zwaal and G. Tans (1986) J. Biol. Chem. 261, 4224–4228).

66

TABLE 3

Effect of accessory components on the kinetic parameters of prothrombin activation

Activator	K_m (μM)	V_{max} (II_a/min/X_a)
X_a	131	0.61
X_a, Ca^{2+}	84	0.68
X_a, Ca^{2+}, PL	0.058	2.25
X_a, Ca^{2+}, V_a	34	373
X_a, Ca^{2+}, V_a, PL	0.21	1919

Data from Rosing et al. [74].
Prothrombin activation was determined at pH 7.5 at 37°C with or without 5 mM $CaCl_2$, saturating amounts of factor V_a and 7.5 μM phospholipid (PL) vesicles (PS/PC, 50/50; mole/mole).

of accessory components in these studies differs considerably. This is most likely caused by the use of different phospholipid and protein concentrations. The important information contained in these experiments is that phospholipids plus Ca^{2+} and factor V_a accelerate prothrombin activation in a multiplicative way independent of each other. In 1980 Rosing et al. [74] showed that the effects of accessory components on the relative rates of thrombin formation could be correlated with changes in the kinetic parameters of prothrombin activation (Table 3). The low rate of prothrombin activation by factor X_a alone appears to be due to the fact that the reaction has very unfavorable kinetic parameters. In the absence of phospholipids and factor V_a prothrombin activation is characterized by a high K_m for prothrombin and a very low V_{max}. The stimulatory effect of phospholipids is due to a dramatic decrease of the K_m for prothrombin, whereas the rate enhancements by factor V_a are caused by an increase of the V_{max}. The physiological importance of these changes in kinetic parameters is obvious. Since the plasma prothrombin concentration is 2 μM, phospholipids lower the K_m to values considerably below the plasma prothrombin level. This means that under physiological conditions saturation of factor X_a with prothrombin is achieved and factor X_a acts at maximal catalytic capacity. Factor V_a subsequently enhances the V_{max} of prothrombinase to a level at which thrombin is formed at a rate sufficiently high to account for rapid clot formation. The effects of phospholipids and factor V_a on the kinetic parameters of factor X_a-catalyzed prothrombin activation give a satisfying explanation for the earlier observed rate enhancements and for their physiological requirement. However, more detailed kinetic and binding studies were necessary to obtain insight in the mechanism by which the accessory components cause these changes of kinetic parameters.

(i) The role of phospholipids in prothrombin activation

It is generally thought that the phospholipid bilayer serves as a surface onto which the proteins bind. Already in 1967 Jobin and Esnouf [72] interpreted the stimulatory effect of phospholipid on the relative rates of prothrombin activation as being due to a proper localization of the interacting proteins on the phospholipid surface and Hemker et al. [75] reported experiments that supported this concept. It was proposed that binding of the proteins to phospholipid results in increased surface concentrations of the reactants which facilitates interactions between the various proteins that participate in prothrombin activation. The early experiments also led to the conclusion that prothrombinase consists of a phospholipid-bound complex of factor X_a and factor V_a. A decennium later more quantitative data regarding the formation of the prothrombinase complex became available. It was shown that the stimulatory effect of phospholipids in prothrombin activation is actually 2-fold: (a) phospholipids promote the interaction between factor X_a and factor V_a and facilitate the formation of a factor X_a–V_a complex and (b) phospholipids promote the interaction of the factor X_a–V_a complex with its substrate prothrombin as judged by the decrease of the K_m.

In 1979 Nesheim et al. [73] inferred from kinetic data the K_d for the interaction between factor V_a and factor X_a in the presence of phospholipid. They estimated a K_d of 7.3×10^{-10} M and concluded that a phospholipid-bound complex between factor X_a and factor V_a with 1:1 stoichiometry is formed (see also Ch. 2A). The K_d value was subsequently confirmed by direct binding measurements using a fluorescent factor X_a derivative [76]. Lindhout et al. [77] also used a kinetic approach to determine the effect of phospholipid on the interaction between factor X_a and factor V_a. In the absence of phospholipid a K_d of 3.3×10^{-9} M and a 1:1 stoichiometry was found. The presence of phospholipid promoted complex formation since apparent K_ds as low as 10^{-11} M were observed. This stimulatory effect of phospholipid on the formation of the factor X_a–V_a complex was dependent on the presence of negatively charged phospholipids in the membrane bilayer. In addition factor X_a has to contain γ-carboxyglutamic acid residues since Skogen et al. [78] reported that the interaction of Gla-domainless factor X_a with factor V_a was not stimulated by phospholipids. Finally, in an independent study, Morisson [79] determined a value of 5.9×10^{-11} M for the apparent dissociation constant of human factor X_a with bovine factor V_a in the presence of phospholipids.

The effect of phospholipid on the K_m is dependent on the amount of phospholipid present since at increasing phospholipid concentrations increasing values for the K_m for prothrombin were observed (Table 4). So a model for the mechanism of action of phospholipids in prothrombin activation has to explain the drastic drop of the K_m for prothrombin and the subsequent increase of the K_m at higher phospholipid concentrations. Since both prothrombin and factor X_a have affinity for phospholipids it was suggested that an increased concentration of reactants at the phospholipid–water interface facilitates the formation of the enzyme–substrate complex which explains the observed decrease of the K_m in the presence of phospholipid [74]. In this what is called the 'bound substrate model', the K_m is determined by the local concentration of prothrombin at the membrane surface [73]. In this model one can easily explain why the K_m increases at increasing phospholipid concentrations. At higher phospholipid concentrations more prothrombin-binding sites are available hence more prothrombin has to be added to attain the local substrate concentration at which surface-bound factor X_a enzyme works at $1/2\ V_{max}$.

TABLE 4

The effect of the phospholipid concentration on the K_m for prothrombin

Phospholipid concentration (μM)	K_m (μM)
4	0.062
8	0.090
16	0.14
40	0.23
80	0.46
240	1.08

Data from Rosing et al. [74].
The phospholipid vesicles contained 50 mole% PS and 50 mole% PC.

Nesheim et al. [80,81] presented a mathematical model, in which the protein concentrations in a shell surrounding the vesicle determine the molecular interactions. This model, which is essentially the same as the 'bound substrate model', could be used to satisfactorily simulate the effect of phospholipid vesicles (25% PS/75% PC) on the rates of prothrombin activation.

In 1978 Nelsestuen [82], however, proposed an alternative model which we will call the 'free substrate model' in which the prothrombinase complex is viewed as a dissociable three-component enzyme (X_a–V_a–phospholipid) that acts on soluble prothrombin. In this model the decreased K_m (interpreted as an increased affinity of prothrombinase for prothrombin) is explained [82,83] to be the result of additive free energies of prothrombin–factor V_a and prothrombin–phospholipid interactions occurring at the active site of prothrombinase. The increase in K_m at increasing phospholipid concentrations is explained by the fact that prothrombin binding to the bilayer decreases the amount of soluble prothrombin available for interactions with the enzymatic unit of the prothrombin-activating complex.

The fundamental difference between the two models is that in the bound substrate model lateral diffusion of prothrombin in a shell surrounding the phospholipid surface is an essential step in the formation of the enzyme–substrate complex whereas in the free substrate model the enzyme–substrate complex is formed by direct interaction of soluble prothrombin with the enzymatic unit.

The bound substrate model predicts that V_{max} and K_m are directly related to the binding parameters of, respectively, factor X_a and prothrombin for phospholipid. Vesicles with increased affinity for factor X_a bind more factor X_a, hence more factor X_a will participate in prothrombin activation and higher V_{max} values will be observed. Vesicles with a high affinity for prothrombin will yield low K_m values since small amounts of prothrombin are required to obtain the prothrombin density at the phospholipid surface at which half of the phospholipid-bound factor X_a is saturated.

These predictions were tested in experiments in which the kinetic parameters of prothrombin activation were determined with vesicles that contained various amounts of different kinds of negatively charged phospholipids [84,85]. In Table

TABLE 5

Kinetic parameters of prothrombin activation for membranes containing various amounts of different negatively charged phospholipids

Membrane phospholipid composition	K_m (μM)	V_{max} (II_a/min/X_a)
−*Factor V_a*		
PS/PC (25/75, M/M)	0.11	2.56
PA/PC (25/75, M/M)	0.10	2.78
PG/PC (25/75, M/M)	1.81	0.17
PS/PC (5/95, M/M)	1.63	0.32
+*Factor V_a*		
PS/PC (25/75, M/M)	0.14	4050
PA/PC (25/75, M/M)	0.11	4184
PG/PC (25/75, M/M)	0.04	3345
PS/PC (5/95, M/M)	0.057	4330

Data from Van Rijn et al. [85].
The phospholipid concentration in this experiment was 50 μM.

5 it is shown that in the absence of factor V_a the K_m and V_{max} indeed correlate with the binding affinities of the phospholipid membranes for factor X_a and prothrombin. Vesicles with a high affinity (PS–PC and PA–PC) for vitamin K-dependent coagulation factors have a low K_m and high V_{max}, whereas vesicles with a low affinity (PG–PC or PS–PC vesicles with low PS content) have unfavorable kinetic parameters. The kinetic parameters determined in the presence for factor V_a do, however, not reflect differences in binding parameters for factor X_a and prothrombin. The V_{max} is hardly dependent on the type of acidic phospholipid present in the membrane bilayer. Since these experiments were carried out at saturating factor V_a concentrations the constant V_{max} can be attributed to the fact that factor V_a promotes the binding of all added factor X_a to the phospholipid vesicles. Moreover, the K_m does not correlate with the binding parameters of prothrombin for the phospholipid vesicles. Membranes containing PG or a low mole percentage PS, which have the lowest affinity for prothrombin, have the most favorable K_m for prothrombin, whereas vesicles with a high affinity (PS–PC and PA–PC) have the most unfavorable K_m. From these experiments it is obvious that in the presence of factor V_a and phospholipid vesicles with a low affinity for prothrombin the K_m for prothrombin and the rate of prothrombin activation are not determined by the prothrombin density at the phospholipid surface. Therefore, it was concluded that the mechanism of action of phospholipid in prothrombin activation in the absence and presence of factor V_a cannot be described in one unique model. In the presence of factor V_a prothrombin activation is most adequately explained in the free substrate model. The effect of phospholipids on the K_m for prothrombin in the absence of factor V_a cannot be satisfactorily explained in either of the two models. Although the K_m for prothrombin measured in the absence of factor V_a varied parallel with the binding affinity of prothrombin for phospholipid (a requirement of the bound substrate model), Van Rijn et al. [85] were not able to reconcile the observed K_m with known binding parameters of prothrombin for phospholipid.

(ii) The role of factor V_a in prothrombin activation

Kinetic studies of prothrombin activation have shown that the effects of factor V_a are 2-fold: (a) factor V_a causes a 2000-fold increase of the V_{max} of prothrombin activation [73,74] and (b) factor V_a lowers the K_m for prothrombin, an effect that is most apparent on procoagulant surfaces with low affinity for prothrombin [84,85].

The increase of the V_{max} by factor V_a is the result of a number of additive effects. Part of the stimulation is caused by the fact that factor V_a promotes the binding of factor X_a to negatively charged phospholipid surfaces (vide supra). Hence in the presence of factor V_a more factor X_a molecules are bound to the phospholipid surface and, therefore, more factor X_a molecules will participate in prothrombin activation. In kinetic measurements this will cause an increase of the observed V_{max}. A second contribution of factor V_a to the increase of the V_{max} was put forward on the basis of experiments in which prothrombin activation with prothrombin-activating mixtures of different compositions was subjected to gel electrophoretic analysis [74]. When factor X_a converts prothrombin in the absence of factor V_a mainly prethrombin 2 is formed irrespective of whether phospholipids plus Ca^{2+} are present or not. With the complete prothrombinase complex (factor X_a, factor V_a, phospholipid and Ca^{2+}) thrombin is the main end product and no prethrombin 2 is detectable. For the explanation of these findings it will be helpful to consider Fig. 5, which depicts a minimal mechanism for the conversion of prothrombin into its activation products. The main pathway occurring during prothrombin activation in the absence of factor V_a is that giving rise to prethrombin 2 (steps 1, 2 and 5) and only a small fraction of prothrombin is directly converted into thrombin (steps 1, 2, 3, 4 or 1, 2', 3', 4). Factor V_a changes the pathway of prothrombin activation from one resulting in prethrombin 2 into one producing thrombin.

Two alternatives can be put forward to explain this effect of factor V_a on the pathway of prothrombin activation:

(1) Factor V_a prevents the dissociation of prethrombin 2 from the prothrombinase complex altering the pathway from 1, 2 and 5 to 1, 2, 3 and 4. The increase

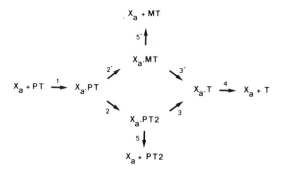

Fig. 5. Possible reaction schemes of prothrombin activation. Xa, factor X_a; PT, prothrombin; PT2, prethrombin 2; T, thrombin; MT, meizothrombin.

in intermediate complex concentration which consequently occurs also increases the rate of thrombin formation.

(2) Factor V_a changes the pathway of activation from one in which prethrombin 2 occurs as intermediate (1, 2, 3, 4) into one with meizothrombin as intermediate (1, 2', 3', 4).

Based on the estimation of the rate constants of prethrombin 2 formation (without factor V_a) and thrombin formation (with factor V_a) Tans et al. [86] concluded that apart from such a possible shift in pathway, factor V_a must also increase at least one forward rate constant in the prothrombin activation pathway. This was indeed shown to be the case by Nesheim and Mann in 1983 (cf. [87] and Ch. 2A). From kinetic experiments with prothrombin and prothrombin activation intermediates they concluded that factor V_a causes a 3000-fold increase of the k_{cat} of factor X_a-catalyzed cleavage of the Arg_{323}–Thr_{324} bond (step 2' or step 3 in Fig. 5).

It is as yet unknown how factor V_a enhances that k_{cat} of peptide bond cleavage. Factor V_a can exert its action through factor X_a by making it a better enzyme with increased catalytic power or via prothrombin by making it a better substrate for factor X_a. In the latter case it would be possible that factor V_a changes the conformation of prothrombin in such a way that the peptide bonds to be cleaved by factor X_a become more susceptible.

The effect of factor V_a on the K_m for prothrombin presumably has physiological importance. Factor V_a causes a profound decrease of the K_m when prothrombin is activated at procoagulant surfaces with a low affinity for prothrombin. It has been proposed that activated blood platelets provide the phospholipid surface at which in vivo prothrombin activation takes place. Since activated platelets expose relatively small amounts of acidic phospholipids [88] factor V_a will likely play an important role in the formation of the enzyme–substrate complex at the platelet surface.

There are several possibilities for the mechanism by which factor V_a can promote the interaction of prothrombin with the prothrombinase complex. This can be accomplished by:

(1) a direct interaction of prothrombin with factor V_a, probably through its fragment 2 region, that provides additional free energy for prothrombin binding to the enzymatic complex or

(2) a factor V_a-induced clustering of negatively charged phospholipid molecules in the enzymatic domain which creates a membrane surface with a higher affinity for prothrombin or

(3) factor V_a-induced increase of a rate constant in the pathway of prothrombin activation that simultaneously increases the k_{cat} and decreases the K_m.

The first possibility is supported by direct binding studies of Van de Waart et al. [89] who showed that factor V_a promotes the binding of prothrombin to negatively charged phospholipid surfaces. Insufficient quantitative data prevent, however, correlation of the effect of factor V_a on prothrombin binding to phospholipids with the effect of this cofactor on the K_m. With respect to the second possibility Mayer and Nelsestuen [90] reported that factor V_a causes a lateral phase separation (clustering) of negatively charged phospholipids in membranes. Although they suggested that this lateral phase separation may be an important process in the formation of the prothrombinase complex, they did not present evidence that this phenomenon can contribute to the binding of prothrombin to the membrane surface. For the understanding of the last possibility it is helpful to consider the simplified reaction scheme for serine proteases:

$$E+S \xrightarrow{K_s} E.S \underset{P_1}{\overset{k_2}{\rightleftharpoons}} EA \xrightarrow{k_3} E+A$$

For such a reaction sequence the kinetic parameters are $k_{cat} = (k_2 \cdot k_3)/(k_2 + k_3)$ and $K_m = (K_s \cdot k_3)/(k_2 + k_3)$. It is obvious that under certain conditions an increase of a single rate constant (k_2) by factor V_a can cause both an increase of k_{cat} and a decrease of the K_m. Whether this occurs depends on the individual rate constants the values of which are presently unknown.

(b) Factor X activation

The activation of factor X in plasma can be accomplished via the so-called extrinsic and intrinsic pathways (cf. Ch. 5A and 5B). Extrinsic factor X activation is catalyzed by factor VII_a, a reaction stimulated by the presence of thromboplastin. Thromboplastin consists of phospholipids and a protein cofactor (tissue factor apoprotein) which is an integral membrane glycoprotein. Factor IX_a is the enzyme responsible for intrinsic factor X activation and this reaction is greatly stimulated by negatively charged phospholipids and the protein cofactor factor VIII_a. The cleavage of one and the same peptide bond by both factor VII_a and factor IX_a results in the activation of factor X [92,93]. Thus the mechanism of factor X activation is simpler than that of prothrombin activation in which reaction two peptide bonds are cleaved. Consequently, enhancements of the rate of factor X_a formation by the accessory components must be explained within this one pathway. We will briefly discuss the role of these accessory components in the activation of factor X

TABLE 6

The effect of tissue factor on the kinetic parameters of factor VII_a-catalyzed factor X activation

	K_m (μM)	k_{cat} (/sec)
Without tissue factor[a]	4.87	3.95×10^{-4}
With tissue factor[b]	0.45	1.15

Data from Silverberg et al. [98].

[a] Experiment carried out in the presence of 10 mM benzamidine with rabbit brain cephalin as phospholipid source.

[b] Experiment carried out in the presence of 10 mM benzamidine with bovine brain thromboplastin as source of phospholipids and tissue factor apoprotein.

and how it relates to the concepts described in the previous paragraph.

Evaluation of kinetic data in extrinsic factor X activation is complicated by the fact that tissue factor apoprotein is an integral membrane protein for which only recently the purification has been reported [94]. Since this protein only functions when reconstituted with phospholipid [95–97] it is difficult to separate the contribution of the protein cofactor from that of the lipid component. Therefore, no full picture is available yet on the kinetics of factor X activation by factor VII_a but the data reported thus far appear similar to prothrombin activation. Silverberg et al. [98] in 1977 reported a combined 10-fold drop in K_m and a 3000-fold increase in k_{cat} of factor VII_a-catalyzed factor X activation upon reconstitution of phospholipids with tissue factor (Table 6). The magnitude of the increase in V_{max} caused by the presence of tissue factor is about the same as the effect of factor V_a on prothrombin activation. Therefore, it seems reasonable to assume that the role of tissue factor apoprotein in factor X activation is similar to the role of factor V_a in prothrombin activation.

The K_m for factor X is dependent on the amount of phospholipid present and increases with increasing phospholipid concentration [99,100]. Nemerson et al. [99] suggested that this increase in K_m was due to binding of factor X to the excess phospholipid-binding sites not adjacent to the enzymatic unit of the factor VII_a–tissue factor–phospholipid complex. In other words it was proposed that the enzymatic unit of the extrinsic factor X activator acts on soluble factor X according to a so-called substrate model (vide supra).

With respect to intrinsic factor X activation it was shown by van Dieijen et al. [101] that in the absence of accessory components the rate of factor X_a formation by factor IX_a is extremely slow. Phospholipids plus $CaCl_2$ stimulate the reaction rate but the resulting rate of activation is still too low to have physiological importance [101–103]. The presence of factor VIII_a finally results in reaction rates that are sufficiently high to be important in vivo [101–106]. Table 7 shows that the effect of the accessory components on the kinetic parameters of the reaction is similar to that in prothrombin activation. Phospholipids stimulate factor X activation by causing a dramatic decrease in the K_m for factor X. Like in prothrombin

TABLE 7

Kinetic parameters of intrinsic factor X activation

Composition of factor X activator	K_m (μM)	V_{max} (X_a/min/IX_a)
IX_a	299	0.0022
IX_a, $CaCl_2$	181	0.0105
IX_a, $CaCl_2$, PL	0.058	0.00247
IX_a, $CaCl_2$, VIII_a, PL	0.063	500

Data taken from van Dieijen et al. [101].
Factor X activation was determined at pH 7.9 at 37°C with or without 7.5 mM $CaCl_2$, 11 clotting units factor VIII/ml and 10 μM phospholipid (PL) vesicles (PS/PC, 25/75; mole/mole).

activation the K_m is dependent on the amount of phospholipid present and increases with increasing phospholipid concentrations [101]. The data obtained thus far on the effect of phospholipid (in the absence of factor VIII_a) do not allow conclusions as to whether phospholipid-bound or soluble factor X is the substrate for factor IX_a bound to the phospholipid vesicles (see also discussion in the previous section). Using binding parameters for factor X obtained under identical conditions as used in the kinetic experiments [107] it was shown that the effects of phospholipid on K_m could be quantitatively accounted for either in a model in which bound factor X is the substrate or in a model in which the bound enzyme acts on soluble factor X [108,109].

The mode of factor VIII_a is most probably the same as that of factor V_a in prothrombinase. There is no doubt that the major function of factor VIII_a is to increase the V_{max} of factor X_a formation. The estimates may vary in the different studies [101,110–112] but van Dieijen et al. [101] showed that when saturation with factor VIII_a is achieved the V_{max} is increased 200 000-fold. Part of this increase by factor VIII_a is likely due to stimulation of factor IX_a binding to the phospholipid bilayer which ensures efficient participation of all enzyme present in the reaction mixture. This is supported by the finding that phospholipid-dependent factor X activation becomes saturable at much lower concentrations of factor IX_a in the presence of factor VIII_a [109,110] than in the absence of this cofactor [109]. However, this cannot explain the total V_{max} increase since it was estimated that even when all factor IX_a participates in factor X activation still factor VIII_a will cause an increase in V_{max} of approximately 6000-fold [101]. Thus apart from stimulating the binding of factor IX_a to phospholipid, factor VIII_a increases the V_{max} by increasing one or more forward rate constants in the reaction sequence of peptide bond cleavage in factor X. The presence of factor VIII_a, like factor V_a, also can result in a decrease in K_m for factor X [110–112]. The estimates on the magnitude of the effect of factor VIII_a on the K_m vary in the different studies from almost no effect [101] to a 10-fold decrease [110]. These differences are, however, likely caused by differences in experimental conditions.

It appears, therefore, that the mode of action of factor VIII_a is almost identical to the mode of action of factor V_a in the prothrombinase complex. No data are as yet available on whether the factor IX_a–factor VIII_a–phospholipid complex acts on soluble factor X as a substrate. However, in view of the data obtained in prothrombin activation this seems likely to be the case.

(c) Other multicomponent enzyme complexes involved in the activation of vitamin K-dependent coagulation factors

A number of other enzyme complexes in which vitamin K-dependent coagulation factors are involved play a role in blood coagulation. These are less well documented than the complexes that have been discussed thus far. We will, however, briefly discuss these complexes in relation to prothrombin and factor X activation.

The role of the accessory components tissue factor apoprotein and phospholipid in the activation of factor IX by factor VII_a appears similar to the role of these components in factor X activation by factor VII_a. During factor IX activation two peptide bonds are cleaved in the zymogen and an internal activation peptide of 9000 dalton is released [113]. Both cleavage sites appear available for proteolytic cleavage [113,114] and only one results in the exposure of the active site [114–116]. Thus in these aspects factor IX activation is more similar to prothrombin activation than to factor X activation. Thus far kinetic data for factor IX activation have been obtained by measurement of the release of the activation peptide and consequently in these experiments, therefore, the final reaction product (factor $IX_{\alpha\beta}$) is quantitated. The kinetic parameters of factor IX activation by factor VII_a in the presence of thromboplastin have been determined and compared with those of factor X activation [99,100,117]. Both reactions show low K_ms for the substrate and high k_{cat}s. Like in factor X activation the K_m for factor IX is a function of the amount of phospholipid present and increases when at constant tissue factor apoprotein concentration the amount of phospholipid is raised [100].

The activations of prothrombin and factor X appear to be under control of negative feedback reactions in which other vitamin K-dependent enzyme complexes are involved. Activated protein C is a vitamin K-dependent serine protease with anticoagulant [26,27,118–123] and profibrinolytic properties [124,125]. The anticoagulant effect of activated protein C is caused by the fact that this enzyme proteolytically degrades factor V_a [121,126,127] and factor VIII_a [128,129]. In these reactions $CaCl_2$, phospholipid and another vitamin K-dependent protein cofactor (protein S) act as accessory components in order to speed up reaction rates sufficiently [26,27]. The activation of protein C itself is also accomplished by a multicomponent enzyme complex consisting of thrombin, a protein cofactor (thrombomodulin) and most likely the endothelial cell surface (cf. [28–30] and Ch. 9B).

5. *Contact activation reactions*

Detailed information concerning the molecular mechanism of the contact activation reactions has become available over the past 10 years but the picture is still far from complete (cf. Ch. 5A). This has in part been due to the fact that purification procedures for the proteins involved have become available only fairly recently. It has also been difficult to find well defined (both chemically and physically) substances promoting contact activation. Contact activation requires a different procoagulant surface than the activation of the vitamin K-dependent clotting factors. The best known activators are glass, kaolin and dextran sulfate. These are, however, not present in the human body and therefore, recent attention has been drawn to the contact activation-promoting activity of sulfatides [35,36], lipopolysaccharides from bacteria [37–40] and heparin [41,42,130] all of which have potential physiological significance. The most potent activator appears to be sulfatides, a sulfated glycosphingolipid, which forms membrane bilayers when dispersed in aqueous environment.

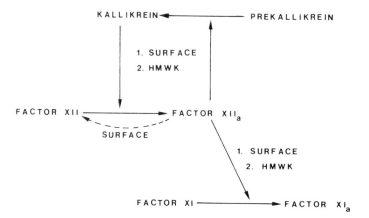

Fig. 6. Zymogen activations during contact activation.

A serious complication in obtaining quantitative data on the various reactions occurring during contact activation is that a number of feedback mechanisms feature prominently. The knowledge gained thus far is schematically summarized in Fig. 6. During the initial stages of contact activation the zymogens factor XII and prekallikrein are involved in a so-called reciprocal activation mechanism in which kallikrein activates factor XII into factor XII_a which in its turn activates prekallikrein. Factor XII_a is the central enzyme in contact activation since (1) it activates prekallikrein into kallikrein, (2) it can activate its own zymogen factor XII into factor XII_a, and (3) factor XII_a is responsible for the activation of factor XI.

It is well accepted that the presence of the negatively charged surface and the protein cofactor HMWK are essential for optimal contact activation. Thus like in the reactions of the vitamin K-dependent coagulation factors the proteins involved in contact activation somehow have to assemble on a surface for optimal interaction. However, the relative importance of the various interactions remains to be established.

(a) Factor XII activation

Factor XII activation is by far the best documented reaction of contact activation. We will primarily discuss the mode of action of the procoagulant surface in this reaction. The zymogen factor XII (80 000 MW) is activated through cleavage of a single peptide bond within a disulfide bridge resulting in a two-chain molecule with a light chain of 28 000 MW that contains the active site. Various other forms of activated factor XII have been described in the literature. We will, however, not discuss these here and refer to Ch. 5A on contact activation and to recent reviews [32–34]. Two reactions contribute to factor XII activation and these are the activation by kallikrein [131–139] and autoactivation [140–148]. For the latter reaction the 80 000 MW form of factor XII (α-factor XII_a) appears to be responsible

[142,145]. In the absence of a procoagulant surface kallikrein dependent activation is very slow (k_{cat}/K_m = 1.57 × 10^3/M/sec [cf. 148], and autoactivation is not detectable [145]. In the presence of surface both reactions are readily detectable since the surface considerably speeds up the reaction rates.

Autoactivation of factor XII has long been a controversial issue. This appears to have been caused by the fact that factor XII from different species was used. Autoactivation was first suggested to occur for rabbit factor XII by Wiggins and Cochrane [140] and subsequently for human factor XII by Silverberg et al. [142]. Bovine factor XII, however, appears to be incapable of autoactivation [149]. Recently, by means of a rigorous kinetic analysis, combined with the use of specific inhibitors, Tans et al. established the mechanism for autoactivation of human factor XII in the presence of sulfatides [145] and this was subsequently confirmed also to occur in the presence of dextran sulfate by Tankersley and Finlayson [146]. For optimal autoactivation both enzyme (factor XII_a) and substrate (factor XII) have to bind to the surface. This is suggested by the fact that the second order rate constant of autoactivation is dependent on the amount of surface present and decreases with increasing surface [145] and by the fact that addition of β-factor XII_a (also known as HF_f, the 28 000 MW form of activated factor XII that lacks the surface-binding site) does not contribute to autoactivation [142,145].

Only recently the first quantitative data concerning factor XII activation by kallikrein have become available. Tankersley and Finlayson [146] showed that the presence of dextran sulfate resulted in a drop in K_m of at least 15-fold and a 500-fold increase in k_{cat}. Thus dextran sulfate increased the catalytic efficiency of kallikrein-dependent factor XII activation approximately 10 000-fold. Moreover, the kallikrein-dependent reaction was much more efficient than autoactivation suggesting that the presence of kallikrein is essential for optimal contact activation in plasma. Tankersley and Finlayson did not evaluate these changes in K_m and k_{cat} in terms of a molecular mechanism. More information concerning the molecular mechanism of factor XII activation was obtained, however, by careful comparison of the kinetics of factor XII activation by kallikrein and the isolated light chain of this enzyme [148]. Kallikrein is a two-chain molecule with a light chain that contains the active site [150]. Van der Graaf et al. [150] showed that the light chain

TABLE 8

Comparison of the catalytic activities of kallikrein and its light chain

Substrate	Rate constants (/M/sec)	
	Kallikrein	Light chain
S 2302	1.45 × 10^6	1.34 × 10^6
Factor XII − sulfatides	1.57 × 10^3	1.51 × 10^3
Factor XII + sulfatides	5.39 × 10^6	4.17 × 10^4

Data from Rosing et al. [148].
S 2302 is H-D-Pro-Phe-Arg-*p*-nitroanilide.

of kallikrein can be separated from the heavy chain by mild reduction and alkyl-ation without loss of enzymatic activity towards the small peptide substrate S 2302 (see also Ch. 5A). The light chain of kallikrein appears to contain all the necessary information for recognition and cleavage of various macromolecular substrates [150–152]. The only difference between kallikrein and its isolated light chains was found when these two enzymes were compared in their ability to shorten the aPTT of prekallikrein-deficient plasma [150]. In this clotting assay kallikrein turned out to be considerably more procoagulant than its light chain. An explanation for this phenomenon was given in a recent study by Rosing et al. [148]. In this study kal-likrein and its light chain were compared in their ability to activate factor XII both in the presence and absence of sulfatides. In the absence of surface kallikrein and its light chain are equally effective in factor XII activation although they have a very low catalytic efficiency (1.57×10^3/M/sec at the optimal pH 7.0). Table 8 shows that the stimulation of factor XII activation due to the presence of surface was vastly different for the two enzymes. The light chain-dependent reaction was stimulated only 30-fold as compared to a 3000-fold stimulation of the rate of factor XII ac-tivation by kallikrein. Binding studies indicated that this difference is due to the fact that kallikrein has affinity for the surface whereas the light chain has not. Ros-ing et al. [148] further observed that both kallikrein-dependent factor XII activa-tion in the presence of sulfatides and the binding of kallikrein to sulfatides were considerably reduced when either the pH or the ionic strength was increased. Since the light chain-dependent reaction was much less affected by variations of pH and ionic strength they concluded that in the kallikrein-dependent reaction surface-bound factor XII is activated by surface-bound kallikrein, whereas in factor XII activation by the light chain, surface-bound factor XII is activated by soluble light chain.

The data reported thus far concerning factor XII activation by kallikrein in the presence of negatively charged surfaces are consistent with a model in which the stimulatory effect of surface is built up of two distinct additive effects (Fig. 7):

(1) Binding of factor XII to the negatively charged surface renders it more sus-ceptible to proteolytic cleavage. This hypothesis was put forward earlier by Griffin [139] and it explains the stimulation of light chain-dependent activation of factor XII in the presence of a surface and part of the stimulation of kallikrein.

(2) The surface, through the fact that both enzyme (kallikrein) and substrate

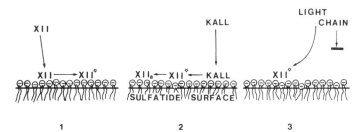

Fig. 7. The effects of negatively charged surfaces in factor XII activation.

(factor XII) have binding affinity, greatly facilitates the formation of productive enzyme–substrate complexes which increases the rate of factor XII_a formation.

The mode of action of the protein cofactor, high molecular weight kininogen, in factor XII activation remains to be established. For optimal factor XII activation in plasma the presence of this cofactor is essential [43–45, 153–155]. HMWK-kininogen forms a tight 1:1 complex with prekallikrein in plasma [156–159] and binds with the same affinity to kallikrein [160]. Since it has been shown that HMWK stimulates binding of prekallikrein and factor XI to negatively charged surfaces [161,162] it is generally thought that this cofactor acts as a carrier bringing prekallikrein (or kallikrein) to the surface for interaction with factor XII_a or factor XII (161–163]. This can explain the stimulation by HMWK of factor XII by kallikrein in the presence of kaolin [136,139,154,155,161–168]. However, further substantiation of such a hypothesis in terms of rate constants has not been reported yet. On the contrary, Espana and Ratnoff [169] recently found that HMWK did not stimulate factor XII activation by kallikrein in the presence of sulfatides, ellagic acid or dextran sulfate. At high concentrations of HMWK they even observed inhibition of factor XII activation. An interesting alternative explanation for the mode of action of HMWK has been put forward by Schapira et al. [170,171]. These authors reported that HMWK protected kallikrein from inhibition by C1-inhibitor and α_2-macroglobulin. Others, however, have failed to find a substantial protective effect of HMWK on the inhibition of kallikrein by these inhibitors [151,152]. Since it is well known that the interactions of contact activation factors can be extremely sensitive to pH and ionic strength it seems that more experimental standardization is required in order to reconcile these different views concerning the mode of action of HMWK in factor XII activation.

(b) Prekallikrein and factor XI activation

The enzyme responsible for the activation of these zymogens is factor XII_a [131,172–185]. Both reactions occur optimally in the presence of a negatively charged surface and the protein co-factor HMWK. The role of these accessory components is generally thought to be the same throughout all the reactions of contact activation. Thus it is assumed that the proteins need to bind to the surface. α-Factor XII_a readily binds via a binding region located in the heavy chain of the molecule [138] and HMWK is thought to be responsible for efficient binding of the substrates factor XI and prekallikrein [156,161,162].

It appears without question that binding of the enzyme factor XII_a is essential. Although β-factor XII_a (the form of factor XII_a lacking the binding site for the surface) is capable of efficient interaction with prekallikrein the most favorable kinetic parameters for prekallikrein activation reported yet are obtained with α-factor XII_a as enzyme in the presence of dextran sulfate [146]. Moreover, β-factor XII_a is also a very poor activator of factor XI and consequently has negligible procoagulant activity.

The mode of action of HMWK in these reactions is still poorly understood. Essentially the same hypotheses as discussed in the previous section have been put forward to explain the effect of HMWK on prekallikrein and factor XI activation. It is generally thought that HMWK facilitates the binding of the reactants to the surface. Recently Sugo et al. [167] reported kinetic parameters of bovine prekallikrein activation by bovine factor XII_a in the presence of kaolin. The remarkable acceleration of the reaction in the presence of HMWK was caused by a reduction of the K_m for prekallikrein from 1 μM to 40 nM which indicates that HMWK strongly promotes the formation of the factor XII_a–prekallikrein complex at the kaolin surface.

6. Concluding remarks

In this chapter we have reviewed the mechanistic data that have become available over the past years concerning the multicomponent enzyme complexes that are involved in blood coagulation. The enzymes that participate in these complexes have a very low catalytic activity towards their natural substrates since without exception substrate conversion by the enzyme alone (in the absence of accessory components) is extremely slow. This is reflected by the unfavorable kinetic parameters observed for these reactions. K_ms as high as 100 μM and k_{cat}s of less than 1 turnover/min are no exception. Yet when the complexes are complete the catalytic efficiency (k_{cat}/K_m for substrate conversion can be increased many orders of magnitude and become as high as 10^7–10^8/M/sec which is close to the values found for diffusion-limited reactions [91]. Thus the multicomponent enzyme complexes show almost the highest efficiency possible for enzyme-catalyzed reactions. The mechanism by which the accessory components bring about this enormous increase of catalytic efficiency has been the subject of this chapter. At the risk of oversimplification we like to summarize in this last section the current views on the mode of action of the multicomponent enzyme complexes of blood coagulation.

The most important contribution of the procoagulant surface is to promote the interactions between the proteins involved. For this stimulatory effect the proteins must be able to bind to the surface. The stimulation by surface is caused by the fact that the proteins have both an affinity for the surface and for each other which ensures efficient interaction at the surface. Thus the surface stimulates coagulation factor activation by facilitating enzyme–substrate complex formation which is reflected in a large drop in K_m and it promotes the formation of enzyme–cofactor complexes which ensures that all enzyme present participates optimally in the reaction. The advantage of such a mechanism for the physiological situation is obvious since coagulation factor activation can only take place at those sites where this procoagulant surface is exposed and where apparently reaction is needed. The surface involved in contact activation appears to have an additional stimulatory effect by rendering the substrate more susceptible to proteolytic cleavage upon binding to the surface. Thus in contact activation both an increase of k_{cat} and a decrease of K_m can be expected in the presence of surface.

The function of the cofactor appears to be the result of three effects. The cofactor causes a decrease in the K_m for the substrate which is most apparent in the presence of surfaces with a low affinity for the proteins involved. In these cases the cofactor also serves as a binding site for the enzyme to the surface which ensures that all enzyme participates in coagulation factor activation. The main function of the cofactor is, however, to cause an increase in the k_{cat} of substrate conversion by the enzyme which must be the result of a large increase in one or more forward rate constants in the reaction pathway. How the cofactor brings about this enhancement is presently unknown. It is as yet also unclear whether the same mechanisms hold for the mode of action of the contact activation cofactor high molecular weight kininogen. The magnitude of the rate enhancements brought about by this cofactor in the various contact activation reactions is much less than those observed for for example factors V_a and VIII_a in prothrombin and factor X activation. Moreover, some disagreement exists whether or not this cofactor protects the active enzymes against the inhibition of natural plasma inhibitors. Therefore, more data will have to become available in the future to gain more insight into the mode of action of this cofactor in the reactions of the contact activation system.

References

1 Macfarlane, R.G. (1964) Nature (London) 202, 498–499.
2 Davie, E.W. and Ratnoff, O.D. (1964) Science 145, 1310–1312.
3 Davie, E.W., Fujikawa, K., Kurachi, K. and Kisiel, W. (1979) Adv. Enzymol. 48, 277–318.
4 Jackson, C.M. and Nemerson, Y. (1980) Annu. Rev. Biochem. 49, 765–811.
5 Blow, D.M., Birktoft, J.J. and Hartley, B.S. (1969) Nature (London) 221, 337–339.
6 Steitz, T.A., Henderson, R. and Blow, D.M. (1969) J. Mol. Biol. 46, 337–345.
7 Henderson, R. (1970) J. Mol. Biol. 54, 341–349.
8 Robertus, J.D., Kraut, J., Alden, R.A. and Birktoft, J.J. (1972) Biochemistry 11, 4293–4297.
9 Fastrez, J. and Fersht, A.R. (1973) Biochemistry 12, 2025–2033.
10 Matthews, D.A., Alden, R.A., Birktoft, J.J., Freer, S.T. and Kraut, J. (1975) J. Biol. Chem. 250, 7120–7127.
11 Hartley, B.S. (1970) Philos. Trans. R. Soc. London, Ser. B 257, 77–87.
12 Titani, K., Hermodson, M.A., Fujikawa, K., Ericsson, L.H., Walsh, K.A., Neurath, H. and Davie, E.W. (1972) Biochemistry 11, 4899–4903.
13 Hartley, B.S. (1974) Sym. Soc. Gen. Microbiol. 24, 152–163.
14 Fujikawa, K., Coan, M.H., Enfield, D., Titani, K., Ericsson, L.H. and Davie, E.W. (1974) Proc. Natl. Acad. Sci. (U.S.A.) 71, 427–430.
15 Enfield, D.L., Ericsson, L.H., Fujikawa, K., Walsh, K.A. and Neurath, H. (1974) FEBS Lett. 47, 132–135.
16 Titani, K., Fujikawa, K., Enfield, D.L., Ericsson, L.H., Walsh, K.A. and Neurath, H. (1975) Proc. Natl. Acad. Sci. (U.S.A.) 72, 3082–3086.
17 Neurath, H. (1975) Cold Spring Harbor Conf. Cell Proliferation, Cold Spring Harbor 2, 51–64.
18 Di Scipio, R.G., Hermodson, M.A., Yates, S.G. and Davie, E.W. (1977) Biochemistry 16, 698–706.
19 Magnusson, S., Sottrup-Jensen, L., Petersen, T.E. and Claeys, H. (1975) in: Prothrombin and Related Coagulation Factors (Hemker, H.C. and Veltkamp, J.J., Eds.) pp. 25–46, Leiden University Press, Leiden.

82

20 Elion, J., Downing, M.R., Butkowski, R.J. and Mann, K.G. (1977) in: Chemistry and Biology of Thrombin (Lundblad, R., Fenton II, J.W. and Mann, K.G., Eds.) pp. 97–111, Ann Arbor Sci. Publ., Ann Arbor, MI.

21 Zwaal, R.F.A. (1978) Biochim. Biophys. Acta 515, 163–205.

22 Marcus, A.J. (1966) Adv. Lipid Res. 4, 1–37.

23 Walsh, P.N. and Biggs, R. (1972) Br. J. Haematol. 22, 743–761.

24 Walsh, P.N. (1978) Br. J. Haematol. 40, 311–331.

25 Rosing, J., van Rijn, J.L.M.L., Bevers, E.M., van Dieijen, G., Comfurius P. and Zwaal, R.F.A. (1985) Blood 65, 319–332.

26 Walker, F. (1980) J. Biol. Chem. 255, 5521–5524.

27 Walker, F. (1981) J. Biol. Chem. 256, 11128–11131.

28 Owen, W.G. and Esmon, C.T. (1981) J. Biol. Chem. 256, 5532–5535.

29 Esmon, C.T. and Owen, W.G. (1981) Proc. Natl. Acad. Sci. (U.S.A.) 78, 2249–2253.

30 Esmon, N.L., Owen, W.G. and Esmon, C.T. (1982) J. Biol. Chem. 257, 859–864.

31 Salem, H.H., Broze, G.J., Miletich, J.P. and Majerus, P.W. (1983) Proc. Natl. Acad. Sci. (U.S.A.) 80, 1584–1588.

32 Griffin, J.H. and Cochrane, C.G. (1979) Semin. Thromb. Hemostas. 5, 254–273.

33 Cochrane, C.G. and Griffin, J.H. (1982) Adv. Immunol. 33, 241–306.

34 Colman, R.W. (1984) J. Clin. Invest. 73, 1249–1253.

35 Fujikawa, K., Heimark, R.L., Kurachi, K. and Davie, E.W. (1980) Biochemistry 19, 1322–1330.

36 Tans, G. and Griffin, J.H. (1982) Blood 59, 69–75.

37 Rodriquez-Erdman (1964) Thromb. Diath. Haemorrh. 12, 471–479.

38 Mason, J.M., Kleeberg, V., Dolan, P. and Colman R.W. (1970) Ann. Intern. Med. 73, 545–556.

39 Kimball, H.R., Melmon, K.L. and Wolff, S.M. (1972) Proc. Soc. Exp. Biol. Med. 139, 1078–1086.

40 Morrison, D.C. and Cochrane, C.G. (1974) J. Exp. Med. 140, 797–803.

41 Moskowitz, R.W., Schwartz, H.J., Michel, B., Ratnoff, O.D. and Astrup, T. (1970) J. Lab. Clin. Med. 76, 790–803.

42 Hojima, Y., Cochrane, C.G., Wiggins, R.C., Austen, K.F. and Stevens, R.L. (1984) Blood 63, 1453–1459.

43 Schiffman, S., Lee, P. and Wladmann, R. (1975) Thromb. Res. 6, 451–454.

44 Schiffman, S., Lee, P., Feinstein, D.I. and Pecci, R. (1977) Blood 49, 935–945.

45 Wuepper, K.D., Miller, D.R. and Lacombe, M.J. (1975) J. Clin. Invest. 56, 1663–1672.

46 Colman, R.W., Bagdasarian, A., Talamo, R.C., Scott, C.F., Seavey, M., Guimaraes, J.A., Pierce, J.V. and Kaplan, A.P. (1975) J. Clin. Invest. 56, 1650–1662.

47 Matheson, R.T., Miller, D.R., Lacombe, M.J., Han, Y.N., Iwanaga, S., Kato, H. and Wuepper, K.D. (1976) J. Clin. Invest. 58, 1395–1406.

48 Donaldson, V.H., Glueck, H.I., Miller, M.A., Movat, H.Z. and Habal, F. (1976) J. Lab. Clin. Med. 87, 327–337.

49 Stenn, K.S. and Blout, E.R. (1972) Biochemistry 11, 4502–4515.

50 Esnouf, M.P., Lloyd, P.H. and Jesty, J. (1973) Biochem. J. 131, 781–783.

51 Jesty, J. and Esnouf, M.P. (1973) Biochem. J. 131, 791–799.

52 Heldebrant, C.M. and Mann, K.G. (1973) J. Biol. Chem. 248, 3642–3652.

53 Fass, D.N. and Mann, K.G. (1973) J. Biol. Chem. 248, 3280–3287.

54 Heldebrant, C.M., Butkowski, R.J., Bajaj, S.P. and Mann, K.G. (1973) J. Biol. Chem. 248, 3642–3652.

55 Heldebrant, C.M., Noyes, C., Kingdon, H.S. and Mann, K.G. (1973) Biochem. Biophys. Res. Commun. 54, 155–160.

56 Morita, T., Nishibe, H., Iwanaga, S. and Suzuki, T. (1973) Proc. Jpn. Acad. 49, 742–747.

57 Kisiel, W. and Hanahan, D.J. (1973) Biochim. Biophys. Acta 329, 221–232.

58 Pirkle, H. and Theodor, I. (1974) Thromb. Res. 5, 511–518.

59 Morita, T., Nishibe, H., Iwanaga, S. and Suzuki, T. (1974) J. Biochem. 76, 1031–1048.

60 Morita, T., Nishibe, H., Iwanaga, S. and Suzuki, T. (1974) FEBS Lett. 38, 345–350.

61 Kisiel, W. and Hanahan, D.J. (1974) Biochem. Biophys. Res. Commun. 59, 570–577.

62 Owen, W.G., Esmon, C.T. and Jackson, C.M. (1974) J. Biol. Chem. 249, 594–605.
63 Esmon, C.T., Owen, W.G. and Jackson, C.M. (1974) J. Biol. Chem. 249, 606–611.
64 Esmon, C.T. and Jackson, C.M. (1974) J. Biol. Chem. 249, 7782–7790.
65 Esmon, C.T. and Jackson, C.M. (1974) J. Biol. Chem. 249, 7791–7797.
66 Esmon, C.T., Owen, W.G. and Jackson, C.M. (1974) J. Biol. Chem. 249, 7798–7807.
67 Esmon, C.T., Owen, W.G. and Jackson, C.M. (1974) J. Biol. Chem. 249, 8045–8047.
68 Franza Jr., B.R., Aronson, D.L. and Finlayson, J.S. (1975) J. Biol. Chem. 250, 7057–7068.
69 Morita, T., Iwanaga, S. and Suzuki, T. (1976) J. Biochem. 79, 1089–1108.
70 Downing, M.R., Butkowski, R.J., Clark, M.M. and Mann, K.G. (1975) J. Biol. Chem. 250, 8897–8906.
71 Kornalik, F. and Blombäck, B. (1975) Thromb. Res. 6, 53–63.
72 Jobin, F. and Esnouf, M.P. (1967) Biochem. J. 102, 666–674.
73 Nesheim, M.E., Taswell, J.B. and Mann, K.G. (1979) J. Biol. Chem. 254, 10952–10962.
74 Rosing, J., Tans, G., Govers-Riemslag, J.W.P., Zwaal, R.F.A. and Hemker, H.C. (1980) J. Biol. Chem. 255, 274–283.
75 Hemker, H.C., Esnouf, M.P., Hemker, P.W., Swart, A.C.M. and MacFarlane, R.G. (1967) Nature (London) 215, 248–251.
76 Nesheim, M.E., Kettner, C., Shaw, E. and Mann, K.G. (1981) J. Biol. Chem. 256, 6537–6540.
77 Lindhout, T., Govers-Riemslag, J.W.P., van de Waart, P., Hemker, H.C. and Rosing, J. (1982) Biochemistry 21, 5494–5502.
78 Skogen, W.F., Esmon, C.T. and Cox, A.C. (1984) J. Biol. Chem. 259, 2306–2310.
79 Morrison, S.A. (1983) Biochemistry 22, 4053–4061.
80 Nesheim, M.E., Tracy, R.P. and Mann, K.G. (1984) J. Biol. Chem. 259, 1447–1453.
81 Nesheim, M.E., Eid, S. and Mann, K.G. (1981) J. Biol. Chem. 256, 9874–9882.
82 Nelsestuen, G.L. (1978) Fed. Proc. 37, 2621–2625.
83 Nelsestuen, G.L. (1980) in: The Regulation of Coagulation (Mann, K.G. and Taylor, F.B., Eds.) pp. 33–42, Elsevier, New York.
84 Pusey, M.L. and Nelsestuen, G.L. (1983) Biochem. Biophys. Res. Commun. 114, 526–532.
85 Van Rijn, J.L.M.L., Govers-Riemslag, J.W.P., Zwaal, R.F.A. and Rosing, J. (1984) Biochemistry 23, 4557–4564.
86 Tans, G., Rosing, J., van Dieijen, G. and Hemker, H.C. (1980) in: The Regulation of Coagulation (Mann, K.G. and Taylor, F.B., Eds.) pp. 173–185, Elsevier, New York.
87 Nesheim, M.E. and Mann, K.G. (1983) J. Biol. Chem. 258, 5386–5391.
88 Bevers, E.M., Comfurius, P., van Rijn, J.L.M.L., Hemker, H.C. and Zwaal, R.F.A. (1982) Eur. J. Biochem. 122, 429–436.
89 Van de Waart, P., Hemker, H.C. and Lindhout, T. (1984) Biochemistry 23, 2838–2842.
90 Mayer, L.D. and Nelsestuen, G.L. (1981) Biochemistry 20, 2457–2463.
91 Fersht, A. (1977) Enzymes, Structure and Mechanism, Freeman, San Francisco, CA.
92 Fujikawa, K., Coan, M.H., Legaz, M.E. and Davie, E.W. (1974) Biochemistry 13, 5290–5299.
93 Fujikawa, K., Titani, K. and Davie, E.W. (1975) Proc. Natl. Acad. Sci. (U.S.A.) 72, 3359–3363.
94 Bach, R., Nemerson, Y. and Koningsberg, W. (1981) J. Biol. Chem. 256, 8324–8331.
95 Chargaf, E., Moore, D.H. and Bendich, A. (1942) J. Biol. Chem. 145, 593–603.
96 Chargaf, E. (1948) J. Biol. Chem. 173, 253–263.
97 Pitlick, F.A. and Nemerson, Y. (1970) Biochemistry 9, 5105–5113.
98 Silverberg, S.A., Nemerson, Y. and Zur, M. (1977) J. Biol. Chem. 252, 8481–8488.
99 Nemerson, Y., Zur, M., Bach, R. and Gentry, R. (1980) in: The Regulation of Coagulation (Mann, K.G. and Taylor F.B., Eds.) pp. 193–203, Elsevier, New York.
100 Zur, M. and Nemerson, Y. (1980) J. Biol. Chem. 255, 5703–5707.
101 van Dieijen, G., Tans, G., Rosing, J. and Hemker, H.C. (1981) J. Biol. Chem. 256, 3433–3442.
102 Suomela, H., Blombäck, M. and Blombäck, B. (1977) Thromb. Res. 267–281.
103 Hultin, M.B. and Nemerson, Y. (1978) Blood 52, 928–940.
104 Østerud, B. and Rapaport, S.I. (1970) Biochemistry 9, 1854–1861.
105 Chuang, T.F., Sargeant, R.B. and Hougie, C. (1972) Biochim. Biophys. Acta 273, 287–291.

106 Varadi, K. and Hemker, H.C. (1976) Thromb. Res. 8, 303–317.

107 van Dieijen, G., Tans, G., van Rijn, J.L.M.L., Zwaal, R.F.A. and Rosing, J. (1981) Biochemistry 20, 7096–7101.

108 Hemker, H.C., van Dieijen, G., Rosing, J., Tans, G. and Zwaal, R.F.A. (1980) in: Protides of Biological Fluids, 28th Colloquium (Peeters, H., Ed.) pp. 265–271.

109 Van Rijn, J.L.M.L., Zwaal, R.F.A., Hemker, H.C. and Rosing, J. Haemostasis, in press.

110 Griffith, M.J., Reisner, H.M., Lundblad, R.L. and Roberts, H.R. (1982) Thromb. Res. 27, 289–301.

111 Hultin, M.B. (1982) J. Clin. Invest. 69, 950–958.

112 Link, R.P. and Castellino, F.J. (1983) Biochemistry 22, 4033–4041.

113 Fujikawa, K., Legaz, M.E., Kato, H. and Davie, E.W. (1974) Biochemistry 13, 4508–4516.

114 Lindquist, P.A., Fujikawa, K. and Davie, E.W. (1978) J. Biol. Chem. 253, 1902–1909.

115 Tans, G., Janssen-Claessen, G., van Dieijen, G., Hemker, H.C. and Rosing, J. (1982) Thromb. Haemostas. 48, 127–132.

116 Byrne, R., Link, R.P. and Castellino, F.J. (1980) J. Biol. Chem. 255, 5336–5341.

117 Jesty, J. and Silverberg, S.A. (1979) J. Biol. Chem. 254, 12337–12345.

118 Mammen, E.F., Thomas, W.R. and Seegers, W.H. (1960) Thromb. Diath. Haemorrh. 5, 218–249.

119 Kisiel, W., Ericsson, L.H. and Davie, E.W. (1976) Biochemistry 15, 4893–4900.

120 Kisiel, W., Canfield, W.M., Ericsson, L.H. and Davie, E.W. (1977) Biochemistry 16, 5824–5831.

121 Walker, F.J., Sexton, P.W. and Esmon, C.T. (1979) Biochim. Biophys. Acta 571, 333–342.

122 Marlar, R.A., Kleiss, A.J. and Griffin, J.H. (1982) Blood 59, 1067–1072.

123 Walker, F. (1981) Thromb. Res. 22, 321–327.

124 Zoltan, R. and Seegers, W. (1973) Thromb. Res. 3, 23–31.

125 Comp, P.C. and Esmon, C.T. (1981) J. Clin. Invest. 68, 1221–1228.

126 Suzuki, K., Stenflo, J., Dahlbäck, B. and Theodorsson, B. (1983) J. Biol. Chem. 258, 1914–1920.

127 Nesheim, M., Canfield, W., Kisiel, W. and Mann, K.G. (1982) J. Biol. Chem. 257, 1272–1275.

128 Vehar, G.A. and Davie, E.W. (1980) Biochemistry 19, 401–410.

129 Fulcher, C.A., Gardiner, J.E., Griffin, J.H. and Zimmerman, T.S. (1984) Blood 63, 486–489.

130 Soulier, J.P. and Gozin, D. (1980) Haematologia 13, 1–4.

131 Kaplan, A.P. and Austen, K.F. (1971) J. Exp. Med. 133, 696–712.

132 Bagdasarian, A., Talamo, R.C. and Colman, R.W. (1973) J. Biol. Chem. 248, 3456–3463.

133 Cochrane, C.G., Revak, S.D. and Wuepper, K.D. (1973) J. Exp. Med. 138, 1564–1583.

134 Revak, S.D., Cochrane, C.G., Johnston, A.R. and Hugli, T.H. (1974) J. Clin. Invest. 54, 619–627.

135 Weiss, A.S., Gullin, J.I. and Kaplan, A.P. (1974) J. Clin. Invest. 53, 622–633.

136 Griffin, J.H. and Cochrane, C.G. (1976) Proc. Natl. Acad. Sci. (U.S.A.) 73, 2554–2558.

137 Chan, J.Y., Habal, F.M., Burrowes, C.E. and Movat, H.Z. (1976) Thromb. Res. 9, 423–434.

138 Revak, S.D. and Cochrane, C.G. (1976) J. Clin. Invest. 57, 852–860.

139 Griffin, J.H. (1978) Proc. Natl. Acad. Sci. (U.S.A.) 75, 1998–2001.

140 Wiggins, R.C. and Cochrane, C.G. (1979) J. Exp. Med. 150, 1122–1133.

141 Miller, G., Silverberg, M. and Kaplan, A.P. (1980) Biochem. Biophys. Res. Commun. 92, 803–810.

142 Silverberg, M., Dunn, J.T., Garen, L. and Kaplan, A.P. (1980) J. Biol. Chem. 255, 7281–7286.

143 Dunn, J.T., Silverberg, M. and Kaplan, A.P. (1982) J. Biol. Chem. 257, 1779–1784.

144 Silverberg, M. and Kaplan, A.P. (1982) Blood 60, 64–70.

145 Tans, G., Rosing, J. and Griffin, J.H. (1983) J. Biol. Chem. 258, 8215–8222.

146 Tankersley, D.L. and Finlayson, J.S. (1984) Biochemistry 23, 273–279.

147 Espana, F. and Ratnoff, O.D. (1983) J. Lab. Clin. Med. 102, 31–45.

148 Rosing, J., Tans, G. and Griffin, J.H. (1985) Eur. J. Biochem. 151, 531–538.

149 Sugo, T., Hamaguchi, A., Shimada, T., Kato, H. and Iwanaga, S. (1982) J. Biochem. 92, 689–698.

150 van der Graaf, F., Tans, G., Bouma, B.N. and Griffin, J.H. (1982) J. Biol. Chem. 257, 14300–14305.

151 van der Graaf, F., Rietveld, A., Keus, F.J.A. and Bouma, B.N. (1984) Biochemistry 23, 1760–1766.

152 van der Graaf, F., Koedam, J.A., Griffin, J.H. and Bouma, B.N. (1983) Biochemistry 22, 4860–4866.

153 Griffin, J.H. and Cochrane, C.G. (1976) Proc. Natl. Acad. Sci. (U.S.A.) 73, 2554–2558.

154 Meier, H.L., Pierce, J.V., Colman, R.W. and Kaplan, A.P. (1977) J. Clin. Invest. 60, 18–31.

155 Revak, S.D., Cochrane, C.G. and Griffin, J.H. (1977) J. Clin. Invest. 59, 1167–1175.
156 Mandle, R.J., Colman, R.W. and Kaplan, A.P. (1976) Proc. Natl. Acad. Sci. (U.S.A.) 73, 4179–4183.
157 Donaldson, V.H., Kleniewski, J., Saito, H. and Sayed, J.H. (1977) J. Clin. Invest. 60, 571–579.
158 Kerbiriou, D.M., Bouma, B.N. and Griffin, J.H. (1980) J. Biol. Chem. 255, 3952–3958.
159 Bouma, B.N., Keribiriou, D.M., Vlooswijk, R. and Griffin, J.H. (1980) J. Lab. Clin. Med. 96, 693–701.
160 Bock, P.E., Tans, G., Griffin, J.H. and Shore, J.D. (1985) J. Biol. Chem. 260, 12434–12443.
161 Wiggins, R.C., Bouma, B.N., Cochrane, C.G. and Griffin, J.H. (1977) Proc. Natl. Acad. Sci. (U.S.A.) 74, 4636–4640.
162 Silverberg, M., Nicoll, J.E. and Kaplan, A.P. (1980) Thromb. Res. 20, 173–189.
163 Saito, H. (1977) J. Clin. Invest. 60, 584–594.
164 Lin, C.Y., Scott, C.F., Bagdasarian, A., Pierce, J.V., Kaplan, A.P. and Colman, R.W. (1977) J. Clin. Invest. 60, 7–17.
165 Sugo, T., Ikari, N., Kato, H., Iwanaga, S. and Fujii, S. (1980) Biochemistry 19, 3125–3220.
166 Sugo, T., Kato, H., Iwanaga, S. and Fujii, S. (1981) Thromb. Res. 24, 329–337.
167 Sugo, T., Kato, H., Iwanaga, S., Takada, K. and Sakakibara, S. (1985) Eur. J. Biochem. 146, 43–50.
168 Shimada, T., Sugo, T., Kato, H., Yoshida, K. and Iwanaga, S. (1985) J. Biochem. 97, 429–439.
169 Espana, F. and Ratnoff, O.D. (1983) J. Lab. Clin. Med. 102, 478–479.
170 Schapira, M., Scott, C.F., James, A., Silver, L., Kuppers, F., James, H. and Colman, R.W. (1982) Biochemistry 21, 567–572.
171 Schapira, M., Scott, C.F. and Colman, R.W. (1981) Biochemistry 20, 2738–2743.
172 Cochrane, C.G. and Wuepper, K.D. (1971) J. Exp. Med. 134, 986–1004.
173 Takahashi, H., Nagasawa, S.and Suzuki, T. (1972) FEBS Lett. 24, 98–100.
174 Mandle, R. and Kaplan, A.P. (1977) J. Biol. Chem. 252, 6097–6104.
175 Heimark, R.L., Kurachi, K., Fujikawa, K. and Davie, E.W. (1980) Nature (London) 286, 456–460.
176 Takahashi, H., Nagasawa, S. and Suzuki, T.(1980) J. Biochem. 87, 23–31.
177 Bouma, B.N., Miles, L.A., Beretta, G. and Griffin, J.H. (1980) Biochemistry 19, 1151–1160.
178 Ratnoff, O.D., Davie, E.W. and Mallet, D.L. (1961) J. Clin. Invest. 40, 803–819.
179 Nossel, H.L. (1964) in: Contact of Phase of Blood Coagulation, Blackwell, Oxford.
180 Wuepper, K.D. (1972) in: Inflammation Mechanism and Control (Lepow, I. and Ward, P.A., Eds.) pp. 93–117, Academic Press, New York.
181 Heck, L.W. and Kaplan, A.P. (1974) J. Exp. Med. 140, 1615–1630.
182 Kurachi, K. and Davie, E.W. (1977) Biochemistry 16, 5831–5839.
183 Bouma, B.N. and Griffin, J.H. (1977) J. Biol. Chem. 252, 6432–6437.
184 Wiggins, R.C., Cochrane, C.G. and Griffin, J.H. (1979) Thromb. Res. 15, 487–498.
185 Kurachi, K., Fujikawa, K. and Davie, E.W. (1980) Biochemistry 19, 1330–1338.

R.F.A. Zwaal and H.C. Hemker (Eds.), *Blood Coagulation*
© 1986 Elsevier Science Publishers B.V. (Biomedical Division)

CHAPTER 4

The role of vitamin K in the post-translational modification of proteins

C. VERMEER

Department of Biochemistry, University of Limburg, P.O. Box 616, 6200 MD Maastricht
(The Netherlands)

1. Introduction

Vitamin K was discovered by Henrik Dam when he tried to investigate the effect of a cholesterol-free diet on chickens [1]. He observed that after about 1 month the chicks had developed hemorrhages and that blood, taken from the animals exhibited a prolonged coagulation time. The addition of purified cholesterol to the food did not reverse these effects and it turned out that, together with the cholesterol, a fat-soluble vitamin had been extracted from the food. This vitamin was called Koagulations-vitamin (coagulation vitamin) or shortly: vitamin K. Until recently blood coagulation was the only process in which vitamin K was thought to be involved.

The bleeding symptoms provoked by vitamin K-deficiency were similar to those described for a hemorrhagic disease in cattle [2] and which were found to be caused by feeding the animals with improperly cured sweet clover hay. The active compound in the clover was identified as dicumarol (4-hydroxycoumarin) [3], which is present in a chemically bound and thus inactive form in the fresh plants, but which may be liberated during the curing of the clover. In its free form dicumarol acts as an antagonist of vitamin K. During the subsequent years numerous coumarin-derivatives have been synthesized and tested for their anticoagulant potency. The drugs most frequently used nowadays include besides dicumarol: phenprocoumon (3-(1-phenyl(propyl)-4-oxycoumarin), difenacoum (3-[3-p-diphenyl-1,2,3,4-tetrahydronaphth-1-yl]-4-hydroxycoumarin) and brodifacoum (3-[3-(4^1-bromodiphenyl-4-yl)-1,2,3,4-tetrahydronaphth-1-yl]-4-hydroxycoumarin. All these compounds serve as anticoagulants either in the form of rodenticides or for the treatment of patients in order to antagonize undesired blood coagulation during thrombogenic episodes.

In this chapter we intend to review our present knowledge concerning the way of action of vitamin K and vitamin K antagonists. We hope to make the readers clear that these drugs affect the synthesis of many proteins and that the blood coagulation factors form only a minor part of this group.

2. The secretion of proteins

Protein biosynthesis starts with the attachment of an mRNA to a ribosome. Proteins destined to remain in the cell are synthesized on free cytoplasmic ribosomes, whereas secretory proteins are exclusively formed on ribosomes bound to the rough endoplasmic reticulum (RER). The question remains: how does the mRNA discriminate between the cytosolic and the membrane-bound ribosomes. Recently the course of events leading to the secretion of a protein has been discovered [4–7] and a summary is given in Fig. 1. After the binding of a ribosome to the mRNA the latter is translated and a growing amino acid chain emerges from the ribosome. Secretory proteins – at least those investigated until now – differ from the cellular proteins in that they are synthesized in the form of precursors consisting of the amino acid residues found in the mature protein and, in addition, a signal sequence. This signal sequence is formed by 15–30 strongly hydrophobic amino acids at the amino-terminal side of the growing peptide chain, so it is the first part of the protein to be synthesized. After the amino acid chain is 60–70 residues long, the signal sequence extends far enough from the ribosome to be recognized by the signal recognition particle (SRP). The SRP then binds to the ribosomal complex, thus causing an immediate stop of any further polypeptide chain elongation.

A second protein involved in the process of protein secretion is located in the RER membrane. It is designated by some authors as 'docking protein' (DP) because it is able to recognize the SRP–ribosome complex and to mediate in its binding to the RER. It is not yet sure whether this interaction leads to a conformational change of SRP or to its removal from the ribosomal complex, but the result of the action of DP is the reinitiation of protein synthesis, whereby the hydrophobic signal sequence rapidly penetrates into the phospholipid membrane, thus facilitating the transport of the growing protein through the membrane to the luminal side of the endoplasmic tubuli. Here are located the enzymes required for the post-translational modifications such as glycosylation, hydroxylation, disulfide bond formation, vitamin K-dependent carboxylation and the proteolytic degradation of the signal sequence by a highly specific enzyme, named signal peptidase. Secretory proteins may undergo one or more of these modifications during their trip down the lumen of the endoplasmic reticulum to the Golgi apparatus, via which the proteins are secreted into the extracellular environment. Since also the proteins present in the outer cellular membrane are secreted via this pathway (they only remain bound to the Golgi membranes during exocytosis) they are generally regarded as secretory proteins. Obviously not all proteins undergo all possible modifications and the way in which the various post-translational enzyme systems are able to discriminate between the different proteins (or parts of the same protein) is still a matter of investigation.

The molecular biology of the blood coagulation factors in particular has been studied by the groups of Davie and MacGillivray. Employing techniques such as immunoprecipitation of polysomes, the mRNA from human liver was enriched in its messenger content coding for either factor IX or prothrombin. Complementary

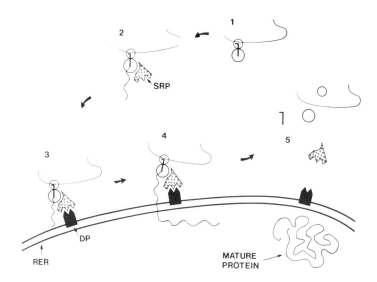

Fig. 1. The synthesis of secretory proteins. Step 1: initiation of protein synthesis and synthesis of the signal sequence. Step 2: recognition of the signal sequence by SRP, binding of SRP to the protein-synthesizing complex and concurrent blockade of further polypeptide chain elongation. Step 3: binding of the ribosome/SRP complex to the RER-bound docking protein (DP) and subsequent re-initiation of the protein synthesis. Step 4: transport of the growing polypeptide chain through the RER membrane and subsequent post-translational modification. Step 5: termination of the protein biosynthesis and dissociation of the protein-synthesizing complex. Transport of the mature protein to the outer cellular environment.

DNA (cDNA) was then synthesized from the enriched mRNA and converted into double-stranded cDNA and incorporated into *E. coli* plasmid DNA. In this way cDNA libraries were prepared and screened for factor IX [8] and prothrombin [9]. When searching for human factor IX-cDNA Kurachi and Davie [8] identified a plasmid containing a cDNA insert of 1466 base pairs, 138 of which coded for a 'leader sequence'. Furthermore the cDNA contained 1248 base pairs coding for the 416 amino acid residues of the mature protein, a stop codon and 48 pairs of non-coding sequence at the 3' end. The previously mentioned leader sequence coded for 46 amino acid residues, which are assumed to constitute the signal sequence (found in all secretory proteins) and a 'pro'-sequence of about 10 amino acid residues length, which is located between the signal and the mature protein.

In a subsequent investigation Degen et al. [9] isolated a cDNA of 2005 base pairs coding for human prothrombin. The cDNA just missed the start of the signal sequence, 27 amino acids of which were coded for, followed by a pro-sequence and the 579 amino acids of prothrombin. A non-coding region of 97 base pairs and a poly A tail of 27 base pairs were found at the 3' end of the genome.

Apart from the fact that these experiments demonstrate that the vitamin K-dependent coagulation factors behave just as the other secretory proteins do, they also inform us about the presence of a pro-insert in between the signal sequence and the mature protein. The function of this pro-insert is not yet clear, but it might be involved in the recognition of the growing polypeptide chain by the enzymes involved in the post-translational modification reactions.

3. The carboxylation of glutamic acid residues

Vitamin K-dependent carboxylase is involved in the conversion of glutamic acid (Glu) residues into γ-carboxyglutamic acid (Gla) residues [10–12]. The structures of these compounds are represented in Fig. 2. Gla may be regarded as a malonic acid derivative, which is stable in base but labile in hot acid. This property explains why Gla had not been detected earlier during amino acid analysis, since all techniques employed include the acid hydrolysis of the peptide bonds. Only after alkaline hydrolysis Gla residues may be identified, for instance by HPLC analysis [13].

Gla residues were discovered in prothrombin and initially it was assumed that this new amino acid exclusively occurred in the classical 'vitamin K-dependent' coagulation factors. Later on Gla residues were also detected in other hepatic proteins (the proteins C, M, S and Z) [14–17] as well as in proteins not related to blood coagulation such as proteins in bone (osteocalcin), dentin, renal stones, hardened atherosclerotic plaque and spermatozoa [18–22]. Gla residues have even been demonstrated in non-mammalian tissues such as corals [23] and the chorioallantoic membrane of chicken eggs [24] so that it may be concluded that the vitamin K-dependent carboxylation reaction is widely spread in nature. Although the functions of the various Gla-containing proteins may vary to a great extent, the only function that could have been attributed to the Gla residues is the strong and selective binding of Ca^{2+}.

When carboxylase is blocked in vivo by the administration of vitamin K antagonists, precursors of the Gla-containing proteins accumulate in the RER [12] and when the blockade is prolonged, the non-carboxylated proteins may be excreted into the extracellular environment. In their excreted form these proteins are designated as descarboxy proteins. These descarboxy proteins are indistinguishable from the corresponding normal proteins with respect to their carbohydrate content. Therefore it is assumed that the vitamin K-dependent carboxylation does not

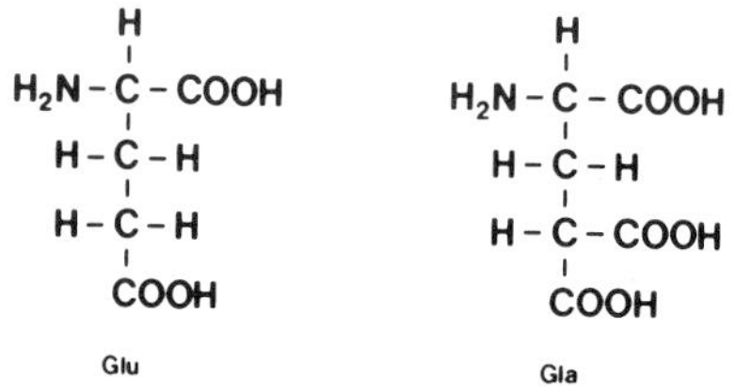

Fig. 2. Structures of Glu and Gla.

influence other post-translational modifications. The hypothesis that blood plasma from anticoagulated patients contained abnormal coagulation factors was put forward as early as in 1963 [25] but it lasted until 1974 before the nature of the abnormality could be identified as the absence of Gla [10,11]. Recently it was shown that also a non-hepatic protein (osteocalcin) is excreted in its descarboxy form during oral anticoagulant treatment [26].

The first in vitro carboxylating enzyme systems were developed in homogenates from rat and cow liver [27,28]. Carboxylase appeared to be present in the rough microsomal fraction and the enzyme could be solubilized with the aid of detergents such as Lubrol, Triton X-100 and CHAPS. When the microsomal fraction was prepared from the livers of animals which had been treated previously with vitamin K antagonists, the accumulated protein precursors (which are present in the same fraction as is carboxylase) could serve as a substrate for carboxylase in vitro, provided that the reaction mixtures were supplemented with vitamin K and $NaH^{14}CO_3$. Under these conditions $^{14}CO_2$ is incorporated into the endogenous substrate proteins, which may subsequently be separated from the bulk of bicarbonate by trichloroacetic acid precipitation.

Although the use of this system has several advantages (e.g. the correct substrate is complexed to carboxylase in such a way that it is readily carboxylated upon adding vitamin K), two drawbacks of the system are that (a) during the purification of carboxylase the substrate may be lost, which inevitably will lead to the loss enzyme activity and (b) kinetic studies may require that the substrate is present in varying and well-defined amounts. Therefore also exogenous substrates have been developed. Two groups of exogenous substrates may be distinguished. In the first place there are the synthetic substrates, which all resemble a short Gla-containing amino acid sequence in one of the coagulation factors, but in which Gla has been replaced by Glu. Examples of these substrates are Phe-Leu-Glu-Glu-Val (sequence homology with bovine factor prothrombin and factor X) [29], Phe-Leu-Glu-Glu-Leu (sequence homology with bovine factor VII and protein C) [30] and Phe-Leu-Glu-Glu-Ile (sequence homology with rat prothrombin) [31]. A second group of substrates is formed by the 'natural' substrates, which are derived from descarboxy proteins or from in vitro decarboxylated Gla-containing proteins. Examples of these substrates are fragment-Su, which is a proteolytic split product of descarboxyprothrombin and which consists of the amino acid residues 13–29 [32], and decarboxylated osteocalcin [33]. Whereas the synthetic substrates are characterized by relatively high K_m values (4–6 mM) in the in vitro carboxylating systems, the K_m values for fragment-Su and decarboxylated osteocalcin were found to be 500–1000 times lower. Remarkably, purified descarboxy coagulation factors or in vitro decarboxylated coagulation factors are very poor substrates for carboxylase. This may be caused by the absence of the leader sequence, which possibly plays a role in the binding between carboxylase and carboxylatable substrates. Alternatively the low affinity between decarboxylated coagulation factors and carboxylase may be the result of the presence of carbohydrates attached to asparagine residues shortly after the Gla-containing region in the various coagulation factors. In vivo these carbohydrates are thought to be attached to the protein backbone after the carboxylation reaction has taken place and in vitro they might hamper the correct binding between carboxylase and its substrate.

4. Occurrence of carboxylase

Prothrombin was the first protein in which Gla residues were detected [10,11]. Soon afterwards the abnormal amino acid was also identified in the other 'vitamin K-dependent' blood coagulation factors. Since no other proteins were known to be synthesized in a vitamin K-dependent way, carboxylase was generally assumed to be uniquely involved in the production of the 4 blood coagulation factors. Consequently it was thought that carboxylase occurred exclusively in the liver. During the last few years, however, vitamin K-dependent enzyme systems have also been identified in non-hepatic tissues such as testis, kidney, lung, spleen, pancreas, thyroid, vessel wall and bone [34,35]. Bone carboxylase resides in the osteoblasts [36]. No carboxylase has been found in white blood cells. It has been demonstrated that at a low intake of vitamin K-antagonists the degree of inhibition of hepatic carboxylase is similar to that of the non-hepatic enzyme systems [37]. Also kinetic constants such as the K_m for vitamin K and the K_i for vitamin K antagonists were similar in all systems examined. It is highly probable therefore, that during the treatment of patients with vitamin K antagonists (oral anticoagulant therapy) not only the synthesis of the blood coagulation factors is inhibited, but also the synthesis of the various non-hepatic Gla-containing proteins. In the light of these findings it is surprising, that the frequent clinical use of coumarin derivatives has revealed only very few side effects. Those reported thus far include skin necrosis and the so-called 'fetal warfarin syndrome' (chondrodysplasia punctata) [38]. Whereas skin necrosis is only seldomly observed, numerous cases of the fetal warfarin syndrome have been reported in the literature. The defect is induced when women take coumarin derivatives during the first trimester of pregnancy and it is characterized by bone abnormalities in the developing fetus. These abnormalities are caused by the excessive and irregular precipitation of calcium phosphate in the rapidly growing parts of the bone [39]. In the calcified areas the growth is stopped in an irreversible way. Women who need anticoagulant treatment and who have a strong wish for progeny are generally treated therefore with heparin during the first 3 months of pregnancy.

Finally, a beneficial side effect of coumarin derivatives seems to be their antimetastatic activity in a number of experimental tumors [40]. Since vitamin K-dependent carboxylase has been found in isolated human tumors as well as in cultivated tumor cells [41], it seems probable that in some cases Gla-containing proteins mediate in the metastasis of tumors. The mechanism of this antimetastatic action is still unclear at this moment.

Besides that carboxylase has been found in a wide variety of tissues also its reaction products (the Gla-containing proteins) have been detected in many different species such as mammals, birds, swordfish and corals. The function of most of these proteins is still unclear, but those that have been characterized to some extent may be classified as follows.

(A) The phospholipid-binding proteins. Except the 4 classical 'vitamin K-dependent' coagulation factors, also the coagulation-inhibiting proteins C [14] and S [15] belong to this category. The function of these proteins is detailed in Ch. 3 and 9B. A considerable sequence homology has been found between all these proteins as well as another Gla-containing protein, protein Z [17]. Therefore it is to be expected that also protein Z is a member of this group. The phospholipid-binding proteins all contain 10–12 Gla residues per molecule. Although in vitro they rapidly bind to insoluble barium and calcium salts, in vivo they exclusively occur dissolved in blood plasma. In the presence of calcium ions these proteins have a high affinity towards negatively charged phospholipid surfaces, the binding to which highly stimulates their enzymatic activity [42].

(B) The calcium salt-binding proteins. These proteins have no detectable affinity towards negatively charged phospholipids [43] and in vivo they are predominantly found in the matrix of calcified tissues. The member of this group most extensively studied is osteocalcin, a Gla-rich protein found in bone [18,44] and it is among the 6 most abundant proteins in man. It comprises over 25% of the non-collagenous proteins in bone and it contains 49 amino acid residues, the sequence of which is known. Three of them are Gla-residues. As was pointed out above, the absence of normal osteocalcin leads to the excessive precipitation of calcium phosphate in rapidly growing bone tissue. Moreover, in vitro studies have demonstrated (1) that osteocalcin has a very high affinity for hydroxylapatite and (2) that low concentrations of osteocalcin are able to efficiently stop the growth of calcium phosphate crystals from supersaturated solutions of calcium and phosphate [45].

Other Gla-containing proteins have been found in dentin [19], in renal stones [20], in hardened atherosclerotic plaque [21] and in corals [23]. The biological function of none of these proteins is fully understood, but a plausible hypothesis is that they are formed to regulate or to reduce the deposition of insoluble calcium salts in the various tissues. A similar function has been proposed for proteins present in the soluble matrix of mollusc shells [46].

(C) The calcium-transporting proteins. An example of these proteins is found in the chorioallantoic membrane of chicken's eggs which is required for the Ca^{2+} transport from the egg shell to the developing embryo. In the embryo the Ca^{2+} is used for the de novo synthesis of bone tissue [24]. When fertilized eggs are injected with warfarin no Gla residues are formed in the transport protein and hence the Ca^{2+} transport through the membrane comes to a halt. Consequently the mineralization of the chicken's bones is very poor. Possibly also the protein synthesized by renal carboxylase belongs to the calcium-transporting proteins, but at this moment we have no experimental evidence to confirm this suggestion.

(D) Other Gla-containing proteins. Several proteins of unknown function have been detected, for instance the sperm Gla protein [47] and a number of tumor Gla proteins [41]. None of these proteins has been characterized to such an extent that

it can be placed in one of the three categories mentioned above or a well-defined separate class.

5. Purification of carboxylase

Since the discovery of carboxylase many attempts have been undertaken to purify the enzyme. The methods employed include the use of various detergents, chaotropic agents, ion exchange and size exclusion columns, sulfhydryl binding and hydrophobic columns as well as affinity chromatography on carrier-bound heparin or lectins. None of these methods has been very successful, however. The procedures leading to an increased specific activity of carboxylase will be shortly discussed below.

(A) Removal of contaminating microsomal proteins. Canfield et al. [48] developed a procedure for the specific extraction of a number of rat liver microsomal membrane proteins. By this procedure the total carboxylase activity increased over 40-fold, indicating that an inhibitor of carboxylase was removed. In parallel about 60% of the microsomal proteins were removed by the extraction, so that a 150-fold increase of specific carboxylase activity was obtained. The preparation thus obtained was called complex A and did not contain reductase activity.

(B) Isolation of the enzyme/substrate complex. Also using livers from warfarin-treated rats, Olson et al. [49] tried to purify the carboxylase-bound prothrombin precursors on a heparin affinity column. Since resin-bound heparin is frequently used for the isolation of normal coagulation factors it was expected that also the coagulation factor precursors would have some affinity towards heparin. In fact the enzyme/substrate complexes could be bound and subsequently eluted with a recovery of about 10%. The total purification was 100-fold, but it is not sure whether this is due to the removal of the inhibitor reported by Canfield et al. (see above) or to the elimination of 99% of the contaminating proteins.

A slightly different approach was followed by De Metz et al. [50] who first determined the identity of the accumulated substrate for carboxylase in the livers of

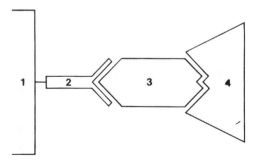

Fig. 3. Structure of solid-phase carboxylase (SPC). From left to right: 1, a Sepharose bead; 2, antibody against plasma coagulation factor; 3, hepatic coagulation factor precursor; 4, carboxylase.

warfarin-treated cows. It resulted that about 60% of the carboxylatable material consists of factor X precursors, whereas only 25% could be identified as prothrombin precursors. Consequently purified antibodies against normal bovine factor X were covalently linked to Sepharose and used for the extraction of enzyme/substrate complexes from solubilized microsomes. By this method part of the carboxylase activity could be bound to the Sepharose beads. After washing away the non-bound material a preparation resulted which was designated as solid-phase carboxylase. The structure of solid-phase carboxylase is represented in Fig. 3. Solid-phase carboxylase is able to incorporate $^{14}CO_2$ into endogenous as well as exogenous substrates and in contrast to solubilized carboxylase it is very stable. Later on Olson et al. [49] prepared in a similar way a solid-phase carboxylase from rat liver using Sepharose-bound antibodies to rat prothrombin.

(C) Column chromatography. Using a new detergent (CHAPS), Girardot has recently described that carboxylase could be isolated from the crude microsomal fraction by low-pressure chromatography on ion exchange and size exclusion columns [51]. The enzyme preparation still contained an endogenous substrate for carboxylase but no reductase and no cytochrome P450 or P420. The degree of purification was 400-fold and the enzyme activity eluted in the inclusion volume of an AcA 34 column, thus indicating that the M_r is lower than 350000. This is the smallest size obtained for the active enzyme complex thus far. Unfortunately the purification procedure described by this group has not yet been confirmed by other laboratories.

6. The mechanism of the carboxylation reaction

In the liver 3 forms of vitamin K have been detected: vitamin K quinone (K), vitamin K hydroquinone (KH$_2$) and vitamin K 2,3-epoxide (KO). Calculations based on the daily requirement for vitamin K relative to the formation of Gla, as measured by its excretion, show that each molecule of the vitamin must be recycled several thousand times before it is metabolized further and excreted [52]. Therefore it has been proposed several years ago, that the 3 forms of vitamin K are interconverted into each other in a cyclic way as is depicted in Fig. 4. Enzymes are required for each step and they will be discussed in more detail consecutively.

Step 1: The conversion of KH$_2$ to KO. In 1974 Willingham and Matschiner described a microsomal enzyme system which was called 'vitamin K epoxidase' and which converts KH$_2$ to KO [53]. Since that time it has been proposed frequently, that the oxidation of KH$_2$ provides the energy required for the γ-carboxylation of glutamyl residues [12]. The evidence that the carboxylation is coupled somehow to the epoxide formation is now overwhelming so that any hypothesis concerning the role of vitamin K must consider the relationship between these two activities. Both reactions mainly occur in the rough endoplasmic reticulum of liver tissue [54,55] and both require the reduced vitamin as a substrate [56]. The K_m values of both enzyme activities for O_2 are closely similar and increasing the number of car-

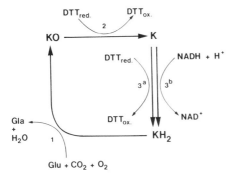

Fig. 4. The vitamin K cycle. The carboxylation reaction is driven by the conversion of KH_2 to KO (step 1). In steps 2 and 3 KO is reduced to K and KH_2 respectively. Step 3 is catalyzed by a DTT-dependent as well as by an NADH-dependent reductase.

boxylation events by increasing either the pentapeptide substrate for carboxylase or adding Mn^{2+} leads to a simultaneous increase of KO formation [52]. In addition, the partly purified solid-phase carboxylase is stimulated about 5-fold by the addition of certain organic solvents. This stimulation is accompanied by a parallel increase of the KO formation [57]. At saturating CO_2 concentrations a 1:1 ratio was found between the number of Gla residues formed and the amount of KO formed. However, at decreased CO_2 concentrations or in the presence of CN^- the two reactions are uncoupled and far more KO is formed than CO_2 is incorporated [58]. The direct vitamin K antagonist 2-chloro-3-phytyl-1,4-naphthoquinone (chloro-K) is an effective inhibitor of both, carboxylase and epoxidase, but the commonly used coumarin derivatives (vide supra) inhibit only at very high concentrations. Their physiological site of action seems to be restricted to the reductases, which are involved in steps 2 and 3 of Fig. 4.

Step 2: the reduction of KO to K. The enzyme involved in this step is KO-reductase and this system is extremely sensitive to coumarin anticoagulants [59]. The hypothesis that KO reductase is the physiological site of action of these drugs is also supported by the observation that in warfarin-resistant rats this reductase has undergone a mutation by which it has become less sensitive to warfarin. In vitro the reducing equivalents required for this reaction are provided by dithiols such as dithiothreitol, but their physiological counterpart has not yet been discovered.

Step 3: the reduction of K to KH_2. Two K reductases are involved in this step, an NADH-dependent one and a DTT-dependent one. Similarly to KO reductase, the DTT-dependent K reductase is strongly inhibited by coumarin derivatives [60]. The NADH-dependent system, on the other hand, is relatively insensitive to these drugs. The NADH-dependent reductase (DT-diaphorase) has been found in the microsomal membranes as well as in the cytosol. The DTT-dependent system occurs exclusively as a membrane-bound activity. It is not known if some of the various reducing systems are identical or partly identical.

Obviously the scheme represented in Fig. 4 does not give any detailed information concerning the mechanism of the carboxylation reaction. Investigations concerning this point are badly hampered by the fact that the enzyme system has not yet been obtained in a purified form. Using the crude microsomal system Jones et al. [61] demonstrated that CO_2 and not HCO^-_3 is the active species in the carboxylation reaction. This seems to be logic, since the hydrophobic nature of the endoplasmic reticulum will protect CO_2 against hydration, thus permitting a sufficient supply of the correct substrate during the carboxylation reaction. The importance of the hydrophobic environment for carboxylase was demonstrated by De Metz et al. [62]. Using the partly purified solid-phase carboxylase these authors showed that phosphatidylcholine is present in the enzyme complex and that neutral phospholipids are an absolute requirement for carboxylase activity. How the CO_2 is exactly exchanged with a proton of glutamic acid is still a matter of debate. Most of the models proposed until now include the formation of radicals via vitamin K hydroquinone. Whereas Friedman et al. [63] and Larson et al. [64] assume that the proton abstraction precedes the addition of the carboxyl group, De Metz et al. [65] proposed a concerted reaction mechanism, via which the proton abstraction, the CO_2 addition and the KO formation all occur by a simple electron shift after the reaction components have been properly aligned on carboxylase (Fig. 5). In the latter model the uncoupling of the carboxylation and epoxidation, which

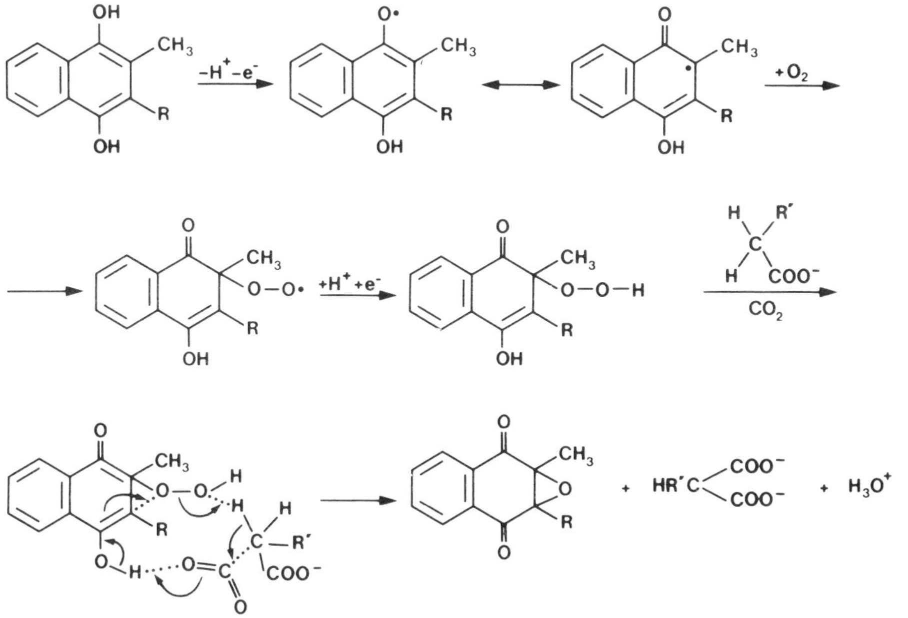

Fig. 5. Proposed mechanism for the carboxylation reaction. In a first step vitamin K is converted into a hydroperoxide. The breakage of the peroxide bond is the driving force for the removal of the γ-C hydrogen, which is then replaced by CO_2. The function of carboxylase is the proper alignment of the various reaction components.

is seen at low CO_2 concentrations, would occur when CO_2 is replaced by H_2O. In fact it remains questionable whether both models are really different from each other.

7. Nutritional aspects of vitamin K

The vitamin K requirement of the human is met by a combination of our dietary intake and the synthesis of the intestinal microflora. Vitamin K_1 (phylloquinone) is present in the plant sources whereas vitamin K_2 (menaquinone) is produced via the microbiologic synthesis. To what extent menaquinone contributes to the production of Gla residues is not sure, but several arguments favor the assumption that phylloquinone is the most important form of vitamin K. In the first place only phylloquinone has been detected in human plasma [66,67]. Secondly, cholates are required for the passage of vitamin K through the intestinal wall, but at the place of the intestinal flora, cholates are hardly present. And last but not least the discovery of vitamin K was made by experiments which clearly demonstrated that a serious vitamin K deficiency occurs after the vitamin has been omitted from the food [1]. For all these reasons we think that phylloquinone is the most important form of vitamin K.

TABLE 1

Vitamin K content of fresh vegetables

Vegetable	Vitamin K_1 (μg/100 g)	
	Shearer et al. [68]	Langenberg [69]
Potato	<1	–
Turnip	<1	–
Mushroom	<1	–
Celery	5	–
Carrot	5	11
Tomato	6	–
Leek	10	18
Cucumber	15	–
Red cabbage	19	–
Cauliflower	27	25
Peas	39	–
Butter beans	46	53
Cress	88	–
White cabbage	83–127	–
Lettuce	120–128	–
Green cabbage	52–189	216
Broccoli	147	–
Brussels sprout	177	175
Spinach	415	385
Kale	724	817

Unfortunately the natural concentration of vitamin K in food and body fluids (plasma, milk) is very low and its detection therein is not an easy task. Recently two groups have developed assay procedures based on high-performance liquid chromatography (HPLC) and they have investigated the amount of vitamin K in various vegetables [68,69]. Although slightly different techniques were employed, there is a fair agreement between their results. The most common foodstuffs investigated are listed in Table 1.

It is know for many years that the concentration of the 'vitamin K-dependent' coagulation factors in the newborn is rather low (about 50% of normal) and the idea that neonates are partially vitamin K deficient has been widely, although not universally accepted [70,71]. Because of the recently developed techniques for vitamin K detection the interest in this subject has strongly revived. It was demonstrated by Shearer et al. [66] that a difference exists between the physiological vitamin K concentration in maternal (0.2 ng/ml) and in cord plasma (not detectable). When 1 mg of vitamin K was given intravenously to the mothers shortly before delivery, the levels in all mothers rose from 0.2 to about 75 ng/ml. The level of vitamin K in the cord plasma was only slightly affected (about 0.1 mg/ml in 4 of 6 babies and not detectable in 2 babies). Therefore, a placental barrier seems to exist which causes the level of vitamin K in neonate plasma to be lower than that in adults. It is not yet sure whether the enzymatic activity of hepatic carboxylase is severely impaired under these conditions.

In addition to the low plasma level immediately after birth it seems that human milk contains 5–6 times less vitamin K than cow's milk [68]. Nevertheless the vitamin K concentration in human milk (about 1.7 ng/ml) is 8–10 fold higher than the physiological plasma concentration. So the vitamin K intake of a breast-fed baby will amount to approximately 1 μg/day. Whether this is sufficient to induce a rapid increase of the vitamin K level in the neonate's plasma remains to be seen.

Acknowledgements

The author wishes to thank Mrs. M. Molenaar-van de Voort for typing this manuscript.

Our research is supported by the following grants: MD 82145 from the Trombosestichting Nederland, 13-30-52 from the Division for Health Research TNO and C 84.463 from the Nier Stichting Nederland.

References

1 Dam, H. (1935) Biochem. J. 29, 127–1285.
2 Schofield, F.W. (1922) Can. Vet. Rec. 3, 74–79.
3 Campbell, M.A. and Link, K.P. (1941) J. Biol. Chem. 138, 21–33.
4 Meyer, D.I. and Dobberstein, B. (1980) J. Cell Biol. 87, 503–508.
5 Meyer, D.I., Krause, E. and Dobberstein, B. (1982) Nature (London) 297, 647–650.

100

6 Gilmore, R., Blobel, G. and Walter, P. (1982) J. Cell Biol. 95, 470–477.

7 Walter, P. and Blobel, G. (1982) Nature (London) 299, 691–698.

8 Kurachi, K. and Davie, E.W. (1982) Proc. Natl. Acad. Sci. (U.S.A.) 79, 6461–6464.

9 Degen, S.J.F., MacGillivray, R.T.A. and Davie, E.W. (1983) Biochemistry 22, 2087–2097.

10 Stenflo, J., Fernlund, P., Egan, W. and Roepstorff, P. (1974) Proc. Natl. Acad. Sci. (U.S.A.) 71, 2730–2733.

11 Nelsestuen, G.L., Zytkovicz, T.H. and Howard, J.B. (1974) J. Biol. Chem. 249, 6347–6350.

12 Suttie, J.W. (1980) CRC Crit. Rev. Biochem. 8, 191–223.

13 Kuwada, M. and Katayama, K. (1983) Anal. Biochem. 131, 173–179.

14 Stenflo, J. (1976) J. Biol. Chem. 251, 355–363.

15 Stenflo, J. and Jönsson, M. (1979) FEBS Lett. 101, 377–381.

16 Seegers, W.H., Gosh, A. and Wu, V.-Y. (1980) in: Vitamin K Metabolism and Vitamin K-Dependent Proteins (Suttie, J.W., Ed.) pp. 96–101, University Park Press, Baltimore, MD.

17 Højrup, P., Roepstorff, P. and Petersen, T.E. (1982) Eur. J. Biochem. 126, 343–348.

18 Hauschka, P.V. and Reid, M.L. (1978) J. Biol. Chem. 253, 9063–9068.

19 Linde, A., Bhown, M., Cothran, W.C., Höglund, A. and Butler, W.T. (1982) Biochim. Biophys. Acta 704, 235–239.

20 Lian, J.B., Prien, E.C., Glimcher, M.J. and Gallop, P.M. (1977) J. Clin. Invest. 59, 1151–1157.

21 Levy, R.J., Lian, J.B. and Gallop, P. (1979) Biochem. Biophys. Res. Commun. 91, 41–49.

22 Vermeer, C. (1984) Mol. Cell. Biochem. 61, 17–35.

23 Hamilton, S.E., King, G., Tesch, D., Riddles, P.W., Keough, D.T., Jell, J. and Zerner, B. (1982) Biochem. Biophys. Res. Commun. 108, 610–613.

24 Tuan, R.S. (1979) J. Biol. Chem. 254, 1356–1364.

25 Hemker, H.C., Veltkamp, J.J., Hensen, A. and Loeliger, E.A. (1963) Nature (London) 200, 589–590.

26 Vermeer, C. (1984) Proc. 2nd Eur. Symp. on Life Sci. Res. in Space, Porz Wahn, 4–6 June 1984, pp. 219–224.

27 Esmon, C.T., Sadowski, J.A. and Suttie, J.W. (1975) J. Biol. Chem. 250, 4744–4748.

28 Vermeer, C., Soute, B.A.M., de Metz, M. and Hemker, H.C., (1982) Biochim. Biophys. Acta 714, 361–365.

29 Suttie, J.W., Hageman, J.M., Lehrman, S.R. and Rich, D.H. (1976) J. Biol. Chem. 251, 5827–5830.

30 Suttie, J.W., Lehrman, S.R., Geweke, C.O., Hageman, J.M. and Rich, D.H. (1979) Biochem. Biophys. Res. Commun. 86, 500–507.

31 Houser, R.M., Carey, D.J., Dus, K.M., Marshall, G.R. and Olson, R.E. (1977) FEBS Lett. 75, 226–230.

32 Soute, B.A.M., Vermeer, C., de Metz, M., Hemker, H.C. and Lijnen, H.R. (1981) Biochim. Biophys. Acta 676, 101–107.

33 Vermeer, C., Soute, B.A.M., Hendrix, H. and de Boer-van den Berg, M.A.G. (1984) FEBS Lett. 165, 16–20.

34 Vermeer, C., Hendrix, H. and Daemen, M. (1982) FEBS Lett. 148, 317–320.

35 Buchtal, S.D. and Bell, R.G. (1983) Biochemistry 22, 1077–1082.

36 Nishimoto, S.K. and Price, P.A. (1979) J. Biol. Chem. 254, 437–441.

37 Roncaglioni, M.C., Soute, B.A.M., de Boer-van de Berg, M.A.G. and Vermeer, C. (1983) Biochem. Biophys. Res. Commun. 114, 991–997.

38 Loeliger, E.A. (1982) in: Side Effects of Drugs Annual (Dukes, M.N.G., Ed.) Vol. 6, pp. 304–314, Excerpta Medica, Amsterdam.

39 Price, P.A., Williamson, M.K., Haba, T., Dell, R.B. and Jee, W.S.S. (1982) Proc. Natl. Acad. Sci. (U.S.A.) 79, 7734–7738.

40 Delaini, F., Colucci, M., De Bellis Vitti, C., Locati, D., Poggi, A., Semeraro, N. and Donati, M.B. (1981) Thromb. Res. 24, 263–266.

41 Buchthal, S.D., McAllister, C.G., Laux, D.C. and Bell, R.G. (1982) Biochem. Biophys. Res. Commun. 109, 55–62.

42 Rosing, J., Tans, G., Govers-Riemslag, J.W.P., Zwaal, R.F.A. and Hemker, H.C. (1980) J. Biol. Chem. 255, 274–283.

43 Vermeer, C. (1984) FEBS Lett. 173, 169–172.

44 Poser, J.W., Esch, F.S., Ling, N.C. and Price, P.A. (1980) J. Biol. Chem. 255, 8685–8691.

45 Price, P.A., Otsuka, A.S., Poser, J.W., Kristaponis, J. and Raman, N. (1976) Proc. Natl. Acad. Sci. (U.S.A.) 73, 1447–1451.

46 Wheeler, A.P., George, J.W. and Evans, C.A. (1981) Science 212, 1397–1398.

47 Soute, B.A.M., Müller-Esterl, W., de Boer-van den Berg, M.A.G., Ulrich, M. and Vermeer, C. (1985) FEBS Lett. 190, 137–141.

48 Canfield, L.M., Sinsky, T.A. and Suttie, J.W. (1980) Arch. Biochem. Biophys. 202, 515–524.

49 Olson, R.E., Hall, A.L., Lee, F.C., Kappel, W.K., Meyer, R.G. and Bettger, W.J. (1983) in: Posttranslational Covalent Modifications of Proteins (Johnson, B.C., Ed.) pp. 295–319, Academic Press, New York.

50 De Metz, M., Vermeer, C., Soute, B.A.M., van Scharrenburg, G.J.M., Slotboom, A.J. and Hemker, H.C. (1981) FEBS Lett. 123, 215–218.

51 Girardot, J.M. (1982) J. Biol. Chem. 257, 15008–15011.

52 Suttie, J.W., Preusch, P.C. and McTigue, J.J. (1983) in: Posttranslational Covalent Modification of Proteins (Johnson, B.C., Ed.) pp. 253–279, Academic Press, New York.

53 Willingham, A.K. and Matschiner, J.T. (1974) Biochem. J. 140, 435–441.

54 Egeberg, K. and Helgeland, L. (1980) Biochim. Biophys. Acta 627, 225–229.

55 Carlisle, T.L. and Suttie, J.W. (1980) Biochemistry 19, 1161–1167.

56 Sadowski, J.A., Schnoes, H.K. and Suttie, J.W. (1977) Biochemistry 16, 3856–3863.

57 De Metz, M., Soute, B.A.M., Hemker, H.C. and Vermeer, C. (1983) Biochem. J. 209, 719–724.

58 De Metz, M., Soute, B.A.M., Hemker, H.C. and Vermeer, C. (1982) FEBS Lett. 137, 253–256.

59 Fasco, M.J., Hildebrandt, E.F. and Suttie, J.W. (1982) J. Biol. Chem. 257, 11210–11212.

60 Fasco, M.J. and Principe, L.M. (1980) Biochem. Biophys. Res. Commun. 97, 1487–1492.

61 Jones, J.P., Gardner, E.J., Cooper, T.G. and Olson, R.E. (1977) J. Biol. Chem. 252, 7738–7742.

62 De Metz, M., Vermeer, C., Soute, B.A.M. and Hemker, H.C. (1981) J. Biol. Chem. 256, 10843–10846.

63 Friedman, P.A., Shia, M.A., Gallop, P.M. and Griep, A.E. (1979) Proc. Natl. Acad. Sci. (U.S.A.) 76, 3126–3129.

64 Larson, A.E., Friedman, P.A. and Suttie, J.W. (1981) J. Biol. Chem. 256, 11032–11035.

65 De Metz, M., Soute, B.A.M., Hemker, H.C., Fokkens, R., Lugtenburg, J. and Vermeer, C. (1982) J. Biol. Chem. 257, 5326–5329.

66 Shearer, M.J., Barkhan, P., Rahim, S. and Stimmler, L. (1982) Lancet 460–463.

67 Langenberg, J.P. and Tjaden, U.R. (1984) J. Chromatogr. 289, 377–385.

68 Shearer, M.J., Allan, V., Haroon, Y. and Barkhan, P. (1980) in: Vitamin K Metabolism and Vitamin K-Dependent Proteins (Suttie, J.W., Ed.) pp. 317–327, University Park Press, Baltimore, M.D.

69 Langenberg, J.P. (1985) Thesis, Leiden.

70 Dam, H., Dyggve, H., Larsen, H. and Plum, P. (1952) Adv. Pediat. 5, 129–153.

71 Van Doorm, J.M., Muller, A.D. and Hemker H.C. (1977) Lancet 852–853.

R.F.A. Zwaal and H.C. Hemker (Eds.), *Blood Coagulation*
© 1986 Elsevier Science Publishers B.V. (Biomedical Division)

Initiation mechanisms:
The contact activation system in plasma

BONNO N. BOUMA and JOHN H. GRIFFIN

*Department of Haematology, University Hospital Utrecht, Utrecht (The Netherlands), and
Department of Immunology, Scripps Clinic and Research Foundation, La Jolla, CA
(U.S.A.)*

1. Introduction

When human plasma is exposed to a variety of negatively charged materials, the intrinsic pathway of blood coagulation is activated. These materials include glass, kaolin, celite, certain connective or collagen preparations, pyrophosphate or urate crystals, endotoxin, and other substances. Central to this pathway is coagulation factor XII (Hageman factor). Activated factor XII (XII_a) activates factor XI which then activates factor IX and thereby propagates the intrinsic coagulation pathway. Moreover factor XII_a is capable of triggering the kinin-forming pathway, plasminogen activation, conversion of factor VII to factor VII_a and the conversion of prorenin to renin. The purpose of this paper is to summarize some current biochemical information and to present several integrated hypotheses for the explanation of the molecular mechanisms that are responsible for activation of the contact system of plasma. Since this review is not particularly clinical the reader is referred for that to several recent review articles [1–5].

The discovery of plasma proteins involved in contact activation reactions has been based on finding human plasmas deficient in specific plasma proteins. It now appears that 4 plasma proteins are involved in normal contact activation reactions: factor XII, factor XI, plasma prekallikrein and high MW kininogen (Table 1). The

TABLE 1

Proteins of the contact activation system

	Molecular weight	pI	Concentration in citrated plasma (μg/ml)
Factor XII	74 000–80 000	6.8	29
Prekallikrein	80 000–85 000	8.5–9.0	50
Factor XI	160 000 (dimer)	8.5–9.0	4
High MW kininogen	110 000	4.5	70

most readily observed property of plasmas deficient in contact activation proteins is the markedly prolonged activated partial thromboplastin time. Prolonged incubation time of prekallikrein-deficient plasma corrects the activated partial thromboplastin time whereas plasmas deficient in factor XII, high MW kininogen, or factor XI preserve a markedly prolonged clotting time. These deficient plasmas also exhibit abnormal surface-initiated fibrinolysis [6–8], kinin formation [6], prorenin activation [9–11] and cold-dependent activation of factor VII [12,13].

A congenital deficiency in any of the contact activation proteins except factor XI has not been conclusively associated with any particular disorder or with an immunity to a specific disease. Thus a deficiency in one of these proteins remains a laboratory curiosity. One group suggests the existence of a factor XII$_a$ inhibitor that exhibits elevated levels in some patients with thrombotic disease, possibly implying that factor XII may be more important for fibrinolysis than for hemostasis [14]. Ratnoff and Saito [3] have reviewed the clinical literature and noted the general absence of hemorrhagic symptoms in patients with deficiencies of factor XII, prekallikrein, or high MW kininogen. Factor XI deficiency may be associated with a mild bleeding diathesis and there is marked variability in clinical bleeding in such patients. In severely affected patients, plasma infusions are an adequate source of factor XI to provide normal hemostasis.

A deficiency in any one of the contact activation proteins is inherited as an autosomal recessive trait [3]. In hepatic disease each of the proteins is reduced, implying that the liver is a major source for synthesis of these proteins. Immunologic studies of factors XII and XI, prekallikrein and high MW kininogen have been recently reviewed [15].

2. Structure–function relationship of components of the contact activation mechanism

(a) Factor XII

Factor XII has been purified from human, bovine and rabbit plasma [16–19]. Factor XII is a glycoprotein that exists as a single polypeptide chain of molecular weight 74 000–80 000. Factor XII is a serine protease zymogen that can be activated by limited proteolysis. Cleavage of the single-chain native molecule within the disulfide loop generates a two-chain enzyme, α-factor XII$_a$; a second cleavage outside the disulfide bond gives a 28 000-dalton active enzyme, β-factor XII$_a$, derived from the carboxy terminal of the molecule [20–22]. The amino-terminal polypeptide of α-factor XII$_a$ contains the major binding site for negatively charged surfaces while the carboxy-terminal 28 000-dalton portion contains the enzymatic active site [23]. Thus α-factor XII$_a$ binds to negatively charged surfaces whereas β-factor XII$_a$ does not. Both α- and β-factor XII$_a$ molecules are potent prekallikrein activators whereas β-factor XII$_a$ is at least 100 times less active than α-factor XII$_a$ in the activation of factor XI (22,24–26]. The differing potencies of different

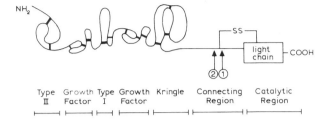

Fig. 1. A tentative alignment of the domain organization of factor XII. Cleavage of factor XII by kallikrein at site 1 generates α-factor XII$_a$, which is composed of $M_r = 52\,000$ and $30\,000$ fragments. A second cleavage at site 2 generates β-factor XII$_a$ which consists of $40\,000$ and $12\,000$ fragments (based on the work of Fujikawa and McMullen [29] and data presented at American Heart Association, Miami, FL, November 1984).

forms of factor XII$_a$ in activating its various substrates may ultimately allow a quantitative description of preferential activation of different factor XII-dependent pathways. Further information about the chemical changes accompanying proteolytic activation of factor XII comes from the amino acid sequence studies of human and bovine factor XII [27–29].

The polypeptide structure of human factor XII is schematically presented in Fig. 1 and is based on the work of Fujikawa and McMullen ([29] and data presented at American Heart Association, Miami, FL, November, 1984). The N-terminal heavy-chain region is connected to the light chain through a connecting region. The light chain contains the catalytic region. The heavy chain of α-factor XII$_a$ contains several folding domains that have been found in other proteins. These are the 'type I' and 'type II' structures that have been found in fibronectin, the 'growth factor' structure found in epidermal growth factor, protein C, factor IX and factor X, and the kringle structure found in plasminogen, tissue plasminogen activator, urokinase and prothrombin (cf. Ch. 8). A tentative alignment of the domain organization of factor XII is shown in Fig. 1. The heavy-chain region of α-factor XII$_a$ that is responsible for binding to negatively charged surface does not contain any sequence rich in basic amino acids, implying that the surface-binding properties of the molecule are based on the juxtapositioning of basic residues by the tertiary structure.

β-Factor XII$_a$ has a two-chain structure [28], a chain of 243 amino acids and a chain of 9 amino acids [29]. The amino acid sequence of the carboxy-terminal chain that contains the active site shows a high degree of homology to the corresponding regions of other plasma serine proteases such as plasmin, thrombin, factor IX$_a$ and factor X$_a$. β-Factor XII$_a$ has 6 internal and 1 interchain disulfide bonds.

The level of factor XII antigen in normal plasma was reported to be 29 μg/ml (range 23–40 μg/ml) by Revak et al. [20]. Saito et al. [31] determined a normal value of 40 μg/ml using a radioimmunoassay for factor XII antigen. Factor XII antigen was found to be reduced in plasmas of patients with disseminated intravascular coagulation and hepatic cirrhosis [31]. Although factor XII deficiency initially was reported to be associated with a total absence of factor XII antigen a

106

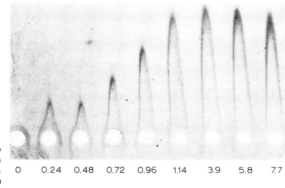

Molar Ratio High Mr Kininogen Versus Prekallikrein   0   0.24   0.48   0.72   0.96   1.14   3.9   5.8   7.7

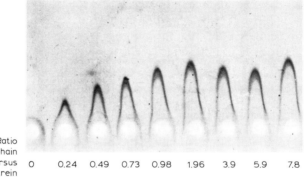

Molar Ratio Light Chain Versus Prekallikrein   0   0.24   0.49   0.73   0.98   1.96   3.9   5.9   7.8

Fig. 2. Titration of prekallikrein with high MW kininogen or its isolated light chain using rocket immunoelectrophoresis with anti-prekallikrein antibodies. Prekallikrein alone does not migrate but it migrates after preincubation with either high MW kininogen or its light chain. The heights of the rocket increase as a function of increasing high MW kininogen or light-chain concentrations until a maximum height is reached (from ref. 40).

more extensive study by Saito [20] indicated that in the plasma of 2 out of 49 subjects with factor XII deficiency, non-functional material immunologically indistinguishable from normal factor XII was present.

(b) Prekallikrein

Plasma prekallikrein has been purified from human, bovine and rabbit plasmas [32–37]. Prekallikrein is a glycoprotein that exists as a single polypeptide chain of approximately 80 000 molecular weight. Prekallikrein isolated from human plasma consists of two very similar forms. In plasma prekallikrein circulates in a complex with high MW kininogen [38]. The formation of this complex can be demonstrated by crossed immunoelectrophoresis and by Laurell rocket immunoelectrophoresis [39,40] (Fig. 2). Under conditions of the electrophoresis, prekallikrein alone does not migrate. Addition of high MW kininogen leads to complex formation and as a result, prekallikrein migrates with an anodal mobility. Using these immunochemical techniques it was shown that high MW kininogen or the light chain derived from it complexes with prekallikrein or with kallikrein [39,40]. These complexes contain equimolar amounts of each molecule [40].

Activation of human prekallikrein by β-factor XII_a is associated with limited proteolysis [32,34,37]. Two slightly different forms of kallikrein are obtained that reflect the presence of two slightly different forms of prekallikrein. Kallikrein molecules are composed of two polypeptide chains linked by disulfide bonds, a heavy chain of 43 000 and a light chain of either 36 000 or 33 000 dalton [32,34,37]. Following reduction and alkylation, the heavy and light chains of kallikrein were isolated by affinity chromatography using insolubilized high MW kininogen [41] (Fig. 3). The alkylated light chain did not bind to high MW kininogen Sepharose while the heavy chain did bind with high affinity and was subsequently eluted. This demonstrated that the heavy chain of kallikrein possesses a high-affinity binding site for high MW kininogen. Binding of prekallikrein or kallikrein to high MW kininogen involves the light-chain region of high MW kininogen [40,42], therefore high-

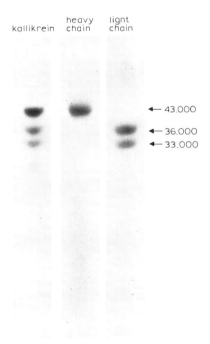

Fig. 3. Human kallikrein and its isolated heavy and light chains on 10% SDS polyacrylamide gels. Kallikrein (10 μg) in the presence of dithiothreitol and 10 μg of isolated heavy chain or light chain were analyzed in the absence of reducing agent (from ref. 41).

affinity interactions between these 2 molecules involves binding sites localized in the heavy-chain region of kallikrein and the light-chain region of high MW kininogen. The enzymatic active site of kallikrein is localized on the light chain. The light chain was as effective as kallikrein in cleaving oligopeptide chromogenic substrates and factor XII in solution, suggesting that the heavy-chain region of kallikrein plays no significant role in forming the enzyme active site. However a major role for the heavy-chain region of kallikrein may be inferred from the observation that the light chain is much less procoagulant than native kallikrein indicating that the heavy-chain region of kallikrein is required for surface-dependent activation of coagulation [41]. Recent studies have indicated that kallikrein can cleave its heavy chain, resulting in two fragments held together by disulfide bonds [43]. This cleavage results in a loss of procoagulant activity, which may be caused by the fact that this form of kallikrein cannot form complexes with high MW kininogen [44]. Other properties of kallikrein such as cleavage of small oligopeptide substrates are retained [40,44].

Prekallikrein exhibits amino acid sequence homology to factor XI [36]. As a protease, kallikrein is capable of liberating kinins from kininogens [45] activating factor XII [25,46,47], activating plasminogen [37] and activating factor IX [48,49]. Kallikrein is particularly potent in its action as a kininogenase and as an activator of surface-bound factor XII.

Based on radioimmunoassay and Laurell rocket immunoelectrophoresis techniques values of approximately 50 μg/ml were found for prekallikrein in normal plasma [39,50]. The absence of prekallikrein antigen in plasma of Fletcher trait patients was reported by several authors [39,50,51]. However in several patients with a prekallikrein deficiency, low levels of prekallikrein antigen were detected using the sensitive radioimmunoassay and the Laurell rocket immunoelectrophoresis [52,53].

Prekallikrein antigen levels were also measured in plasmas of patients with high MW kininogen deficiency. Using the radial immunodiffusion technique values were reported of 0.4 and 0.71 units/ml [54,55], although the last value was reported to be 0.32 units/ml using a radioimmunoassay [55]. In studies using rocket immunoelectrophoresis no prekallikrein rocket was observed in plasmas of patients with high MW kininogen deficiency unless the plasmas were reconstituted with normal levels of high MW kininogen. Prekallikrein antigen levels in such deficient plasmas were found to be 30% of normal [39]. These levels are in agreement with the prekallikrein clotting activity levels in these plasmas.

Prekallikrein antigen levels were reported to be decreased in hepatic cirrhosis, DIC, chronic renal failure, and nephrotic syndrome [50]. During typhoid fever, a decrease in prekallikrein clotting activity was found [50]. Prekallikrein antigen levels, however, apparently remained the same, and crossed immunoelectrophoretic analysis of these plasmas showed complexes of kallikrein with C1-inhibitor [56].

(c) Factor XI

Human factor XI is a glycoprotein with an apparent molecular weight of 160000. It consists of two very similar or identical polypeptide chains that are held together by disulfide bonds [57–60]. Factor XI is present in plasma in a complex with high MW kininogen [61–63]. The binding site for factor XI was shown to be localized in the light-chain region of high MW kininogen [62,63]. During the activation of factor XI by factor XII$_a$ or trypsin an internal peptide bond in each of the two chains is cleaved giving rise to a pair of disulfide-linked heavy and light chains with molecular weights of 48000 and 35000 respectively [57,58] (Fig. 4). Studies using diisopropylphosphofluoridate or antithrombin III showed that each of these inhibitors bound to the light chain of factor XI$_a$ in a stoichiometry of 2 moles of inhibitor/1 mole of enzyme suggesting that each light chain of factor XI$_a$ bears one active site [58]. Direct evidence that the light chain contained the enzymatically active site derived from studies in which factor XI$_a$ was first reduced and alkylated and subsequently subjected to affinity chromatography on high MW kininogen–Sepharose [64]. The alkylated light chain did not bind while the heavy chain bound with high affinity. The isolated light chain retained the specific amidolytic activity of native factor XI$_a$ against an oligopeptide chromogenic substrate. However in clotting assays using factor XI-deficient plasma in the presence of kaolin, the light chain was only 1% as active as native factor XI$_a$. From these studies it was concluded that the light-chain region of factor XI$_a$ contains the entire enzymatic active site. The heavy-chain region contains the high-affinity binding site for high MW kininogen. In addition it was found that the heavy chain of factor XI$_a$ was involved in calcium-dependent mechanisms that accelerate the activation of factor IX [64].

The major activity of factor XI$_a$ is the proteolytic activation of factor IX in a calcium-dependent two-step mechanism. Initially, an internal peptide bond in factor IX is cleaved giving rise to two-chain disulfide-linked inactive intermediates. This intermediate is then converted to factor IX$_a$ by a second cleavage due to factor XI$_a$, resulting in the release of an activation peptide [65,66].

An antibody neutralization assay was used by Forbes and Ratnoff [67] and by Rimon et al. [68] to study the presence of factor XI antigen in plasma from pa-

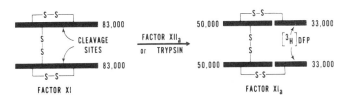

Fig. 4. Schematic model of the polypeptide chain structure of factor XI and factor XI$_a$. Activation of factor XI by activated factor XII or by trypsin can occur by limited proteolytic cleavage at the sites designated by the small arrows. The polypeptide chains of factor XI$_a$ that take up [^{3}H]diisopropyl phosphorofluoridate ([^{3}H]DFP) and that contain the enzymatic active site are indicated (from ref. 57).

tients with factor XI clotting deficiency. Both studies indicated the absence of factor XI antigen in plasma from these patients. The level of factor XI antigen in normal plasma was determined by radioimmunoassay to be approximately 6 μg/ml [69]. In an extensive study of 125 patients with congenital factor XI deficiency of different ethnic background the level of factor XI antigen was shown to be reduced in proportion to the reduction in factor XI clotting activities [70]. A reduction of factor XI antigen was also detected in plasma from patients with hepatic cirrhosis [69].

(d) High and low MW kininogens

Human plasma contains at least two distinct kininogens, high MW kininogen and low MW kininogen that are single polypeptide chains of 110 000 and 50 000–78 000, respectively (Fig. 5). High MW kininogen is a non-enzymatic cofactor that is central to contact activation reactions [71–74]. Low MW kininogen plays no known role in coagulation activation reactions, although it is highly homologous in its amino acid sequence with the N-terminal 60% of the high MW kininogen [75–77]. Cleavage of low MW kininogen with trypsin gives a kinin-free molecule with a

STRUCTURE AND FUNCTION OF HUMAN HIGH MW KININOGEN AND ITS FRAGMENTS

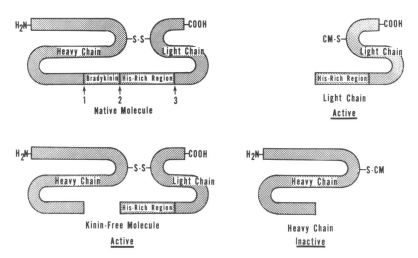

Fig. 5. Structural models for the polypeptide chain structure of high molecular weight and low molecular weight kininogens. These schematic models represent both molecules as single polypeptide chains and are based on the studies of human and bovine kininogens. Cleavage by plasma kallikrein at arrows 1 and 2 liberates kinin. In the case of high molecular weight kininogen, the kinin-free molecule can be reduced and alkylated to yield isolated heavy and light chains as indicated in the figure. The alkylated heavy chains of high and low molecular weight kininogens are not procoagulant. These heavy chains share identical immunologic determinants and are homologous in amino acid sequence. These chains are thiol protease inhibitors [79]. The alkylated light chain in high molecular weight kininogen is unique to this molecule and possesses the entire procoagulant activity of the parent molecule (from ref. 40).

62 000 MW heavy chain and a light chain of about 4000 MW. The heavy chain corresponds to the amino-terminal part of the original kininogen molecule and the light chain to the carboxy-terminal part.

Cleavage of high MW kininogen by plasma kallikrein liberates bradykinin to give a kinin-free molecule with a 65 000 MW heavy chain and 44 800 MW light chain [75,77]. The kinin-free molecule retains its procoagulant activity. After reduction and alkylation the heavy and light chains were isolated. The alkylated heavy chain in high and low MW kininogen is not procoagulant. These heavy chains share identical immunologic determinants and are highly homologous in amino acid sequence [78]. Recent data [79] indicate that the heavy-chain regions of high and low MW kininogen have an inhibitory effect on thiol proteases. The light chain of high MW kininogen is unique to this molecule and possesses the entire procoagulant activity of the parent molecule [78,80,81]. High MW kininogen has been shown to contain an unusual and unique region of amino acid sequence that is rich in histidine, lysine and glycine [75–77]. In a sequence of approximately 50 amino acids, approximately 30% are histidine, 30% are glycine and 10% are lysine. Moreover this portion of the carboxy-terminal region of the high MW kininogen molecule has been shown to be essential for the contact activation cofactor activity [77,81,82]. It may be speculated that this highly positively charged region of the molecule is responsible for the binding of the molecule to negatively charged sur-

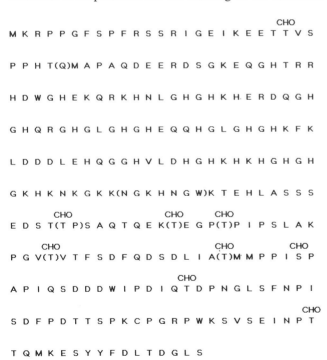

Fig. 6. The amino acid sequence of human high MW kininogen light chain (from ref. 83).

face. Recently the complete amino acid sequences of the light chains of human high and low MW kininogen were reported [83,84] (Fig. 6). The light chain of low MW kininogen contains 38 amino acids of which the first 11 residues show complete identity with the light chain of high MW kininogen. The complete gene structure for high and low MW kininogen was also recently reported [85]. High and low kininogens were shown to originate from one single gene, but different splicing mechanisms result in mRNAs specific for high and low MW kininogen [85].

Antisera against the isolated heavy chain precipitate both high and low MW kininogens [78]. Anti-light-chain antisera exclusively precipitate high MW kininogen [78]. These antisera were used to measure the levels of high and low MW kininogen in normals and in patients with high MW kininogen deficiency [39]. Laurell rocket immunoelectrophoresis gave a level of high MW kininogen in 20 normal subjects of 70 μg/ml [39]. Based on hemagglutination inhibition assays [86] or radioimmunoassays [87] a normal level of 90 μg/ml has been reported. High MW kininogen antigen was absent from plasma of patients with high MW kininogen deficiency [39,55,86]. Low MW kininogen was present in reduced amounts in plasmas of 2 patients with high MW kininogen deficiency and absent from 3 other plasmas [39,54,88].

3. Roles of negatively charged surfaces

Data collected in recent years allow a coherent series of hypotheses for the contributions of negatively charged surfaces to the activation of factor XII and to the expression of the activities of factor XII$_a$ [89]. Available evidence indicates that the 3 major roles of negatively charged surfaces are: (1) to induce a structural change in factor XII such that surface-bound factor XII is highly susceptible to proteolytic activation, (2) to promote high MW kininogen-dependent interactions between factor XII and prekallikrein that result in reciprocal proteolytic activation of each molecule, and (3) to promote the high MW kininogen-dependent activation of factor XI by surface-bound α-factor XII$_a$.

(a) Surface-dependent activation of factor XII

Studies employing highly purified factor XII indicated that the surface-bound molecule is much more susceptible to proteolytic activation by plasma and cellular proteases [46]. Evidence for such a hypothesis was obtained from kinetic studies of the cleavage of radiolabeled human factor XII by plasma kallikrein, plasmin, trypsin in the presence and absence of high MW kininogen and a variety of negatively charged surfaces. The data indicate that surface-bound factor XII is 500 times more susceptible to proteolytic activation by kallikrein than is factor XII in solution. Similar data have been accumulated for purfied bovine factor XII [47,90]. Support for the importance of proteolytic activation of factor XII was derived from studies of radiolabeled factor XII in human plasmas that are subjected to contact activation [21]. Radiolabeled factor XII was added to normal or various deficient plasmas that were then put into glass tubes. Factor XII in normal plasma rapidly binds to the glass surface and is then cleaved to give polypeptide fragments representative of α-factor XII_a and β-factor XII_a. In plasma deficient in prekallikrein or high MW kininogen, a rapid binding of factor XII to the glass surface occurs, however, no rapid cleavage of the surface-bound molecules occurs. These initial observations of the binding and cleavage of radiolabeled factor XII in human plasma have been extended to include studies of radiolabeled bovine as well as human factor XII in both bovine and human plasmas. Such studies showed that the initial observations of Revak et al. [21] are applicable to both the human and bovine molecules in either human or bovine plasmas. Although such studies are consistent with an emphasis on the proteolytic activation of factor XII, they do not rule out the possibility that the surface-bound factor XII in its single-polypeptide-chain form functions as an active enzyme.

For many years it was assumed, but never proven, that factor XII is maximally activated by binding to negatively charged surfaces. Such a simple and attractive hypothesis is not consistent with the fact that surface-bound factor XII does not react with diisopropylfluorophosphate and does not exhibit enzymatic activity against small peptide or ester substrates [27,90,91]. These studies show that surface binding of factor XII, per se, does not result in the formation of a detectable number of active factor XII_a single-chain molecules. Nonetheless, this question remains controversial. It was suggested that single-chain factor XII is as potent as α-factor XII_a in the dextran sulfate-dependent activation of prekallikrein and factor XI [47,92]. Related but not identical studies in our laboratories provide no support for this hypothesis but rather support the suggestion that factor XII may exhibit much weaker (5% of maximum) enzymatic activity than α-factor XII_a [90]. Further kinetic studies will be necessary to determine how much enzymatic activity the single polypeptide chain of factor XII may exhibit in comparison to the activities of α-factor XII_a and β-factor XII_a.

(b) Reciprocal proteolytic activation of factor XII and prekallikrein

Cochrane et al. [24] first proposed that a reciprocal proteolytic activation may be important in the activation of factor XII and prekallikrein when they observed that kallikrein could activate factor XII by limited proteolysis in the fluid phase. Previously, it was understood that factor XII_a could activate prekallikrein in an enzymatic reaction [26,32]. Subsequently, the concept of reciprocal proteolytic activation was adapted to describe the surface-dependent reactions of the contact system [46,73,74]. Localizing reciprocal proteolytic activation on the surface followed from kinetic evidence that high MW kininogen accelerates the activation of prekallikrein by surface-bound α-factor XII_a as well as the proteolytic activation of surface-bound factor XII by kallikrein [73]. This led to the following hypothesis, factor XII binds to a negatively charged surface where it is highly susceptible to proteolytic activation by kallikrein. Prekallikrein is associated non-covalently

114

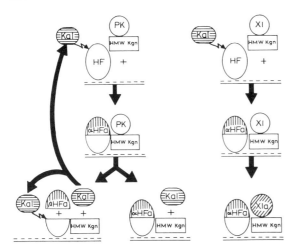

Fig. 7. Representation of surface-dependent assembly of molecules responsible for contact activation reactions. The following abbreviations were used: Kal, kallikrein; PK, prekallikrein; HMW Kgn, high MW kininogen; XI, factor XI; HF, Hageman factor (factor XII). Subscript 'a' designates active enzymes. The dashed lines represent a negatively charged surface.

with high MW kininogen in the fluid phase, but in the presence of a negatively charged surface, high MW kininogen links prekallikrein to this surface. Prekallikrein is then converted to kallikrein by limited proteolysis by surface-bound α-factor XII_a (Fig. 7). Studies of radiolabeled prekallikrein and kallikrein suggest that these molecules dissociate readily from their surface-binding sites [93]. Dissociation of kallikrein from surface-binding sites and subsequent action on surface-bound factor XII at distant sites to propagate this reciprocal proteolytic cycle have been experimentally demonstrated [94]. α-Factor XII_a is converted to β-factor XII_a by a secondary cleavage by kallikrein. β-Factor XII_a does not bind to negatively charged surfaces and can further propagate the reciprocal reactions in the fluid phase by activating prekallikrein.

Current data support the hypothesis that reciprocal proteolysis involving factor XII and prekallikrein is the major normal pathway for activation of factor XII. Nonetheless, the ability of prekallikrein-dependent plasma to undergo autocorrection upon prolonged incubation with kaolin shows that prekallikrein is not absolutely essential for surface-deficient activation of factor XII, factor XI, or plasminogen. This observation suggests that other much less potent mechanisms exist for the activation of surface-bound factor XII. Recent evidence has raised the possibility that either factor XII or prekallikrein zymogen molecules may possess low levels of inherent enzymatic activity [37,90]. Neurath and his colleagues [95] have shown that trypsinogen and chymotrypsinogen exhibit weak enzymatic activities and this challenges the idea that serine protease zymogens are totally inactive [95–97]. If either factor XII or prekallikrein might function as weakly 'active zymogens' in analogy to trypsinogen or chymotrypsinogen, then activation of either prekallikrein or of factor XII might take place when these molecules are brought into close proximity by binding to a negative surface. In this situation, the role of a negatively charged surface would be to assemble these molecules into productive enzyme–substrate complexes where a weak activity could be expressed. In this case surface binding essentially lowers K_m for the reaction. Dissociation of kallikrein or of β-factor XII_a from the surface could then propagate reciprocal proteolytic activation. The binding of factor XII and kallikrein to sulfatide surfaces has been shown to augment greatly the rate of factor XII activation by kallikrein (Rosing, Tans and Griffin, unpublished data). Another possible contribution for initiating reciprocal proteolysis might be the autoactivation of the zymogen factor XII by its own enzymatic form, α-factor XII_a (cf. [98–100] and Ch. 3). Although the occurrence of autoactivation of factor XII was confirmed, the catalytic efficiency of kallikrein-dependent factor XII activation is much greater than that of autoactivation indicating that factor XII activation by kallikrein is the more important process under physiologic conditions [101; Rosing, Tans and Griffin, unpublished data]. Another possible trigger for initiating reciprocal proteolysis might involve proteases such as plasmin. Proteases derived from damaged tissue or cells such as basophils [102] or endothelial cells [103] may function in this role. Another possibility involves the theory that surface binding alters factor XII such that it undergoes substrate-induced activation and then cleaves prekallikrein or factor XI [92]. Depending upon the nature of the initiating surface and the local fluid phase contents, any one or all of these possibilities may function as the trigger of reciprocal activation.

(c) Activation of factor XI

Factor XI is activated by limited proteolysis by factor XII_a. Factor XI circulates in plasma in a complex with high MW kininogen. This high MW kininogen links factor XI to a negatively charged surface. Factor XII which binds directly to the surface is converted to α-factor XII_a by proteolytic activation by kallikrein. α-Factor XII_a activates factor XI by limited proteolysis to generate surface-bound factor XI_a, which remains surface-bound. This hypothesis is derived from a variety of experiments. In kinetic studies of the activation of factor XI, high MW kininogen was shown to function as a non-enzymatic stoichiometric cofactor that increased the rate of activation by surface-bound α-factor XII_a[73,74,105,106]. Factor XI complexes with high MW kininogen in the fluid phase [61]. Wiggins et al. [93] studied the binding and cleavage of radiolabeled factor XI in normal and various deficient plasmas subjected to contact activation and obtained data showing that in normal plasma factor XI is bound to kaolin and cleaved to give polypeptide chains typical of factor XI_a. However, in high MW kininogen-deficient plasma containing kaolin, radiolabeled factor XI remains in the fluid phase and is not cleaved, thus demonstrating the necessity of high MW kininogen for the binding of factor XI to negative surfaces. Factor XII is required for the cleavage of factor XI but not for its binding to negative surfaces.

Sugo et al. [108] showed that when bovine high MW kininogen was activated by limited proteolysis by bovine plasma kallikrein, it became a much more efficient cofactor of factor XII activation than the intact form. This observation was further extended by Scott et al. [109] for human high MW kininogen. They demonstrated that cleavage of high MW kininogen by kallikrein enhances its association with a clot-promoting surface, which is necessary for expression of its cofactor activity. These studies suggest that high MW kininogen exists as a procofactor.

4. The role of the contact activation mechanism in the intrinsic fibrinolytic system

A role for the proteins of the contact activation system in fibrinolysis was proposed because euglobulin clot lysis activity is enhanced by the presence of negatively charged surface [110] and because plasmas deficient in factor XII [110,111], high MW kininogen [112] and prekallikrein [113–115], show defective generation of fibrinolytic activity after incubation with negatively charged surfaces (see Ch. 8 for general discussion of fibrinolysis). Early studies of factor XII-dependent fibrinolysis reported that activated factor XII did not activate plasminogen directly [116–118] but later reports have implicated factor XII$_a$ as a plasminogen activator with weak activity [119]. Kallikrein was also reported to have plasminogen activator activity [12,20], but on a molar basis its activity was 1650 times less than urokinase [37]. Mandle and Kaplan [120] reported that the γ-globulin fraction of a prekallikrein-deficient plasma contained one third of the plasminogen activator activity of the γ-globulin fraction of normal plasma. They suggested that this residual factor XII-dependent plasminogen proactivator activity was factor XI since the factor XI procoagulant activity and plasminogen proactivator activities co-eluted during sulfopropyl Sephadex chromatography. These investigators also reported that factor XI$_a$ has plasminogen activator activity when assayed on fibrin plates and that it has an activity 25 000-fold less than that of urokinase [122]. Saito [123] has suggested that the autocorrection of the defective fibrinolytic activity in prekallikrein-deficient plasma may be due to the activity of factor XI$_a$ as a plasminogen activator. However other investigators did not observe any plasminogen activator activity in γ-globulin fractions of prekallikrein-deficient plasma [124,125] and also other workers observed normal kaolin stimulated euglobulin lyses times in factor XI-deficient plasma [111,126,127]. In a direct study the relative potencies of plasma kallikrein, β-factor XII$_a$, factor XI$_a$ and urokinase were compared as plasminogen activators using a radiolabeled fibrin plate assay [128]. Urokinase was approximately 20 000 times more active than kallikrein or factor XI$_a$ and 300 000 times more active than β-factor XII$_a$. Kallikrein and factor XI$_a$ were approximately equal in plasminogen activator activity and were 20 times more potent than β-factor XII$_a$ [128].

The isolation of urokinase-related enzymes was recently reported by two different groups of investigators. Wun et al. [129] isolated an urokinase-like enzyme from human plasma and found this enzyme to be essentially identical to the 53 000 component of human urinary urokinase. Wijngaards et al. [130] found anti-urokinase antibodies capable of quenching a part of the plasma fibrinolytic activity. Dooijewaard et al. [131] described their plasma urokinase to be a two- or more-chain polypeptide with a molecular weight of 110 000, while subsequently the isolation of the fibrinolytically inactive single-chain pre-urokinase was also reported [132]. The identity of the enzyme which converts the zymogen form of urokinase into the active form has not yet been established. Wijngaards et al. [130] and later Kluft et al. [133] demonstrated that urokinase-related fibrinolytic activity is present in dextran sulfate euglobulin fractions of factor XII- or prekallikrein-deficient plasmas in a similar concentration to that present in normal plasma, and that this urokinase-related fibrinolytic activity can be quenched with anti-urokinase antibodies. They conclude that the quenching involved the factor XII-independent portion of activator activity [133].

Miles et al. [134] used dextran sulfate to stimulate fibrinolysis in whole plasma. After pretreating the plasma with N-flufenamyl β-alanine a component known to inactivate α_2-antiplasmin and C1-inhibitor defective dextran sulfate-dependent fibrinolysis was demonstrated in factor XII-deficient and prekallikrein-deficient plasma [135]. In addition, a requirement for plasma molecules immunologically related to urokinase was demonstrated. When plasma was preincubated with an immunopurified γ-globulin fraction of goat antiserum to urokinase, 80% of dextran sulfate-dependent fibrinolytic activity was inhibited. A component of the uro-

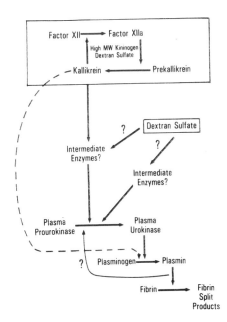

Fig. 8. Dextran sulfate-dependent fibrinolysis in whole human plasma (from ref. 134).

kinase-dependent fibrinolytic activity is independent of the contact activation system since the low fibrinolytic plasmas were inhibited by antibodies to urokinase. Fig. 8 shows a model for dextran sulfate-dependent fibrinolysis based on these observations. In the presence of dextran sulfate and high MW kininogen, kallikrein and factor XII_a are generated. Factor XII_a and kallikrein are weak plasminogen activators. Factor XII_a was also shown to increase the urokinase-like activities of urokinase-like material purified from normal plasma by antibody affinity chromatography [136]. Therefore activation of factor XII and prekallikrein also may lead to activation of plasma pro-urokinase which may then activate plasminogen. In addition the activation of plasma pro-urokinase can be stimulated independently of factor XII and prekallikrein. Part of the discrepancies described above may be explained by the fact that whole plasma or plasma fractions were used, and by the fact that the antibodies used to block the urokinase activity were added either before or after the activation of the contact system by dextran sulfate.

5. Regulation by inhibitors

Plasma contains several protease inhibitors that are able to inactivate proteolytic enzymes. These plasma proteins regulate and modulate the involvement of several interrelated enzyme systems in various hemostatic and inflammatory reactions. Table 2 gives a list of the major inhibitors and their effect on the components of the contact system.

(a) Inactivation of factor XII_a

The relative importance of plasma protease inhibitors in the inhibition of factor XII_a was established by studying the kinetics of inactivation of factor XII_a using purified inhibitors, normal plasma and plasmas deficient in inhibitors.

Using purified plasma protease inhibitors, the second-order rate constant for the reaction of β-factor XII_a with C1-inhibitor was 18.5×10^4/M/min, compared to 0.91 and 0.32×10^4/M/min for the reactions involving β-factor XII_a and α_2-antiplasmin

TABLE 2

Plasma inhibitors of activated components of the contact activation system

	Mol. wt.	Concentration (mg/ml)	Factor XII_a	Factor XI_a	Kallikrein
C$\bar{1}$-Inhibitor	110 000	0.2	+ +	+	+ +
α_2-Macroglobulin	720 000	2	−	−	+
α_1-Antitrypsin	55 000	3	−	+ +	±
Antithrombin III	65 000	0.2	+	+	+
α_2-Antiplasmin	70 000	0.07	±	±	−

The inactivation of the enzymes by the inhibitors is qualitatively indicated by + +, major inhibitor; +, inhibitor; ± minor inhibitor; − no inhibitory effect.

or antithrombin III [137]. No reaction was detected between the enzyme and plasma concentrations of α_1-antitrypsin or α_2-macroglobulin. Thus on a molar basis C1-inhibitor was the most efficient plasma inhibitor of β-factor XII_a. These results are in agreement with previous studies [138–142]. SDS analysis of the enzyme–inhibitor complexes resulting from the inactivation of [^{125}I]β-factor XII_a by purified C1-inhibitor, α_2-antiplasmin, and antithrombin III indicated that complexes are generated with a molecular weight in agreement with a 1:1 stoichiometry between β-factor XII_a and the 3 inhibitors [137,140,142]. In the plasma milieu the rate constant for β-factor XII_a inactivation was 14.4×10^{-2}/M/min [137], well in agreement with the results obtained with the purified proteins. The dominant role of C1-inhibitor in inactivating β-factor XII_a in the plasma milieu was further demonstrated by the observation that the rate constant for β-factor XII_a inactivation by plasma deficient in C1-inhibitor was reduced to 13%. Also, inactivation of [^{125}I]β-factor XII_a in various plasmas and analysis of the reaction mixtures by SDS–polyacrylamide gel electrophoresis followed by autoradiography indicated that 74% of [^{125}I]β-factor XII_a was complexed to C1-inhibitor, whereas the 26% was complexed to α_2-antiplasmin and antithrombin III [137]. In agreement with the results obtained with purified proteins, no other complexes were detected.

The inactivation of α-factor XII_a (80 000 MW) was studied by plasma protease inhibitors in purified systems and in plasma. C1-Inhibitor, α_2-antiplasmin, α_2-macroglobulin and antithrombin III inhibited factor XII_a with second-order rate constants of 2.2×10^5, 1.1×10^4, 5.0×10^3 and 1.3×10^3/M/min [143]. The relative effectiveness of each inhibitor at plasma concentration in percent is 91, 3, 4.3 and 1.5 for C1-inhibitor, α_2-antiplasmin, α_2-macroglobulin and antithrombin III respectively. This confirms the predominant role of C1-inhibitor in the inactivation of α-factor XII_a as was also observed for β-factor XII_a (factor XII_f). α-Factor XII_a and β-factor XII_a have virtually identical light chains, indicating that the heavy chain does not play an important role in inhibiting α-factor XII_a in plasma. α-Factor XII_a formed 1:1 stoichiometric complexes with C1-inhibitor, antithrombin III and α_2-antiplasmin. No conclusive data are available for α_2-macroglobulin but the results suggest that α_2-macroglobulin can inhibit more than one α-factor XII_a molecule [143].

(b) Inactivation of kallikrein

The relative importance of plasma protease inhibitors in the inhibition of kallikrein in plasma was established by studying the kinetics of inactivation of kallikrein in normal plasma and plasmas deficient in inhibitors [144]. In normal plasma a pseudo-first-order rate constant of 0.68/min was obtained. The absence of C1-inhibitor resulted in a markedly decreased rate of kallikrein inactivation and a 90% reduction in the pseudo-first-order rate constant whereas the rate constant was reduced to 63% in the absence of α_2-macroglobulin. The absence of antithrombin III appeared to have a minor influence on the rate of kallikrein inactivation. Thus C1-inhibitor and α_2-macroglobulin are the major inhibitors of kallikrein. Lewin et

120

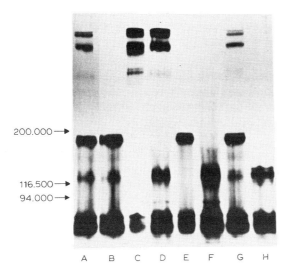

$200.000 \rightarrow$

$116.500 \rightarrow$
$94.000 \rightarrow$

A B C D E F G H

Fig. 9. Autoradiogram of a SDS 3–25% gradient polyacrylamide slab gel containing mixtures of [^{125}I]kallikrein incubated for different times at 37°C with A, normal human plasma; B, α_2-macroglob-ulin-deficient plasma (20 min); C, purified α_2-macroglobulin; D $\overline{\text{C1}}$, inhibitor-deficient plasma; E, pur-ified $\overline{\text{C1}}$-inhibitor; F, plasma deficient in both α_2-macroglobulin and $\overline{\text{C1}}$-inhibitor; G, antithrombin III-deficient plasma; H, purified antithrombin III (from ref. 144).

al. [145] developed an enzyme-linked immunosorbent assay for the quantification of C1-inhibitor–kallikrein complexes. This assay provided insight in the regulation of kallikrein formation and inactivation in plasma at 37°C. Addition of kaolin to plasma induced the formation of C1-inhibitor–kallikrein complexes, after an ap-preciable delay, whereas addition of factor XII$_a$ fragments directly induced the formation of these complexes.

In plasma, kallikrein forms a number of complexes with apparent molecular weights in the range of 400 000–1 000 000, 185 000 and 125 000–135 000 [144]. By using purified proteins and plasmas deficient in inhibitors, the complexes were identified (Fig. 9). The complexes with molecular weights in the range of 400 000–1 000 000 were due to the formation of complexes between α_2-macroglob-ulin and kallikrein, the complex at $M_r = 185 000$ was the C1-inhibitor–kallikrein complex, the complexes at $M_r = 125 000$–135 000 were shown to be due to com-plex formation with antithrombin III and another inhibitor. Calculation of the in-corporation of radiolabeled kallikrein in the different complexes indicated that 35% of kallikrein formed a complex with α_2-macroglobulin, 52% with C1-inhibitor and 13% with antithrombin III and another inhibitor [144]. Similar data based on ki-netic studies were reported by Schapira et al. [146]. These quantitative data con-firm previous reports that suggested that C1-inhibitor and α_2-macroglobulin are the major inhibitors of kallikrein in plasma [138,146–154].

Inactivation of kallikrein or its light chain by C1-inhibitor occurs with a second-order rate constant of 2.7×10^6/M/min or 4.0×10^6/M/min, respectively [155].

Similar values were reported by Schapira et al. [153]. High MW kininogen was reported to protect kallikrein from inactivation by C1-inhibitor [152]. However, in contrast to this, no detectable effect of high MW kininogen on the rate of inactivation of kallikrein by C1-inhibitor was reported in another study [155] (Fig. 10). This latter observation complements the observation that the heavy chain of kallikrein, which provides the high-affinity binding site for high M_r kininogen [41], does not significantly affect the rate of kallikrein inactivation by C1-inhibitor. Kallikrein [148,153,155,156] or its light chain [155] forms a 1:1 stoichiometric complex with C1-inhibitor that is stable in SDS [148,153,155,156] indicating that the functional binding site for C1-inhibitor is localized in the light chain of kallikrein. During the inactivation of kallikrein or its light chain, a 94000 MW fragment of C1-inhibitor is formed which is unable to inactivate or bind kallikrein or its light chain [155]. Plasmin also generated a 96000 MW fragment from C1-inhibitor which was inactive with regard to CĪS binding [156]. Recently CĪS was shown to release a fragment from C1-inhibitor during the inactivation of CĪS [157]. This fragment was demonstrated on SDS gels.

Human α_2-macroglobulin (MW 726000) is a tetramer of 4 identical subunits (MW 185000) formed by the non-covalent association of 2 disulfide-linked pairs of subunits [158]. α_2-Macroglobulin is capable of forming complexes with endopeptidases from all known classes of proteases [159]. Only active proteases appear to be bound by α_2-macroglobulin. It was argued that the process was initiated by the

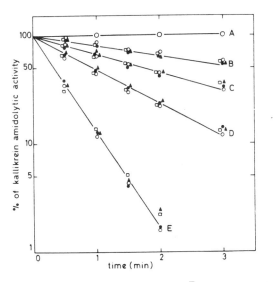

Fig. 10. Inactivation of kallikrein by CĪ-inhibitor. Kallikrein at 85 nM was preincubated with different concentrations of high MW kininogen for 5 min in 0.05 M Tris at pH 7.4, 1 mg/ml BSA. CĪ-inhibitor was then added at a final concentration of 0 μM (A), 0.11 μM (B), 0.21 μM (C), 0.42 μM (D) and 1.0 μM (E) and kallikrein amidolytic activity was determined at various times. High MW kininogen was present at 0 μM (○), 0.42 μM (●), 1.05 μM (□) and 2.10 μM (△) (from ref. 155).

cleavage of a vulnerable region near the middle of the α_2-macroglobulin subunit chain, followed by a conformational change resulting in steric entrapment of the enzyme [159]. The active site of the bound protease is not involved in maintaining the complex, since activity toward small substrates is usually partly impaired or not impaired at all. The demonstration of Harpel [160] that the residual kallikrein esterolytic activity, present in normal plasma after activation with kaolin, was resistant to inhibition by soybean trypsin inhibitor was the first indication of kallikrein inactivation by α_2-macroglolublin.

Inactivation of kallikrein or its light chain by α_2-macroglobulin occurs with a second-order rate constant of 3.5×10^5/M/min or 4.8×10^5/M/min, respectively [160]. This suggests that the heavy-chain region of kallikrein does not affect the rate of kallikrein inactivation by α_2-macroglobulin. The presence of high MW kininogen decreases the inactivation rate of kallikrein by α_2-macroglobulin [154,161], due to its high affinity binding to the heavy chain of kallikrein [161]. This is in agreement with the observation that the rate of inactivation of the light chain is unaffected by high MW kininogen [161]. α_2-Macroglobulin-bound kallikrein or α_2-macroglobulin-bound kallikrein light chain retain considerable activity on low MW substrates [144, 154], but very low reactivity towards high MW substrates [161–163]. The binding of kallikrein and its light chain to α_2-macroglobulin is associated with a decrease in the apparent K_m and k_{cat} for the hydrolysis of the low M_r substrate, H-D-Pro-Phe-Arg-p-nitroanilide [161]. In analogy Rinderknecht et al. [164] found a lower apparent K_m for the hydrolysis of 2-Gly-Gly-Arg-NNAP by α_2-macroglobulin-bound trypsin as compared to the free enzyme. The kinetic effects of entrapment of an enzyme within α_2-macroglobulin are likely to be complex and probably depend to a large degree on the altered microenvironment created by the 'trap'. SDS gradient polyacrylamide gel electrophoresis indicated that the interaction between kallikrein and α_2-macroglobulin results in the formation of a number of complexes with approximate molecular weight of 400 000–1 000 000. Although the nature of these complexes seems rather complicated and at present unclear, the M_r of the complexes suggest that one or more kallikrein molecules are linked to one or more α_2-macroglobulin dimers. The fact that the interactions are stable in SDS implies that the formed bonds possess a stability normally characteristic of covalent bonds. The reaction of kallikrein with α_2-macroglobulin leads to a cleavage of some of the α_2-macroglobulin subunits, producing a 85 000 M_r fragment which is only detected after reduction [158]. Under reducing conditions 4 kallikrein–α_2-macroglobulin complexes were observed. Three of these complexes consisted of α_2-macroglobulin and the light chain of kallikrein and one complex contained α_2-macroglobulin and the heavy chain of kallikrein.

High MW kininogen decreases the inactivation rate of kallikrein by α_2-macroglobulin. In contrast high MW kininogen fails to protect kallikrein from inactivation by C1-inhibitor in one study, whereas others did find a protective effect of high MW kininogen on the inactivation of kallikrein by C1-inhibitor. Recent studies, however, demonstrated that high MW kininogen, present at normal plasma concentrations, had no effect on the rate of kallikrein inactivation in plasma. This can be explained by the observation that high MW kininogen does not affect the rate of kallikrein inactivation by C1-inhibitor which is the major inhibitor of kallikrein in plasma, and also relatively high concentrations of high MW kininogen to kallikrein were necessary to demonstrate the protective effect of high MW kininogen.

(c) Inactivation of factor XI_a

Four different plasma proteins have been found to have inhibitory activity for factor XI_a; C1-inhibitor [165], α_1-protease inhibitor (α_1-antitrypsin) [166], antithrombin III [167] and α_2-antiplasmin [141], whereas α_2-macroglobulin did not inactivate factor XI_a [168]. The relative importance of plasma protease inhibitors in the inhibition of factor XI_a in plasma was established by studying the kinetics of inactivation of factor XI_a in normal plasma, and plasma deficient in inhibitors. In normal plasma a pseudo-first-order rate constant of 0.034/min was obtained [169]. The absence of C1-inhibitor or α_1-antitrypsin reduced the rate constant to respectively 0.026 and 0.022/min. The absence of antithrombin III had only a minor effect on the pseudo-first-order reaction rate constant. Thus, α_1-antitrypsin appears to be the major inhibitor of factor XI_a in normal plasma.

Using purified plasma protease inhibitors the second-order rate constants for the reaction of factor XI_a and α_1-antitrypsin, C1-inhibitor and antithrombin III were reported to be 4, 10, and 14.6/M/min $\times 10^3$ respectively [170]. These kinetic data predict that α_1-antitrypsin accounts for 68%, antithrombin III for 16% and C1-inhibitor for 8% of the total inhibitory activity of plasma against factor XI_a. The α_2-antiplasmin inhibitor accounts for the remaining 8% of inhibitory activity.

High MW kininogen was reported to protect factor XI_a for inactivation by C1-inhibitor and α_1-antitrypsin [170]. In another study no effect of high MW kininogen on the rate of inactivation of factor XI_a by α_1-antitrypsin and C1-inhibitor was detected [169]. The inactivation rates of factor XI_a and its isolated light chain by C1-inhibitor, α_1-antitrypsin and antithrombin III were very similar, indicating that the heavy-chain region of factor XI_a is not significantly involved in the inactivation of factor XI_a by these inhibitors. The heavy-chain region provides the high-affinity binding for high MW kininogen, whereas the light chain of factor XI_a contains the enzymatically active site. Complex formation of factor XI_a with C1-inhibitor and α_1-antitrypsin was shown to occur with the light chain. This indicates that the light-chain region contains the binding site for C1-inhibitor and α_1-antitrypsin.

Acknowledgements

The excellent secretarial assistance of Annemiek Beyer and Maeyken Hoeneveld is gratefully acknowledged.

124

References

1 Kaplan, A.P. (1978) Progr. Haemostas. Thromb. 4, 127–175.
2 Movat, H. (1979) in: Bradykinin, Kallidin and Kallikrein (Erdos, E.G., Eds.) pp. 1–9, Springer, Berlin.
3 Ratnoff, O.D. and Saito, H. (1979) in: Current Topics in Haematology, Vol. 2, pp. 1–57, Liss, New York.
4 Cochrane, C.G. and Griffin, J.H. (1982) Adv. Immunol. 33, 241–306.
5 Fritz, H., Back, N., Dietze, G. and Haberland, G.L., Eds. (1983) Kinins III, Advances in Experimental Medicine and Biology.
6 Margolis, J. (1963) Ann. N.Y. Acad. Sci. 104, 133–145.
7 Niewiarowski, S. and Prou-Wartelle, P. (1959) Thromb. Diath. Haemorrh. 3, 593–603.
8 Ratnoff O.D. (1969) Adv. Immunol. 10, 146–228.
9 Derkx, F.H.M., Bouma, B.N., Schalekamp, M.P.A. and Schalekamp, M.A.D.H. (1979) Nature (London) 280, 315–316.
10 Sealey, J.E., Atlas, S.A., Laragh, J.H., Silverberg, M. and Kaplan, A.P. (1979) Proc. Natl. Acad. Sci. (U.S.A.) 76, 5914–5918.
11 Yokosawa, N., Takahashi, Inagami, T. and Page, D.L. (1979) Biochim. Biophys. Acta 569, 211–219.
12 Seligsohn, U., Østerud, B., Griffin, J.H. and Rapaport, S.I. (1978) Thromb. Res. 13, 1049–1056.
13 Seligsohn, U., Østerud, B., Brown, S.F., Griffin, J.H. and Rapaport, S.I. (1979) J. Clin. Invest. 64, 1056–1065.
14 Hedner, U. and Martinsson, G. (1978) Thromb. Res. 12, 1015–1023.
15 Bouma, B.N. and Griffin, J.H. (1980) in: Immunoassays: Clinical Laboratory Techniques for the 1980's: Laboratory and Research Methods in Biology and Medicine (Nakamura, R., Dito, W.R. and Tucker III, E.S., Eds.) Vol. 4, pp. 325–337, Liss, New York.
16 Griffin, J.H. and Cochrane, C.G. (1976) Meth. Enzymol. 45, 56–65.
17 Fujikawa, K., Walsh, K.A. and Davie, E.W. (1977) Biochemistry 16, 2270–2278.
18 Claeys, H. and Collen, D. (1978) Eur. J. Biochem. 87, 69–74.
19 Movat, H.A. and Ozge-Anwar, A.H. (1974) J. Lab. Clin. Med. 84, 861–877.
20 Revak, S.D., Cochrane, C.G., Johnson, A.R. and Hugli, T.H. (1974) J. Clin. Invest. 54, 619–627.
21 Revak, S.D., Cochrane, C.G. and Griffin, J.H. (1977) J. Clin. Invest. 59, 1167–1175.
22 Revak, S.D., Cochrane, C.G. Bouma, B.N. and Griffin, J.H. (1978) J. Exp. Med. 147, 719–729.
23 Revak, S.D. and Cochrane, S.G. (1976) J. Clin. Invest. 57, 852–860.
24 Cochrane, C.G., Revak, S.D., Aikin, B.S. and Wuepper, K.D. (1972) in: Inflammation: Mechanisms and Control (Lepow, I.H. and Ward, P.A., Eds.) pp. 119–138, Academic Press, New York.
25 Cochrane, C.G., Revak, S.D. and Wuepper, K.D. (1973) J. Exp. Med. 138, 1564–1583.
26 Kaplan, A.P. and Austen, K.F. (1971) J. Exp. Med. 133, 696–712.
27 Fujikawa, K., Kurachi, K. and Davie, E.W. (1977) Biochemistry 16, 4182–4188.
28 Dunn, J.T. and Kaplan, A.P. (1982) J. Clin. Invest. 70, 627–631.
29 Fujikawa, K. and McMullen, B.A. (1983) J. Biol. Chem. 258, 10924–10933.
30 Saito, H., Ratnoff, O.D. and Pensky, J. (1976) J. Lab. Clin. Med. 88, 506–514.
31 Saito, H., Scott, J.G., Movat, H.Z. and Scialla, S.J. (1979) J. Lab. Clin. Med. 94, 256–265.
32 Wuepper, K.D. and Cochrane, C.G. (1972) J. Exp. Med. 35, 1–20.
33 Kaplan, A.P. and Austen, K.F. (1972) J. Exp. Med. 136, 1378–1393.
34 Mandle, R. and Kaplan, A.P. (1977) J. Biol. Chem. 252, 6097–6104.
35 Takahashi, H., Nagasawa, S. and Suzuki, T. (1972) J. Biochem. 71, 471–483.
36 Heimark, R.L. and Davie, E.W. (1979) Biochemistry 18, 5743–5750.
37 Bouma, B.N., Miles, L.A., Beretta, G. and Griffin, J.H. (1980) Biochemistry 19, 1151–1160.
38 Mandle, R.J., Colman, R.W. and Kaplan, A.P. (1976) Proc. Natl. Acad. Sci. (U.S.A.) 11, 4179–4183.
39 Bouma, B.N., Kerbiriou, D.M., Vlooswijk, R.A.A. and Griffin, J.H. (1980) J. Lab. Clin. Med. 96, 693–709.
40 Kerbiriou, D.M., Bouma, B.N. and Griffin, J.H. (1980) J. Biol. Chem. 255, 3952–3958.

41 Van der Graaf, F., Tans, G., Bouma, B.N. and Griffin, J.H. (1982) J. Biol. Chem. 23, 14300–14305.

42 Thompson, R.E., Mandle, Jr., R. and Kaplan, A.P. (1978) J. Exp. Med. 147, 488–499.

43 Colman, R.W., Wachtfogel, Y.T., Kucich, U., Weinbaum, G., Hahn, S., Pixley, R.A., Scott, C.F., de Agostini, A., Burger, D. and Schapira, M. (1985) Blood 65, 311–318.

44 Bouma et al. Unpublished results.

45 Fujii, S., Moriya, H. and Suzuki, T. (1979) Adv. Exp. Med. Biol. 120AB.

46 Griffin, J.H. (1978) Proc. Natl. Acad. Sci. (U.S.A.) 75, 1998–2002.

47 Fujikawa, K., Heimark, R.L., Kurachi, K. and Davie, E.W. (1980) Biochemistry 19, 1322–1330.

48 Østerud, B., Bouma, B.N. and Griffin, J.H. (1978) J. Biol. Chem. 253, 5946–5951.

49 Seligsohn, U., Østerud, B., Brown, S.F., Griffin, J.H. and Rapaport, S.I. (1979) J. Clin. Invest. 64, 1056–1065.

50 Saito, H., Poon, M.C., Vicic, W., Goldsmith, G.H. and Menitove, J.E. (1978) J. Lab. Clin. Med. 92, 84–95.

51 Wuepper, K.D. (1973) J. Exp. Med. 138, 1345–1355.

52 Saito, H., Goodnough, L.T., Soria, J., Soria, C., Aznar, J. and Espana, F. (1981) New Engl. J. Med. 305, 910–914.

53 Bouma, B.N., Kerbiriou, D.M., Baker, J. and Griffin, J.H. (1986) J. Clin. Invest. 78, 170–176.

54 Colman, R.W., Bagdasarian, A., Talamo, R.C., Scott, C.F., Seavey, M., Guimaraes, J.A., Pierce, J.V. and Kaplan, A.P. (1975) J. Clin. Invest. 56, 1650–1662.

55 Donaldson, V.H., Kleniewski, J., Saito, H. and Sayed, J.U. (1979) J. Clin. Invest. 60, 571–583.

56 Colman, R.W., Edelman, R., Scott, C.F. and Gilman, R.M. (1978) J. Clin. Invest. 61, 287–296.

57 Bouma, B.N. and Griffin, J.H. (1977) J. Biol. Chem. 252, 6432–6437.

58 Kurachi, K. and Davie, E.W. (1977) Biochemistry 16, 5831–5839.

59 Wuepper, K.D. (1972) in: Inflammation: Mechanism and Control (Lepow, J. and Ward, P.A., Eds.) pp. 83–117, Academic Press, New York.

60 Heck, L.W. and Kaplan, A.P. (1974) J. Exp. Med. 140, 1615–1630.

61 Thompson, R.E., Mandle Jr., R. and Kaplan, A.P. (1977) J. Clin. Invest. 60, 1376–1380.

62 Thompson, R.E., Mandle Jr., R. and Kaplan, A.P. (1979) Proc. Natl. Acad. Sci. (U.S.A.) 76, 4862–4866.

63 Bouma, B.N., Vlooswijk, R.A.A. and Griffin, J.H. (1983) Blood 62, 1123–1131.

64 Van der Graaf, F., Greengard, J.S., Bouma, B.N., Kerbiriou, D.M. and Griffin, J.H. (1983) J. Biol. Chem. 258, 9669–9675.

65 Fujikawa, K., Legaz, M.E., Kato, H. and Davie, E.W. (1974) Biochemistry 13, 4500–4516.

66 Østerud, B., Bouma, B.N. and Griffin, J.H. (1978) J. Biol. Chem. 253, 5946–5941.

67 Forbes, C.D. and Ratnoff, O.D. (1972) J. Lab. Clin. Med. 79, 113–127.

68 Rimon, A., Schiffman, S., Feinstein, D.I. and Rapaport, S. (1976) Blood 48, 165–174.

69 Saito, H. and Goldsmith, G. (1977) Blood 50, 377–385.

70 Saito, H., Ratnoff, O.D., Bouma, B.N. and Seligsohn, U. (1985) J. Lab. Clin. Med. 106, 718–722.

71 Colman, R.W., Bagdasarian, A., Talamo, R.C., Scott, C.F., Seavey, M., Guimaraes, J.A., Pierce, J.V. and Kaplan, A.P. (1975) J. Clin. Invest. 56, 1650–1662.

72 Wuepper, K.D., Miller, D.R. and Lacombe, M.J. (1975) J. Clin. Invest. 56, 1663–1672.

73 Griffin, J.H. and Cochrane, C.G. (1976) Proc. Natl. Acad. Sci. (U.S.A.) 73, 2554–2558.

74 Meier, H.K., Webster, M.E., Mandle, R., Colman, R.W. and Kaplan, A.P. (1977) J. Clin. Invest. 60, 18–31.

75 Han, Y.N., Kato, H., Iwanaga, S. and Komiya, M.J. (1978) Biochemistry 83, 223–235.

76 Han, Y.J., Komiyo, M., Iwanaga, S. and Suzuki, T. (1975) J. Biochem. 77, 55–68.

77 Kato, H., Han, Y.N., Iwanaga, S., Hashimoto, N., Sugo, T., Fujii, S. and Suzuki, R. (1977) in: Kininogenases (Haberland, G., Rohen, J.W. and Suzuki, T., Eds.) Vol. 4, Schattauer, Stuttgart.

78 Kerbiriou, D.M. and Griffin, J.H. (1979) J. Biol. Chem. 254, 12020–12027.

79 Ohkubo, J., Kurachi, K., Takasawa, T., Shiokawa, H. and Sasak, M. (1984) Biochemistry 23, 5691–5697.

80 Thompson, R.E., Mandle, R. and Kaplan, A.P. (1978) J. Exp. Med. 147, 488–499.

81 Sugo, R., Ikari, N., Kato, H., Iwanaga, S. and Fujii, S. (1980) Biochemistry 19, 3215–3220.

126

82 Kato, H., Sugo, T., Ikari, N., Hashimoto, I.S. and Fujii, S. (1979) Thromb. Haemostas. 42, 262.
83 Lottspeich, F., Kellermann, J. and Müller-Esterl, W. (1985) submitted for publication.
84 Lottspeich, F., Kellermann, J., Henschen, A., Rauth, G. and Müller-Esterl, W. (1984) Eur. J. Biochem. 142, 227–232.
85 Kitamura, N., Takagaki, Y., Furuto, S., Tanaka, T., Nawa, H. and Nakanishi, S. (1983) Nature (London) 545–549.
86 Kleniewski, J. and Donaldson, V.H. (1977) Proc. Soc. Exp. Biol. Med. 156, 113–116.
87 Proud, D., Pierce, J.V., Peyton, M.P. and Pisano, J.J. (1979) Fed. Proc. 38, 686.
88 Oh-Ishi, S., Keno, A., Uchida, Y., Katori, M., Hayishi, H., Koya, H., Kitajima, K. and Kimura, I. (1979) in: Kinins II (Fujji, S., Moriya, H. and Susuki, T. Eds.) pp. 93–99, Plenum, New York.
89 Griffin, J.H. and Cochrane, C.G. (1979) Thromb. Haemostas. 5, 254–273.
90 Griffin, J.H. and Beretta, G. (1979) in: Kinins II (Fujji, S., Moriya, H. and Suzuki, T., Eds.) pp. 39–51, Plenum, New York.
91 Claeys, H. and Collen, D. (1978) Eur. J. Biochem. 87, 69–74.
92 Heimark, R.L., Kurachi, K., Fujikawa, K. and Davie, E.W. (1980) Nature (London) 286, 456–460.
93 Wiggins, R.C., Bouma, B.N., Cochrane, C.G. and Griffin, J.H. (1977) Proc. Natl. Acad. Sci. (U.S.A.) 74, 4636–4640.
94 Cochrane, C.G. and Revak, S.D. (1980) J. Exp. Med. 152, 608–619.
95 Neurath, H. and Walsh, K.A. (1976) in: Proteolysis and Physiological Regulation (Ribbons, D.W. and Brew, K., Eds.) Academic Press, New York.
96 Morgan, P.H., Robinson, N.C., Walsh, K.A. and Neurath, H. (1972) Proc. Natl. Acad. Sci. (U.S.A.) 69, 3312–3316.
97 Lonsdale-Eccles, J.D.L., Neurath, H. and Walsh, K.A. (1978) Biochemistry 17, 2803–2805.
98 Wiggins, R.C. and Cochrane, C.G. (1979) J. Exp. Med. 150, 1122–1133.
99 Silverberg, M., Dunn, J.T., Garen, L. and Kaplan, A.P. (1980) J. Biol. Chem. 255, 7281–7286.
100 Tans, G., Rosing, J. and Griffin, J.H. (1983) J. Biol. Chem. 258, 8215–8222.
101 Tankersley, D.L. and Finlayson, J.S. (1984) Biochemistry 23, 273–279.
102 Newball, H., Revak, S., Cochrane, C.G., Griffin, J.H. and Lichtenstein, J. (1979) in: Kinins II (Suzuki, T. and Moriya, H., Eds.) pp. 139–153, Plenum, New York.
103 Wiggins, R.C., Loskutoff, D.F., Cochrane, C.G., Griffin, J.H. and Edgington, T.S. (1980) J. Clin. Invest. 65, 197–206.
104 Kurachi, K.,Fujikawa, K. and Davie, E.W. (1980) Biochemistry 19, 1330–1338.
105 Schiffman, S. and Lee, P. (1973) J. Clin. Invest. 56, 1082–1092.
106 Saito, H. (1977) J. Clin. Invest. 60, 584–593.
107 Sugo, T., Kato, H., Iwanaga, S. and Fujii, S. (1981) Thromb. Res. 24, 329–337.
108 Kato, H.J., Sugo, T., Ikari, N., Hashimoto, N., Maruyama, I., Han, Y.N., Iwanaga,S. and Fujii, S. (1979) in: Kinins II, Adv. in Exp. Med. Biol. (Fujii, S., Moriya, H. and Susuki, T., Eds.) Vol. 120B, pp. 19–37, Plenum, New York.
109 Scott, C.F., Silver, L.D., Schapiro, M. and Colman, R.W. (1984) J. Clin. Invest. 73, 954–962.
110 Niewiarowski, S. and Prou-Wartelle, O. (1959) Thromb. Diath. Haemorrh. 3, 593–603.
111 Iatridis, S.G. and Ferguson, J.H. (1961) Thromb. Diath. Haemorrh. 6, 411–423.
112 Saito, H., Ratnoff, O.D., Waldmann, R. and Abraham, J.P. (1975) J. Clin. Invest. 55, 1082–1089.
113 Saito, H., Ratnoff, O.D. and Donaldson, V.H. (1974) Circ. Res. 34, 641–651.
114 Weiss, A.S., Gallin, J.I. and Kaplan, A.P. (1974) J. Clin. Invest. 53, 622–633.
115 Wuepper, K.D. (1973) Clin. Res. 21, 484.
116 Ratnoff, O.D. and Davie, E.W. (1962) Biochemistry 1, 967–974.
117 Iatridis, S.G. and Ferguson, J.H. (1962) J. Clin. Invest. 41, 1277–1287.
118 Schoenmakers, J.G.G., Kurstjens, R.M., Haanen, C. and Zilliken, F. (1963) Thromb. Diath. Haemorrh. 9, 546–569.
119 Goldsmith, G., Saito, H. and Ratnoff, O.D. (1978) J. Clin. Invest. 62, 54–60.
120 Mandle, R. and Kaplan, A.P. (1972) J. Biol. Chem. 252, 6097–6104.
121 Colman, R.W. (1969) Biochem. Biophys. Res. Commun. 35, 273–279.
122 Mandle, R.J. and Kaplan, A.P. (1979) Blood 54, 850–862.

123 Saito, H. (1980) in: The Regulation of Coagulation (Mann, K.G. and Taylor, F.B., Eds.) pp. 555–562, Elsevier/North Holland, Amsterdam.

124 Bouma, B.N. and Griffin, J.H. (1978) J. Lab. Clin. Med. 91, 148–155.

125 Vennerod, A.M. and Laake, K. (1976) Thromb. Res. 8, 519–522.

126 Ogston, D., Ogston, C.M., Ratnoff, O.D. and Forbes, C.D. (1969) J. Clin. Invest. 48, 1786–1801.

127 Kluft, C., Trumpi-Kalshoven, M.M., Jie, A.F.N. and Veldhuyzen-Stolk, E.C. (1979) Thromb. Haemostas. 41, 756–773.

128 Miles, L.A., Greengard, J.S. and Griffin, J.H. (1983) Thromb. Res. 9, 407–417.

129 Wun, T.C., Schleuning, W.D. and Reich, E. (1982) J. Biol. Chem. 257, 3276–3283.

130 Wijngaards, C., Kluft, C. and Groeneveld, E. (1982) Br. J. Haematol. 51, 165–169.

131 Dooijewaard, G., van Iersel, J.J.L., Wijngaards, G. and Kluft, C. (1983) Thromb. Haemostas. 50, 82.

132 Wun, T.E., Ossowski, L. and Reich, E. (1982) J. Biol. Chem. 257, 7262–7268.

133 Kluft, C., Wijngaards, C. and Jie, A.F.H. (1984) J. Lab. Clin. Med. 103, 408–419.

134 Miles, L.A., Rothschild, Z. and Griffin, J.H. (1983) in: Progress in Fibrinolysis (Davidson, J.F., Bachmann, F., Bouvier, C.A. and Kruithof, E.K.O., Eds.) pp. 58–61, Churchill Livingstone, Edinburgh.

135 Miles, L.A., Rothschild, Z. and Griffin, J.H. (1983) J. Lab. Clin. Med. 101, 214–225.

136 Grasl, B., Jörg, M. and Binder, B.R. (1983) in: Progress in Fibrinolysis VI (Davidson, J.F., Bachmann, F., Bouvier, C.A., Kruithof, E.K.O., Eds.) Vol. VI, pp. 50–53, Churchill Livingstone, Edinburgh.

137 De Agostini, A., Lijnen, H.R., Pixley, R.A., Colman, R.W. and Schapira, S. (1984) J. Clin. Invest. 73, 1542–1549.

138 Ratnoff, O.D., Pensky, J., Ogston, D. and Naff, G.B. (1969) J. Exp. Med. 129, 315–331.

139 Schreiber, A.D., Kaplan, A.P. and Austen, K.F. (1973) J. Clin. Invest. 52, 1402–1409.

140 Stead, N., Kaplan, A.P. and Rosenberg, R.D. (1976) J. Biol. Chem. 251, 6481–6488.

141 Saito, H., Goldsmith, G.H., Moroi, M. and Aoki, N. (1979) Proc. Natl. Acad. Sci. (U.S.A.) 76, 2013–2017.

142 Ratnoff, O.D. (1981) Blood 57, 55–58.

143 Pixley, R.A., Schapira, M. and Colman, R.W. (1985) J. Biol. Chem. 260, 1723–1729.

144 Van der Graaf, F., Koedam, J.A. and Bouma, B.N. (1983) J. Clin. Invest. 71, 149–158.

145 Lewin, M.F., Kaplan, A.P. and Harpel, P.C. (1983) J. Biol. Chem. 258, 6415–6421.

146 Schapira, M., Scott, C.F. and Colman, R.W. (1982) J. Clin. Invest. 69, 462–468.

147 Harpel, P.C. (1970) J. Exp. Med. 132, 329–352.

148 Gigli, J., Mason, J.W., Colman, R.W. and Austen, K.F. (1970) J. Immunol. 104, 574–581.

149 McConnell, D. (1972) J. Clin. Invest. 51, 1611–1623.

150 Fritz, H.G., Wunderer, K.K., Heimburger, N. and Werle, E. (1972) Hoppe-Seyler's Z. Physiol. Chem. 353, 906–910.

151 Trumpi-Kalshoven, M.M. and Kluft, C. (1978) in: Current Concepts in Kinin Research (Haberland, G.L. and Hamberg, U., Eds.) pp. 93–101, Pergamon, New York.

152 Gallimore, M.J., Amundsen, E., Larsbraaten, M., Lyngaas, K. and Fareid, E. (1979) Thromb. Res. 16, 695–703.

153 Schapira, M., Scott, C.F. and Colman, R.W. (1981) Biochemistry 20, 2738–2743.

154 Schapira, M., Scott, C.F., James, A., Silver, L.D., Kuepper, S.F., James, H.L. and Colman, R.W. (1982) Biochemistry 21, 567–572.

155 Van der Graaf, F., Koedam, J.A., Griffin, J.H. and Bouma, B.N. (1983) Biochemistry 22, 4860–4866.

156 Harpel, P.C. and Cooper, N.R. (1975) J. Clin. Invest. 55, 593–604.

157 Weiss, V. and Engel, J. (1983) Hoppe-Seyler's Z. Physiol. Chem. 364, 295–301.

158 Harpel, P.C. (1973) J. Exp. Med. 138, 508–521.

159 Barrett, A.J. and Starkey (1973) Biochem. J. 133, 709–724.

160 Harpel, P.C. (1970) J. Exp. Med. 132, 329–352.

161 Van der Graaf, F., Rietveld, A., Keus, F.J.A. and Bouma, B.N. (1984) Biochemistry 23, 1760–1766.

162 Harpel, P.C. and Mosesson, M.W. (1973) J. Clin. Invest. 52, 2175–2184.

163 Harpel, P.C. and Rosenberg, R.D. (1976) in: Progress in Hemostasis and Thrombosis (Spaet, T.H., Ed.) Vol. 3, pp. 145–189, Grune and Stratton, New York.

164 Rinderknecht, H., Fleming, R.M. and Geokas, M.C. (1975) Biochim. Biophys. Acta 377, 158–165.

165 Forbes, C.D., Pensky, J. and Ratnoff, O.D. (1970) J. Lab. Clin. Med. 76, 809–815.

166 Heck, L.W. and Kaplan, A.P. (1974) J. Exp. Med. 140, 1615–1630.

167 Damus, D.S., Hicks, M. and Rosenberg, R.D. (1973) Nature (London) 246, 355–357.

168 Harpel, D.C. (1971) J. Clin. Invest. 50, 2084–2090.

169 Bouma et al., unpublished results.

170 Scott, C.F., Schapira, M., James, H.L., Cohen, A.B. and Colman, R.W. (1982) J. Clin. Invest. 69, 844–852.

R.F.A. Zwaal and H.C. Hemker (Eds.), *Blood Coagulation*
© 1986 Elsevier Science Publishers B.V. (Biomedical Division)

CHAPTER 5B

Initiation mechanisms:
Activation induced by thromboplastin

BJARNE ØSTERUD

Department of Clinical Chemistry, Institute of Medical Biology, University of Tromsø,
9000 Tromsø (Norway)

1. Introduction

The induction of clotting is a crucial event in the hemostatic mechanism. Based on observations in vitro the intrinsic activation pathway of the coagulation system was thought to be the major pathway in thrombin generation. However, three or possibly four of the clotting factors essential for normal clotting through the intrinsic pathway, factor XII, prekallikrein, high molecular weight kininogen (HMWK) and factor XI did not seem to play a key role in the hemostatic mechanism. This conception stemmed from the observation that patients lacking one of these factors, have normal hemostatic functions, even after severe surgical procedures (see Ch. 5A for extensive discussion).

The existence of the extrinsic pathway has been acknowledged for a long time. Severe factor VII deficiency is closely associated with hemostatic defects similar to those seen in hemophilia. The extrinsic pathway, however, was not believed to be physiologically important despite the potent activation of factor X by factor VII and thromboplastin seen in vitro, because of the severe bleeding problems observed in hemophiliacs. That thrombotic episodes could occur, associated with moderate factor VII deficiency, was another reason for believing that the extrinsic system was not important in hemostasis. About 7 years ago, however, this concept was abandoned, when the factor VII–thromboplastin complex was clearly shown to activate factor IX as well as factor X [1,2]. Based on this knowledge, the classical hemophilias can be viewed as diseases of the coagulation system operating via the extrinsic pathway. Thromboplastin may therefore together with factor VII be the physiological inducer of blood clotting.

2. The biochemistry of thromboplastin

The existence of thromboplastin has been known for a long time [3]. Many years after the first registration of thromboplastin as a procoagulant substance, Chargaff et al. [4,5] demonstrated that it was located in subcellular particles. They also showed that it consisted of a lipid part and a protein part both of which were necessary for the expression of procoagulant activity. Thromboplastin has recently been purified, and has been shown to consist of one species of protein, called apoprotein III, in a complex with a mixture of phospholipids [6,7]. Bovine apoprotein III was reported to be a single-chain glycoprotein with apparent molecular weight of 45 000 [7], whereas a molecular weight of 52 000 [6] was indicated for human apoprotein III.

Apoprotein III alone is devoid of any procoagulant activity, but will regain its full potency upon recombination with the appropriate phospholipids. In the human system, the most potent phospholipid mixture was shown to be phosphatidyl choline, phosphatidyl ethanolamine and phosphatidyl serine in a ratio of 1:1:0.2 [6]. Due to the hydrophobic character of apoprotein III, such recombination is only accomplished in the presence of detergents as deoxycholate or sodium dodecyl sulfate. Upon removal of detergent by dialysis, the phospholipids recombine with the apoprotein III molecule to form multilayered vesicles with procoagulant activity [6].

3. The localization of thromboplastin and its availability

(a) Tissue

Thromboplastin activity is probably present in almost all tissues [8]. Specially high activities of thromboplastin are observed in lungs, brain, bone marrow, kidney, placenta and mesenteral fat. Many cell types (i.e. endothelial and smooth muscle cells and fibroblasts) have a low activity of thromboplastin, but thromboplastin synthesis appears to be inducible in almost all cell types [9–15]. The only exception so far are mouse trophoblasts [16] and sperm cells (Østerud, unpublished) that apparently synthesize apoprotein III constitutively, i.e. the synthesis is uninfluenced by exogenous inducers.

(b) Blood cells

Blood cells were shown to generate thromboplastin activity upon incubation with endotoxin (lipopolysaccharides of Gram-negative bacteria). Both neutrophils and lymphocytes [17–21] were suggested to be responsible for the increased procoagulant activity identified as thromboplastin. In 1975, Rivers et al. [22] demonstrated that monocytes possessed thromboplastin activity after being exposed to endotoxin. Today it is established that monocytes are the only blood cells with this property [23–28]. It is also recognized that normal circulating monocytes possess weak but significant thromboplastin activity in their plasma membranes, whereas granulocytes, lymphocytes, red cells and blood platelets are totally devoid of this activity [29].

(c) Vessel wall

In the vessel wall, one .finds that the cell layer in close contact with blood, the endothelial cells (EC) have low but significant thromboplastin activity in the cell membranes [30]. This activity is under normal conditions protected from the blood, but may upon cell damage or endothelial cell activation become available and trigger the clotting cascades. Upon more extensive damage of the vessels, other subendothelial cells such as smooth muscle cells, known to contain substantial amount of thromboplastin [13], may play a role in the hemostatic mechanism as well. Furthermore, fibroblasts and macrophages in the vessel wall are also known to contain thromboplastin activity. Thus the vessel wall seems to provide sufficient thromboplastin for potent activation of the clotting system. Evidence supporting this hypothesis was recently documented by the observation that the vessels of placenta which has a relatively high thromboplastin activity, contained the major part of the apoprotein III antigen (Bjørklid, personal communication).

Although the endothelial cells possess relatively weak thromboplastin activity in their native condition [15–30], blood may get in contact with rather large surfaces of endothelial cells. In the microcirculation for example, 200 μl of blood is in direct contact with 1 m^2 endothelial surface [29]. Small injuries of the endothelial cell layer may therefore induce here a significant clotting activation. In a thrombotic situation, the endothelial cells may provide substantial trigger activity of the clotting system, as the thromboplastin synthesis is also inducible here [13–15]. Its

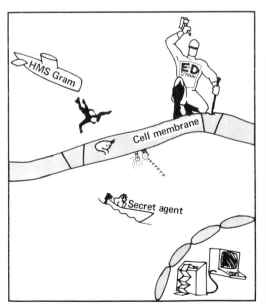 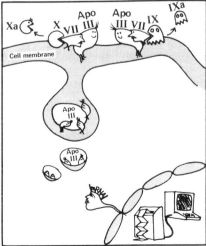

Figs. 1 and 2. A cartoon of a model for stimulation of cells to produce and expose apo III, the protein entity of thromboplastin lipoprotein.

activity may increase up to 250-fold when exposed to certain inducing agents. Such agents are thrombin and endotoxin [15]. Low levels of thrombin are capable of enhancing thromboplastin synthesis in endothelial cell cultures and in whole umbilical cord veins [15]. The effect of thrombin is accelerated manyfold by the presence of platelets. A comparable inducing effect is also obtained by exposing endothelial cells to endotoxin [15]. Recently we showed that the effect of endotoxin in endothelial cell cultures with human plasma medium, is complement dependent [30]. This might indicate that the vessel wall may become thrombotic in conditions where complement is activated. It should also be emphasized that when cells are induced to produce more thromboplastin, the newly synthesized thromboplastin becomes exposed on the surface of the cells, and thereby in direct contact with plasma coagulation factors [15] (see Figs. 1 and 2).

4. Role of thromboplastin in pathology

(a) Sepsis

Blood clotting may also be triggered by thromboplastin in the cell membranes of monocytes. This source of thromboplastin is probably not involved in the hemostatic process, but may play a significant role under thrombotic conditions, especially in patients with sepsis. We have observed very high levels of thromboplastin in monocytes of patients with meningococcal infection, and the high content of thromboplastin appeared to be correlated with an unfavorable prognosis [31]. The acceleration of thromboplastin synthesis of blood monocytes is also complement dependent [32]. This supports the earlier observation by Garner et al. [33], who found increased factor VII activity in decomplemented dogs given endotoxin shock, whereas factor VII in normal dogs in septic shock was rapidly removed from the circulation. This last phenomenon is probably caused by the stimulation of monocytes to produce surface-exposed thromboplastin to which factor VII binds [34,35]. Upon cell stimulation the monocytes and granulocytes are removed from the circulation, and in this way factor VII in the plasma will be withdrawn from the circulation.

(b) Shwartzman reaction

It has generally been accepted that the white cells play an important role in the Shwartzman reaction [36,37]. Recently we found that by inducing Shwartzman reaction in rabbits by injecting intravenously a dose of endotoxin a relatively small (but significant) rise (7-fold increase) of thromboplastin activity of the circulating monocytes resulted [38]. In contrast, a second dose of endotoxin, given 24 h after the first dose, caused a tremendous rise (70-fold) in the thromboplastin activity of the circulating monocytes. Interestingly, pretreatment of the rabbits with prior doses of corticosteroids, promoted a striking response to an endotoxin injection. The thromboplastin activity of the monocytes was comparable to the thromboplastin activity induced by giving the animals two doses of endotoxin without pretreatment with steroids. There is therefore reason to believe that steroids may provoke disseminated intravascular coagulation (DIC), and that part of the Shwartzman reaction is caused by an extreme increase in and exposure of thromboplastin activity from blood monocytes.

5. Factor VII

(a) Properties and function

Factor VII is a single-chain glycoprotein with a molecular weight of 54 000 [39,40] for bovine factor VII and an apparent molecular weight of 50 000 [41] or 47 000 [42] for human factor VII. Similar to other vitamin K-dependent factors IX, X, prothrombin and protein C, factor VII contains γ-carboxyglutamic acid residues that are required for a calcium-mediated binding in the activation of factor IX and factor X. In contrast to all the other clotting factors in blood, factor VII circulates in a zymogen form that possesses strong esterase activity [43]. Fortunately, this form of factor VII has only very limited ability to induce clotting by itself. To exert its function in promoting clotting, factor VII has to interact with thromboplastin.

The current concept of this interaction is that the thromboplastin acts as a cofactor for factor VII (cf. [44] and Ch. 3). The lipid part of the thromboplastin molecule is an essential part in this reaction. In the same way apoprotein III is mandatory for the function of thromboplastin as shown by neutralization of the thromboplastin activity when thromboplastin is allowed to interact with an antibody raised against purified apoprotein III antigen [45].

Native plasma factor VII is neutralized slowly when incubated with high concentrations of diisopropylfluorophosphate (DFP) [42,46,47]. However, after factor VII has been allowed to interact with thromboplastin, the factor VII in the reaction product is much more readily inactivated by DFP, suggesting a conformational change in the factor VII molecule. No molecular cleavage of factor VII occurs in forming the complex with thromboplastin.

(b) Factor VII–phospholipid interaction

Some years ago we proposed a model whereby factor VII, after interaction with thromboplastin, might be separated from thromboplastin and still retain its ability to activate factor X by itself [48]. This was based on experiments where factor VII incubated with thromboplastin, still retained its ability to activate factor X even after the phospholipid part of thromboplastin in the reaction mixture was broken down by phospholipase C. The activation product appeared, however, to be phospholipid dependent as further treatment with phospholipase C, abolished the procoagulant activity.

134

The role of phospholipid in the activation of factor IX and factor X by factor VII and thromboplastin has gained new interest after the recent observation by Dalaker and Prydz [49], who found that the elevated level of factor VII activity in pregnant women (about 2.5 times greater than in non-pregnant women) may stem from a complex of factor VII and phospholipid rather than an increased factor VII synthesis. By subjecting the plasma samples from pregnant women to phospholipase treatment, the factor VII level was reduced to normal level, strongly suggesting that the increased factor VII probably was reflecting a phospholipid involvement. The same authors have now also shown that factor VII, in the plasma of pregnant women, is much more readily susceptible to inactivation by DFP than factor VII in the plasma of non-pregnant women (Dalaker and Prydz, personal communication). It was suggested that such a phospholipid–factor VII may arise from the interaction of factor VII with, for example, exposed thromboplastin from the placenta. This complex of factor VII and phospholipid requires thromboplastin for its activating function on factors IX and X, but there is reason to believe that smaller amounts of thromboplastin will be needed for the expression of this type of factor VII. It certainly may be a thrombogenic factor during pregnancy.

Many of the details of the interaction between factor VII and thromboplastin are still unknown. For example, what is the role of apoprotein III in the thromboplastin molecule? Whether there is any direct interaction between factor VII and apoprotein III, or a complex of factor VII and lipid requiring the presence of the apoprotein, or a complex with phospholipid alone, is unknown.

Most probably there is a formation of a complex of factor VII bound to the lipid part of thromboplastin, so that the whole factor IX- and factor X-activating complex is constituted of a factor VII–phospholipid–apoprotein III complex. However, the very high activity of factor VII in pregnant women [50], and our earlier results [48], may imply complexes of factor VII–phospholipids can be formed as a result of an interaction between factor VII and thromboplastin. In pregnant women this may occur as a result of exposure of blood to large amounts of thromboplastin in the placenta, and subsequent slow release of factor VII–lipid complexes. This complex is probably not itself efficient in activating factors IX and X, but, in the presence of thromboplastin, will exert a much more potent activating effect than factor VII and thromboplastin alone. Nevertheless, it is possible that such a factor VII-lipid complex may be able to activate sufficiently factors IX and X, even in the absence of thromboplastin, to account for the increased thrombogenicity during pregnancy.

6. The activity state of factor VII and its potency to trigger clotting

(a) The inherent activity of factor VII

As already indicated above, factor VII circulates as a zymogen, a single-chain molecule with strong esterase activity. This form of factor VII can, however, be converted into a two-chain molecule factor VII$_a$, by the cleavage of a single bond. Both forms of factor VII participate actively in the clotting process, but the activated form has been reported to be from 25- to 120-fold more active than the zymogen [41,51–53]. Zymogen activation results in the formation of a two-chain protein consisting of polypeptide chains with molecular weights of 29 500 and 23 500, that are held together by disulfide bonds [40]. Based on these observations, it was suggested that factor VII zymogen itself possesses low activity, of approximately 0.8% that of the enzyme form [53]. However, the K_m of the cleavage of a synthetic enzyme, benzoyl-o-carbonyl-arginine-p-nitrobenzyl ester, was approximately 17-fold higher for factor VII than for factor VII$_a$, whereas k_{cat} was only 2-fold lower [43]. Since factor VII is nearly absolutely dependent on thromboplastin for proteolytic activity, and thromboplastin is not normally exposed in the blood, the blood does not clot despite the fact that factor VII is circulating in a partially active form.

(b) Factor VII$_a$ activation of factor X in the absence of thromboplastin

Recent evidence seems to imply a role of factor VII in the activation of factor X even in the absence of thromboplastin. Thus, purified factor VII activated by incubation with purified factor X$_a$ in the presence of phospholipids, to yield a 30–40-fold increase in factor VII activity, caused a slow but significant activation of factor X in the absence of thromboplastin [54]. A concentration of 55 ng factor VII$_a$ (about 1 nM) induced 2% (200 ng) factor X$_a$ formation in 20 min incubation time. This activation process was also dependent on phospholipids. Whether factor VII$_a$ may play a physiological role in the absence of thromboplastin is not yet known. Under in vivo conditions it may not seem likely to form so much factor VII$_a$ that it can cause a significant factor X activation. It may, however, account for the factor VIII bypassing effect in activated factor IX concentrates used to treat factor VIII-deficient patients with acquired factor VIII inhibitor. The activated factor IX concentrates have been shown to contain large concentrations of activated factor VII [55]. Furthermore, factor VII$_a$ has been shown to persist in the blood circulation for some hours before it is removed, which gives the activated form enough time to interact with its substrates, factor IX and factor X [55].

(c) Factor VII and ischemic heart disease

In a prospective study by Meade [56,57], it became clear that there was an increasing risk of cardiovascular death with increasing level of factor VII, factor VIII and cholesterol. The association seemed to be specific for cardiovascular disease, as no significant association was found between clotting factors at recruitment and later death from cancer. The rise in factor VII might stem from increased factor VII synthesis, but may also reflect an activation process that could play a direct, causal role in ischemic heart disease (IHD), or reflect other processes which are the direct causes. Some evidence for an activation process was indicated in this study by the finding that there was a discrepancy between factor VII clotting activity and factor VII antigen [56]. This phenomenon strongly suggests that factor VII in these patients may have been subject to activation.

Meade [57] also proposes an association between raised factor VII levels with increasing age, diabetes, obesity, the use of oral contraceptives and the occurrence of menopause, and increased risk of IHD. On the other hand, low levels of factor VII are associated with black ethnic groups and vegetarianism. These are known to have low risk of IHD.

(d) The activation of factor VII

The conversion of the one-chain factor VII into the two-chain form, factor VII_a, is probably a crucial mechanism in hemostasis and thrombosis. Several coagulation enzymes have been shown to have the ability to activate factor VII. These are thrombin [40], plasmin [58], factor XII_a [58–60], factor IX_a [58,61,62] and factor X_a [40–42,52,62]. In the recalcification and clotting of plasma, factor IX_a appeared to be the most effective in converting factor VII to VII_a [62]. In other studies however, it has become evident that factor X_a in the presence of phospholipids is the most potent activator of factor VII [52,61]. It is therefore reasonable to believe that factor X_a bound to the surface of activated platelets or white cells will cleave factor VII to VII_a, and thereby accelerate the formation of more factor IX_a and factor X_a when thromboplastin is exposed on the surface of activated or disrupted cells. The very rapid activation of factor VII by factor X_a in the presence of phospholipids or activated platelets, may in vivo be essential for a normal hemostatic mechanism. But is may also cause severe enhancement of the coagulation activation in a thrombotic situation, e.g. disseminated intravascular coagulation.

7. The function of factor VII–thromboplastin complex

When thromboplastin is exposed on disrupted or activated cells, it binds factor VII. The newly formed complex of factor VII–thromboplastin will slowly initiate the activation of factors IX and X, and the resultant generated enzymes, factors IX_a and X_a, can then proteolytically activate factor VII to the 40–120-fold more active enzyme. If there is excess of thromboplastin present, a rapid activation of more of factors IX and X will take place. However, normally only limited amounts of thromboplastin are likely to be exposed to blood plasma. Since native factor VII and factor VII_a have the same affinity to thromboplastin [44], and factor VII is largely unconverted, factor VII zymogen will act as an inhibitor of factor VII_a by competing with factor VII_a for the available thromboplastin, and prevent full expression of the activity of the factor VII_a present. This positive feedback activation of factor VII and the control of the expression of factor VII–thromboplastin complex, is probably essential for normal hemostasis and may be required to prevent thrombosis as a result of an unnecessarily strong reaction.

The above model for factor VII function and expression appears also to agree with the older observations that patients with moderate factor VII deficiency may experience thrombotic episodes [63,64]. Under these conditions there are low levels of factor VII zymogen, so when factor VII$_a$ is formed, a much larger portion of this factor VII$_a$ will be expressed when thromboplastin becomes available. Due to the failure of the system to dampen the factor VII$_a$ formed, an overreaction that may lead to thrombosis may take place despite the low level of plasma factor VII. However, when the total level of factor VII gets too low, serious bleeding similar to that observed in hemophilia can be observed. This again demonstrates that factor VII is important and essential for normal hemostasis. It is tempting to suggest that the discrepancy seen in bleeding tendency in moderate factor VII deficiency, may stem from the great variance in cellular concentrations and availability of thromboplastin between different individuals, indicated by measurements of thromboplastin in various blood cells as well as in cell cultures.

8. Factor VII association with blood cells and its potency in triggering clotting

Cells stimulated to synthesize and expose thromboplastin activity on their surfaces bind factor VII as mentioned earlier. Thus, when heparinized blood is incubated with endotoxin, an increase in factor VII associated with the isolated monocytes parallels the increase in thromboplastin activity [65]. This factor VII was shown to be activated (factor VII$_a$, probably through a first interaction between factor VII zymogen and the exposed thromboplastin, followed by the activation of factors IX and X and subsequent feedback activation of factor VII by the activation products, factors IX$_a$ and X$_a$. Since this even occurred in blood anticoagulated with heparin one may propose that factors IX$_a$ and X$_a$ are protected on the monocyte cell surface from being neutralized immediately by heparin–antithrombin III. Similar protection of these factors has been observed on activated platelets [66]. Recently it was shown that the number of factor VII-binding sites on stimulated monocytes paralleled the procoagulant activity of the cells [67].

Further evidence for a cellular expression of procoagulant activity was recently documented by Tracy et al. [68]. They showed that isolated peripheral blood monocytes and lymphocytes interact with factor V$_a$ and factor X$_a$ to form a functional catalytic complex which proteolytically activates prothrombin to thrombin. The rate of thrombin generation by monocytes exceeded that of lymphocytes and increased as monocytes adhered to a surface. The monocyte prothrombinase activity appeared to be mediated through factor V$_a$ receptors for factor X$_a$ on the monocyte surface. Interestingly, the rate of thrombin generation per cell exceeded that previously obtained with either bovine or human platelets.

Obviously, the availability of thromboplastin activity on cell surfaces or disrupted cells may be crucial in inducing activation of the coagulation system. The availability of thromboplastin at the site of an injury is probably essential for a normal hemostatic mechanism. There is also reason to believe that thromboplastin exposure to blood is the major source of coagulation activation in diseases associated with intravascular coagulation.

References

1 Østerud, B. and Rapaport, S.I. (1977) Proc. Natl. Acad. Sci. (U.S.A.) 74, 5260–5264.
2 Zur, M. and Nemerson, Y. (1978) J. Biol. Chem. 255, 5703–5707.
3 Morawitz, P. (1905) Ergebn. Physiol. 4, 307–422.
4 Chargaff, E., Moore, D.H. and Bendich, A.A. (1942) J. Biol. Chem. 145, 593–603.
5 Chargaff, E., Bendich, A.A. and Cohen, S.S. (1944) J. Biol. Chem. 156, 161–178.
6 Bjørklid, E. and Storm, E. (1977) Biochem. J. 65, 89–96.
7 Bach, R., Nemerson, Y. and Koningsberg, W. (1981) J. Biol. Chem. 256, 8324–8331.
8 Astrup, T. (1965) Thromb. Diath. Haemorrh. 14, 401–416.
9 Zacharski, L.R. and McIntyre, O.R. (1971) Nature (London) 232, 338–339.
10 Zeldis, S.M., Nemerson, Y., Pitlick, F.A. and Leutz, T.L. (1972) Science 175, 766–768.
11 Zacharski, L.R. and McIntryre, O.R. (1973) J. Med. 4, 118–131.
12 Maynard, J.R., Heckman, C.A., Pitlick, F.A. and Nemerson, Y. (1976) Lab. Invest. 35, 550–557.
13 Maynard, J.R., Dreyer, B.E., Stemerman, M.B. and Pitlick, F.A. (1977) Blood 50, 387–396.
14 Lyberg, T., Galdal, K.S., Evensen, S.A. and Prydz, H. (1983) Br. J. Haematol. 53, 85–95.
15 Brox, J.H., Østerud, B., Bjørklid, E. and Fenton II, J.W. (1984) Br. J. Haematol. 57, 239–246.
16 Dalaker, K., Kaplun, A., Lyberg, T. and Prydz, H. (1983) Gynecol. Obstet. Invest. 15, 325–336.
17 Lerner, R.G., Goldstein, R. and Cummings, G. (1971) Proc. Soc. Exp. Biol. Med. 138, 145–148.
18 Niemetz, J. (1972) J. Clin. Invest. 51, 307–313.
19 Niemetz, J. and Fani, K. (1973) Blood 42, 47–59.
20 Rikles, F.R., Hardin, J.A., Pitlick, F.A., Hoyer, L.W. and Conrad, M.E. (1973) J. Clin. Invest. 52, 1427–1434.
21 Lerner, R.G., Goldstein, R. and Cummings, G. (1977) Thromb. Res. 11, 253–261.
22 Rivers, R.P.A., Hathaway, W.E. and Weston, W.L. (1975) Br. J. Haematol. 30, 311–316.
23 Hiller, E., Saal, J.G. and Riethmüller, G. (1977) Haemostasis 6, 347–350.
24 Prydz, H. and Allison, A.C. (1978) Thromb. Haemostas. 39, 582–591.
25 van Ginkel, C.J.W., Thorig, L., Thompson, J., Oh, J.I.H. and van Aken, W.G. (1979) Infect. Immunol. 25, 388–395.
26 Edwards, R.L., Rickles, F.R. and Bobrove, A.M. (1979) Blood 54, 359–370.
27 Levy, G.A., Schwartz, B.S. and Edgington, T.S. (1981) J. Immunol. 127, 357–363.
28 Østerud, B. and Bjørklid, E. (1982) Scand. J. Haematol. 29, 175–184.
29 Busch, C., Cancilla, P., DeBault, L., Goldsmith, J. and Owen, W. (1982) Lab. Invest. 47, 498–504.
30 Østerud, B., Olsen, J.O. and Welle Benjaminsen, A. (1984) Haemostasis 14, 386–392.
31 Østerud, B. and Flægstad, T. (1983) Thromb. Haemostas. 49, 5–7.
32 Østerud, B. and Eskeland, T. (1982) FEBS Lett. 149, 75–79.
33 Garner, R., Chater, B.R. and Brown, D.L. (1974) Br. J. Haematol. 28, 393–401.
34 Brooze Jr., G.J. (1982) J. Clin. Invest. 70, 526–535.
35 Østerud, B. and Bjørklid, E. (1982) Biochem. Biophys. Res. Commun. 108, 620–626.
36 Horn, R.S. and Collins, R.D. (1968) Lab. Invest. 18, 101–107.
37 Lerner, R.G., Rapaport, S.I., Siemens, J.K. and Spitzer, J.M. (1968) Am. J. Physiol. 214, 532–537.
38 Østerud, B., Olsen, J.-O. and Tindall, A., in: Mononuclear Phagocytes (van Furth, R., Ed.) Nijhoff, The Hague, in press.
39 Kisiel, W. and Davie, E.W. (1975) Biochemistry 14, 4928–4934.
40 Radcliffe, R. and Nemerson, Y. (1975) J. Biol. Chem. 250, 388–395.
41 Bajaj, S.P., Rapaport, S.I. and Brown, S.F. (1981) J. Biol. Chem. 256, 253–258.
42 Broze, G.J. and Majerus, P.W. (1980) J. Biol. Chem. 255, 1242–1247.

43 Zur, M. and Nemerson, Y. (1978) J. Biol. Chem. 253, 2203–2209.

44 Nemerson, Y. (1983) Haemostasis 13, 150–155.

45 Bjørklid, E., Giercksky, K.E. and Prydz, H. (1978) Br. J. Haematol. 39, 445–458.

46 Østerud, B., Bjørklid, E. and Brown, S.F. (1979) Biochem. Biophys. Res. Commun. 85, 59–67.

47 Prydz, H. and Lyberg, T. (1980) in: Protides of the Biological Fluid (Peters, H., Ed.) Vol. 28, pp. 241–244, Pergamon, Oxford.

48 Østerud, B., Berre, Å., Otnaess, A-B., Bjørklid, E. and Prydz, H. (1972) Biochemistry 11, 2853–2857.

49 Dalaker, K. and Prydz, H. (1984) Br. J. Haematol. 56, 233–241.

50 Øian, P., Omsjø, I., Maltau, J.M. and Østerud, B. (1985) Br. J. Haematol. 59, 133–137.

51 Broze, G.J. and Majerus, P.W. (1980) J. Biol. Chem. 255, 1242–1247.

52 Østerud, B. (1980) in: Protides of the Biological Fluids (Peters, H., Ed.) Vol. 28, pp. 245–248, Pergamon, Oxford.

53 Bach, B., Oberdick, J. and Nemerson, Y. (1984) Blood 63, 393–398.

54 Østerud, B. (1983) Haemostasis 13, 161–168.

55 Seligsohn, U., Kasper, C.K., Østerud, B. and Rapaport, S.I. (1979) Blood 53, 828–837.

56 Meade, T.W., Chakrabarti, R., Haines, H.P., North, W.R.S., Stirling, Y. and Thompson, S.G. (1980) Lancet 1, 1050–1054.

57 Meade, T.W. (1983) Haemostasis 13, 178–185.

58 Laake, K. and Østerud, B. (1974) Thromb. Res. 5, 759–772.

59 Radcliffe, R., Bagdasarian, A., Colman, R. and Nemerson, Y. (1977) Blood 50, 611–617.

60 Kiesiel, W., Fujikawa, K. and Davie, E.W. (1977) Biochemistry 16, 4189–4194.

61 Masys, D.R., Bajaj, S.P. and Rapaport, S.J. (1982) Blood 60, 1143–1150.

62 Seligsohn, U., Østerud, B., Brown, S.F., Griffin, J.H. and Rapaport, S.I. (1979) J. Clin. Invest. 64, 1056–1065.

63 Godal, H.C., Madsen, K. and Nissen-Meyer, R. (1962) Acta Med. Scand. 171, 325–327.

64 Gersheim, M.E. and Gude, J.K. (1983) New Engl. J. Med. 288, 141–142.

65 Østerud, B. and Bjørklid, E. (1982) Biochem. Biophys. Res. Commun. 108, 620–626.

66 Miletich, J.P., Jackson, C.M. and Majerus, P.W. (1978) J. Biol. Chem. 253, 6908–6916.

67 Rodgers, G.M., Broze, G.J. and Shuman, M.A. (1984) Blood 63, 434–438.

68 Tracy, P.B., Rohrbach, M.S. and Mann, K.G. (1983) J. Biol. Chem. 258, 7264–7267.

R.F.A. Zwaal and H.C. Hemker (Eds.), *Blood Coagulation*
© 1986 Elsevier Science Publishers B.V. (Biomedical Division)

CHAPTER 6

Platelets and coagulation

R.F.A. ZWAAL, E.M. BEVERS and P. COMFURIUS

University of Limburg, Biomedical Centre, Maastricht (The Netherlands)

1. Introduction

Formation of a hemostatic plug at sites of vascular injury requires the participation of blood platelets. This they do by clumping together into an aggregate and by promoting efficient coagulation which consolidates the plug with strands of fibrin. Apart from this, platelets participate in a number of other physiological processes, such as phagocytosis, inflammation, immunological reactions, and interactions with tumor cells. To perform these functions, platelets show a wide variety of cellular reactions which also make them attractive research tools in biochemistry. It is evident that cellular organization and integrity is required for adequate platelet function. This organization critically depends on the presence and architecture of both plasma membrane and intracellular organelles. The plasma membrane plays a crucial role in the binding of external stimuli, in the transduction of the signal into the cell, and in the execution of the platelet response. Part of this response consists of a secretory event [1], releasing components that interfere with coagulation such as factor V, von Willebrand factor, fibrinogen, and a heparin-neutralizing protein referred to as platelet factor 4. Moreover, coagulation is accelerated by virtue of binding of clotting factors to the plasma membrane, resulting in the assembly of multi-enzyme complexes with great catalytic efficiency.

This essay will deal mainly with the participation of platelets in the coagulation process. Particular attention will be paid to the involvement of the platelet plasma membrane in prothrombin and factor X activation. Some information on platelet structure and function will be given first to set the scope for further discussions.

2. Structural and functional aspects of platelets

(a) Non-activated platelet

Blood platelets are formed in the bone marrow from cytoplasmic fragments of megakaryocytes [2]. In the absence of vessel wall injury, platelets circulate in the

142

blood for 8–11 days as smooth, disk-shaped cells that are non-adherent to each other or to vascular endothelium.

(i) Plasma membrane

The platelet is surrounded by a trilaminar plasma membrane of 70–80 Å in diameter [3]. This membrane displays a number of peculiar invaginations to form a sponge-like system of channels that burrow their way through the cytoplasm. This open canalicular system significantly increases the surface area of the cell in contact with its aqueous environment, and serves as a channel in which intracellular granules discharge their contents upon platelet activation. The plasma membrane is coated on the exterior with an electron-dense glycocalyx, representing carbohydrate-rich domains of more than 30 membrane glycoproteins exposed to the outside of the cell [4]. A schematic representation of the essential features of the platelet plasma membrane is shown in Fig. 1. The most abundant of these glycoproteins are Ib, IIb, III and IV, their functional roles including that of glycoprotein V are beginning to be understood (vide infra). At the cytoplasmic surface, the membrane contains cytoskeletal proteins that undergo structural changes during platelet activation [5]. These alterations involve polymerization of actin into filaments that associate with myosin. This interaction between myosin and actin filaments is regulated by the level of phosphorylation of the myosin light chains. Actin polymerization is regulated by a number of proteins, such as profilin [6] and gelsolin [7], while α-actinin has been implicated as the membrane attachment site for actin filaments [8]. Branching of actin filaments into a network is brought about by actin-binding protein [9]. The core of the membrane is formed by a lipid bilayer to which peripheral membrane proteins (such as cytoskeletal proteins) are at-

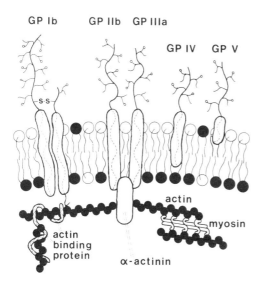

Fig. 1. Schematic representation of the platelet plasma membrane. GP, glycoprotein.

tached via polar interactions, and which is interrupted to allow hydrophobic interactions with integral membrane proteins (e.g. the hydrophobic domains of glycoproteins). The lipid bilayer contains 70% phospholipids by weight, while the remainder consists predominantly of cholesterol plus a small amount of glycolipids. Five major phospholipid classes have been identified in human platelets [10,11]: phosphatidylcholine (38%), phosphatidylethanolamine (27%), sphingomyelin (19%), phosphatidylserine (10%) and phosphatidylinositol (5%). The lipid composition of the plasma membrane resembles that of the intracellular membranes although it contains more sphingomyelin and cholesterol. As in red cells, the phospholipids are asymmetrically distributed over the bilayer [11–14]. The exterior half of the plasma membrane contains most of the sphingomyelin, whereas phosphatidylserine and phosphatidylinositol are mainly confined to the interior leaflet of the membrane. Phosphatidylcholine and phosphatidylethanolamine are present on either side of the membrane, though not to the same extent.

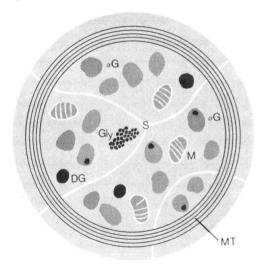

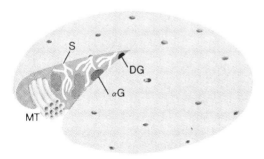

Fig. 2. Schematic view of the blood platelet. S, open canalicular system; MT, microtubules; G, α-granules; DG, dense bodies; M, mitochondria, Gly, glycogen granules.

(ii) Intracellular structures

Several subcellular structures have been recognized in the platelet by the use of electron microscopy [2,3] (Fig. 2). Below the surface membrane and not in contact with the open canalicular system, platelets contain a dense tubular system which is presumably derived from the smooth endoplasmic reticulum of the parent megakaryocyte. Both the dense tubular system and the open canalicular system have been proposed to serve similar functions as the sarcotubules and the transverse tubuli of the sarcoplasmic reticulum of muscle cells [15]. Indeed, vesicles which are thought to be derived from the dense tubular system are able to accumulate Ca^{2+} as efficiently as sarcoplasmic reticulum of muscle [16,17]. The dense tubular system has been shown to contain amongst others the enzyme system required for the formation of thromboxane A_2 from arachidonic acid [18]. It may also contain the site of the de novo synthesis of fatty acids and phospholipids, considering that it is derived from the megakaryocyte's smooth endoplasmic reticulum. The discoid form of resting platelets is regulated by a circumferential bundle of hollow cylindrical structures, similar in appearance to microtubules found in a wide variety of other mammalian cells. Together with microfilaments of polymerized actin, these tubules assemble in highly organized structures during cell activation. During platelet activation, they contract toward the center of the cell, thereby trapping the randomly dispersed storage granules to concentrate them into a tightly packed mass [3]. These storage granules can be divided in at least 3 sub-classes, dense bodies, α-granules, and lysosomal enzyme storage organelles [19–23], their abundance and mutual ratio being variable among different mammalian species. The α-granules are the most abundant in human platelets, and contain a number of non-enzymatic proteins, part of which interfere with coagulation such as fibrinogen, factors V and XIII, von Willebrand factor, and heparin-binding protein platelet factor 4. It is also the locus of platelet-derived growth factor, which is a low molecular weight cationic protein that stimulates the proliferation of arterial smooth muscle cells and fibroblasts in tissue culture [24]. The lysosomal fraction contains a number of acid hydrolases, such as hyaluronidase, α-N-acetyl-glucosaminidase and β-glucuronidase. The dense bodies contain calcium and low molecular weight compounds, the most prominent of which are serotonin, ATP, ADP and pyrophosphate. The energy-rich phosphates in these granules do not actively participate in cell metabolism, and are distinguished from the metabolic pool of ATP and ADP [25], which is regulated by a few small-sized mitochondria and by active glycolysis in conjunction with abundant glycogen granules in the cytoplasm. Platelets do not contain a cell nucleus and are devoid of DNA. A small amount of RNA is present and ribosomal structures have occasionally been observed. Protein synthesis is almost negligible, and presumably serves no function in platelet physiology.

(b) Activated platelet

Platelets can be activated by a variety of structurally non-related compounds to execute a number of cellular responses. Among these stimulators are collagen, thrombin, ADP, epinephrine, platelet-activating factor (PAF), Ca-ionophores, immune complexes, serotonin, arachidonic acid and prostaglandin intermediates. Evidence is accumulating that most of these activators exert their action by binding to specific receptors of the platelet surface membrane [4]. A possible exception concerns the activation by thrombin, one of the most potent platelet activators known. Activation is initiated by a rapid proteolytic cleavage of glycoprotein V at the platelet outer surface [4]. Although thrombin also binds to glycoprotein Ib without splitting it, this is not sufficient to evoke platelet activation. The molecular mechanisms that are implicated in platelet activation are intricate and not completely understood. A critical level of metabolic ATP is required and platelets respond to stimulation with an increase in glycolysis and tricarboxylic acid cycle to replenish ATP supplies [25]. Most of the data are consistent with the notion that a prerequisite for platelet activation is an increase of the cytoplasmic Ca^{2+} level of the cell [26]. Two different pathways have been distinguished in the regulation of the cytoplasmic Ca^{2+} concentration [27], i.e. an efflux of Ca^{2+} from the dense tubular system which is thought to sequester Ca^{2+} from the cytoplasm in resting platelets, and an influx of Ca^{2+} from the cell environment resulting from an increased permeability of the plasma membrane during interaction with different stimulators. Both pathways are presumably regulated by cAMP levels of the cell. Platelet stimulators can exert their action by decreasing the activity of adenylate cyclase or by increasing phosphodiesterase activity, whereas the reverse effect usually results in inhibition of the platelet response [28]. cAMP might be involved in maintaining membrane integrity [27], and in the accumulation of Ca^{2+} by the dense tubular system controlled by a cAMP-dependent protein kinase [16]. Increase of cytoplasmic Ca^{2+} concentration has a number of effects that contribute to platelet activation. These include activation of phospholipases [29], inhibition of adenylate cyclase [30], activation of contractile proteins of microfilaments [5,31], depolymerization of microtubules [32], activation of Ca-dependent protease [5] and facilitation of fusion between granule membranes and the plasma membrane during the secretory process [12,33].

(i) Platelet adhesion

The initial reaction in hemostasis following injury to vascular endothelium is adhesion of platelets to subendothelial structures which comprise microfibrils of elastin, basement membrane-like amorphous material, and collagen fibrils [34]. Of these structures, collagen is required to achieve full release and aggregation following adhesion. Platelet adhesion to subendothelium is mediated by a high molecular weight plasma protein usually referred to as the von Willebrand factor [35]. For adhesion to collagen a specific receptor in the platelet membrane has been described [36]. Since resting platelets demonstrate low-affinity binding of von Willebrand factor [37] while the amount of this protein bound to subendothelium correlates with the extent of platelet adhesion [38], it has been suggested that von Willebrand factor initially interacts with a subendothelial structure in a calcium-dependent process leading to an alteration such that it will recognize specific receptors on platelets [39]. This receptor has been identified as glycoprotein Ib mainly through studies on platelets from patients with Bernard–Soulier syndrome [40,41]. These platelets are deficient in glycoprotein Ib and this hereditary bleeding disorder can be considered the mirror image of von Willebrand's disease where the plasma protein required for adhesion is missing. In both syndromes, ristocetin-induced platelet aggregation as well as platelet adhesion to subendothelium are absent or disturbed [42,43].

(ii) Shape change

Most of the known platelet activators, except for epinephrine, produce shape change of the platelet from a disk to a sphere with pseudopod formation [44]. This process, which occurs directly after addition of platelet activators in vitro, is accompanied by increased exposure of sialic acid residues at the membrane outer surface [45]. It also involves increased actin polymerization [5] and collection of storage granules by a ring of microtubules near the cell center [3]. Although extracellular Ca^{2+} is not required, an influx of Ca^{2+} from the dense tubular system into the cytoplasm is suspected, the more so as platelet shape change is inhibited by cAMP.

(iii) Release reaction

The release reaction is the secretory process which involves discharge of granular contents into the open canalicular system of the platelet after fusion of the granular membrane with the plasma membrane. All known platelet stimulators can evoke the release reaction in vitro. Secretion of the contents of α-granules and dense bodies occurs almost simultaneously [46], while lysosomal release is delayed and less complete [47]. Secretion of lysosomal enzymes is absent upon triggering of platelets with ADP or epinephrine [19]. Although it is generally assumed that the release reaction involves platelet contractile proteins, the precise molecular interactions involved are poorly understood. With a number of stimulators, release is mediated by the formation of prostaglandin endoperoxides and thromboxane A_2 [48]. These compounds are formed from free arachidonic acid, liberated from phospholipids by Ca^{2+}-dependent phospholipases [49–54]. Thromboxane A_2 production is inhibited by aspirin which acetylates and blocks cyclo-oxygenase [55]. Nevertheless, thromboxane-stimulated release (and aggregation) can be bypassed, since activation of platelets by thrombin or higher concentrations of collagen is not inhibited by aspirin [46]. The suggestion that thromboxane A_2 may act as a Ca-ionophore [56], thus enlarging the cytoplasmic Ca^{2+} concentration to a level required for the secretory event, is still a matter of debate. Although there is still controversy whether or not thromboxane A_2 reduces the basal level of platelet cyclic AMP, it is generally accepted that it inhibits hormone-stimulated adenylate cyclase activity [57]. Platelet release and aggregation by all stimuli so far tested are completely inhibited by prostacyclin produced by endothelial cells [58]. This is presumably due to elevation of platelet cAMP levels, resulting in complete inhibition of the platelet response [59,60]. The release reaction is diminished or disturbed in platelets with storage-pool deficiencies [61]. These deficiencies have been observed for dense granules (Hermansky–Pudlak syndrome) as well as for α-granules (gray platelet syndrome).

(iv) Aggregation

During activation, platelets interact with each other to form a tightly packed mass which functions as the primary hemostatic plug. In vitro, this process can be followed by measuring the increase in light transmission in a platelet aggregometer. Aggregation requires extracellular Ca^{2+}, while extracellular fibrinogen is a required cofactor for ADP-induced aggregation [62,63]. Moreover, when platelets are activated without stirring they do not aggregate but shape change and release still occur. ADP and epinephrine at low concentrations produce primary reversible aggregation without release, while this process is followed by release and secondary aggregation with higher concentrations of these activators [25,64]. With potent platelet stimulators like collagen, thrombin, and PAF, this biphasic aggregation pattern is virtually not observed and full aggregation and release occur in parallel. Platelet aggregation is one of many examples of direct interaction between cells, mediated by specific surface receptors. Recent studies have implicated two surface membrane glycoproteins, IIb and III, in platelet aggregation and fibrinogen receptor function. These two glycoproteins with apparent molecular weights of 136 000 and 95 000 [65] form a non-covalent complex in the presence of calcium [66–68]. In Glanzmann's thrombasthenia, platelets are deficient in both glycoproteins [5,40,41]. These platelets do not aggregate in response to any stimulus in spite of normal release reaction [61], and fail to express increased binding of fibrinogen [69] as occurs with normal platelets in the presence of Ca^{2+} and ADP [70]. Antibodies directed against glycoproteins IIb and III prevent fibrinogen binding and aggregation of normal platelets [71]. It seems plausible that calcium induces the formation of the glycoprotein IIb–III complex, which becomes the receptor for fibrinogen on the platelet membrane surface [70]. Subsequent aggregation would then occur by bridging of platelets via fibrinogen, which due to its symmetric structure is thought to have two interaction sites.

(v) Clot-promoting activity

Unlike resting platelets, activated platelets have been shown to accelerate clot formation in a variety of coagulation assays. Thus, ADP-treated platelets could shorten clotting times of non-contacted plasma in the presence of factor XII [72], while collagen-treated platelets promote clot formation in factor XII-deficient plasma provided that factor XI is present [73]. It has been shown that both activities are related to the ability of activated platelets to promote proteolytic activation of factor XII by kallikrein and of factor XI by both factor XII-dependent and factor XII-independent mechanisms [74]. The most powerful clot-promoting activity of activated platelets, often referred to a platelet factor 3, concerns their ability to shorten the Russell's viper venom (RVV) clotting time [for reviews: refs. 13,75].

Since RVV activates both factors V and X [76], platelet factor 3 refers to the capacity of platelets to promote the activation of prothrombin by the factor X_a–factor V_a complex. Although it was originally proposed that this was due to certain platelet lipoproteins [75], it has become evident that the reduction of the clotting time can be attributed to a combined effect of exposed procoagulant phospholipid and factor $V(V_a)$ [77,78] released from activated platelets [79,80]. In other coagulation assays, accessibility of procoagulant phospholipid will contribute to shorten the clotting time also by promoting activation of factor X by factor IX_a and VIII_a [81,82]. Indirect clot-promoting effects of platelets can be expected from release of certain α-granula proteins, such as heparin-neutralizing protein (platelet factor 4), factor VIII-related antigen and fibrinogen [23].

3. Prothrombin- and factor X-converting activities of platelets

The interaction between the platelet surface membrane and various plasma proteins plays an essential role in several reactions which are necessary for normal hemostasis. Thus, adhesion of platelets at the site of vascular injury requires subendothelial-bound von Willebrand factor that recognizes glycoprotein Ib at the platelet outer surface [38,39]. Platelet aggregation requires binding of fibrinogen with an induced complex of glycoprotein IIb and III [69–71]. Furthermore, minor quantities of thrombin formed early in hemostasis [83] bind to platelet receptors (presumably glycoprotein Ib) and produce splitting of glycoprotein V to elicit release and aggregation [4]. The platelet surface membrane also interacts with factors X_a and V_a to form the prothrombinase complex, as well as promoting the assembly of the factor IX_a–VIII_a complex required for factor X activation [13]. These interactions dramatically enhance enzymatic formation of both thrombin and factor X_a, in a way which strongly resembles the powerful catalytic activity of a negatively charged phospholipid surface in both reactions. At a phospholipid–water interface, binding of factors IX, X and prothrombin is brought about by Ca^{2+} which forms a complex between negative charges on the phospholipid molecules and γ-carboxyglutamic acid residues that are introduced in the proteins by post-ribosomal vitamin K-dependent carboxylation of a number of glutamic residues near the N-terminus of the polypeptide (cf. [84] and Ch. 4). The two non-enzymatic protein cofactors V_a and VIII_a are thought to interact with lipids by hydrophobic bonding. This interaction does not depend on Ca^{2+} but requires negatively charged phospholipids, which suggests that direct electrostatic interactions are also essential [85–87]. The reader is referred to Ch. 3 for a detailed discussion on the function of phospholipids and cofactors in proteolytic conversions occurring during blood coagulation.

(a) Activity of non-stimulated platelet

Unstimulated platelets are able to bind factor V_a with high affinity, and once factor V_a is bound it forms a locus on the platelet membrane which specifically binds factor X_a with high affinity [88–91]. Thrombin-induced platelet activation is not required for, nor has any effect on the binding of factor V_a and its subsequent interaction with factor X_a. With human platelets, there are approximately 2000–3000 binding sites for factor V_a and binding does not require, but is stimulated by factor X_a and prothrombin [91]. The number of factor V_a-binding sites exceeds that of factor X_a. Binding of factor X_a to unstimulated human platelets requires exogenous factor V_a and is limited by some platelet component other than factor V_a. At saturating levels of factor V_a, there are approximately 200–300 factor X_a-binding sites with an apparent K_d of 30–70 pM, while binding correlates precisely with rates of factor X_a-dependent prothrombin activation at the platelet surface [89]. The binding is specific for factor X_a since neither the zymogen factor X nor other coagulation factors displace bound factor X_a. Bovine platelets show minor differences with respect to human platelets [88,90]. They have about 800–900 factor V_a-binding sites with an apparent K_d of 400 pM. In contrast to human platelets, all the high-affinity bound factor V_a participates in the receptor site of factor X_a on bovine platelets, since at saturating concentrations of factor X_a, the ratio of platelet-bound factor X_a to platelet-bound factor V_a was found to be unity. Factor X_a binding occurs with an apparent K_d of 600 pM, and kinetic experiments indicate that this high-affinity binding is functional in prothrombin activation at the platelet surface.

Whether measuring the binding of a ligand to a cell surface has physiological importance is often difficult to ascertain. Relevance is inferred when binding correlates with some functional response. However, binding of factor V_a, and to a lesser extent also of factor X_a, to platelets is complex in that it is not simply hyperbolic, saturation is not reached, and a significant amount binds non-specifically and with low affinity (cf. Ch. 2A). Therefore, the number of physiological important binding sites can only be estimated from determining the number of functional prothrombinase complexes at the platelet surface using conditions approaching maximal velocity of prothrombin conversion by factor X_a–V_a in the presence of optimal calcium concentrations. Assuming that the turnover number (k_{cat}) of the enzymatic prothrombinase unit (factor X_a, V_a and Ca^{2+}) is the same when it is bound to negatively charged phospholipids or to platelets, the number of functional units on unstimulated platelets can be calculated from the rate of thrombin formation (Table 1). Taking into account that the number of enzymatic units at saturating prothrombin concentration equals the number of functional binding sites, there appear to be 2500 sites for prothrombinase at the outer surface of human platelets [92]. This is in good agreement with the number of high-affinity sites for factor V_a derived from binding experiments [91]. The same approach can be used to calculate the number of binding sites for the factor X-activating complex composed of factor IX_a and VIII_a in the presence of optimal Ca^{2+} concentrations. A maximal number of about 900 functional sites can be derived for the factor X-activating complex on unstimulated human platelets [92] (Table 1). At present, no binding parameters for these coagulation factors and platelets are available from binding measurements.

TABLE 1

Non-activated human platelets: procoagulant activity and functional binding sites

	Rate/5×10^6 platelets/ml	Functional sites/platelet
Prothrombin activation	34.4 nM thrombin/min	2550 X_a–V_a sites
Factor X activation	2.3 nM X_a/min	920 IX_a–VIII_a sites

The number of functional procoagulant sites per platelet is calculated with the formula:

$$\text{number of sites/platelet} = \frac{\text{rate}}{k_{cat}} \times 10^{-9} \times N/\text{platelets} \cdot l^{-1}$$

k_{cat} prothrombin activation = 2700/min [92]; k_{cat} factor X activation = 500/min [92]; N = Avogadro's number.

The fact that the number of sites for the factor X-activating complex is smaller than that for the prothrombinase complex does not necessarily exclude that there may be gross similarities in the nature of both sites. Both complexes assemble on phospholipid surfaces but the optimal phospholipid requirement has been shown to be somewhat different for the two enzymatic complexes, and to depend on the concentration of the non-enzymatic cofactors V_a or VIII_a [92]. Also, prothrombinase activity at the platelet surface is reduced when factors VIII_a and IX_a are added and vice versa, suggesting competition for similar binding domains at the outer surface of the membrane. Since factor V_a promotes the binding of factor X_a to the platelet surface, factor V_a has been proposed to be the receptor for factor X_a [89]. The term 'receptor' may be confusing, however, since it differs from the classical concept of a membrane receptor in that factor V_a is not a conventional membrane protein but associates with platelets (or negatively charged phospholipids) with high affinity after being formed from its precursor factor V. Although the dissociation constant of factor V_a for negatively charged phospholipid has been reported to be 2 orders of magnitude larger than that for platelets [85], these data have been questioned in a recent study [86] showing a dissociation constant of 50 pM for phospholipid vesicles containing 20% phosphatidylserine, i.e. binding properties similar if not identical to those for platelets. Moreover, factor V_a bound to phospholipid promotes binding of factor X_a with an apparent dissociation constant that is indistinguishable from binding of factor X_a to platelet-bound factor V_a [93]. Regardless of whether the enzymatic complex was composed of factor X_a, Ca^{2+} and plasma factor V_a plus negatively charged phospholipid, or activated platelets instead of the latter two components, similar specific activities were observed. It has also been mentioned that des(1–44)factor X_a, which lacks 44 amino acid residues at the NH_2-terminal end including all of the γ-carboxyglutamic acids, has a more than 100 times weaker affinity than factor X_a for factor V_a associated to platelets [91]. Since des(1–44)factor X_a is equivalent to factor X_a in its ability to interact with factor V_a in free solution and in its catalytic activity towards prothrombin, this indicates that binding of factor X_a to its platelet receptor not only involves binding to platelet-bound factor V_a but also requires interaction between the γ-carboxyglutamic acid-rich domain near the NH_2-terminus and some platelet membrane component. Conflicting evidence has been proposed to claim that this component would be a specific protein receptor at the platelet surface (cf. [89,91] and Ch. 2A). It was shown that a monoclonal antibody reactive towards negatively charged phospholipid inhibited prothrombin activation in the presence of phospholipids, but not when platelets were substituted for phospholipids [94]. It went apparently unnoticed [91] that this antibody failed to react with negatively charged phospholipids when presented in the form of lysed platelets or red cells, invalidating it as evidence against the involvement of phospholipids in platelet prothrombinase activity. Moreover, in a recent study [95] prothrombinase activity in the presence of platelets as well as phospholipids was shown to be completely blocked by a particular lupus antibody with specificity for negatively charged phospholipids, supporting the notion that negatively charged phospholipids are important for the activation of prothrombin on the surface of platelets. Another argument that has been forwarded to indicate that a membrane protein component would be required stems from studies with platelets from a patient with a moderately severe bleeding disorder, who had normal plasma coagulation factors and platelet factor V but prolonged clotting times in the presence of platelets [96]. This patient's platelets showed abnormal binding of factor X_a accompanied by lower factor X_a-catalyzed prothrombin activation [97]. It remains unclear, however, why this would be caused by a deficiency of a certain membrane protein receptor, since these platelets have been shown to be equally impaired in their ability to promote the other 'lipid-dependent' reaction, i.e. factor X activation [142].

Involvement of phospholipid in platelet prothrombinase activity would require the presence of negatively charged phospholipids at the platelet outer surface. The major negatively charged phospholipid, phosphatidylserine, is predominantly confined to the cytoplasmic surface of the plasma membrane, although minor amounts of this lipid may be present in the exterior leaflet of the membrane [11,12,77,98]. We have demonstrated that prothrombinase activity in the presence of unstimulated platelets can be completely blocked by treatment of platelets with certain phospholipases using conditions where cell lysis is negligible [99]. Only those phospholipases that can exert their activity towards intact cells and are able to degrade phosphatidylserine (i.e. phospholipase A_2 from *N. naja* and bee venom), inhibit platelet prothrombinase activity (Fig. 3). In contrast, phospholipases which cannot exert their action towards intact cells (*B. cereus* phospholipase C and *C. adamanteus* phospholipase A_2), or attack the membrane but do not degrade phosphatidylserine (*S. aureus* sphingomyelinase), fail to produce any inhibition of platelet prothrombinase activity. Similarly, both phospholipase A_2 from *N. naja* and bee venom also completely abolish factor X-converting activity of non-stimulated platelets [92]. Proteolytic pretreatment of platelets is, however, without effect on both procoagulant activities. Since phospholipases have no effect on prothrombin and factor X activation in free solution, these observations strongly suggest that minor amounts of phosphatidylserine are implicated in the assembly of both complexes at the surface of unstimulated platelets. Therefore, there is at

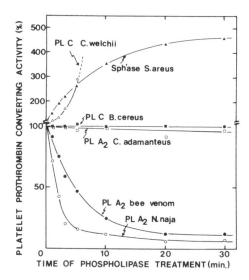

Fig. 3. Prothrombinase activity of unstimulated platelets treated with different phospholipases. PL, phospholipase (PLC from *C. welchii* produces cell lysis).

present no necessity to postulate that prothrombin and factor X activation at the platelet surface would be essentially different from that at the surface of phospholipid vesicles.

(b) Activity of stimulated platelet

It was originally proposed that platelet stimulation by thrombin was required to induce the high-affinity factor X_a-binding sites at the outer surface [100–102]. Apparently, this is due to release and activation of factor V from the platelets, thereby promoting the binding of factor X_a to the outer surface. This requirement for platelet factor V was inferred from experiments showing that thrombin-stimulated platelets treated with an antibody to factor V as well as stimulated factor V-deficient platelets had decreased factor X_a binding and factor X_a-catalyzed prothrombin activation [103]. Activation of human platelets with thrombin expresses the same number of high-affinity binding sites for factor X_a as unstimulated platelets to which exogenous factor V_a is added. This strongly suggests that activation by thrombin does not result in the formation of new membrane domains that promote assembly of the prothrombinase complex. Also, sufficient factor V is released and activated to saturate factor X_a binding [91]. In contrast, bovine platelets contain less factor V molecules than high-affinity sites for factor V_a at the outer surface, and thrombin-induced release does therefore not saturate factor X_a binding unless exogenous factor V_a is available [88,90].

It will be clear from the foregoing that platelets can be considered to provide a phospholipid-like surface to which factor V_a binds thereby promoting high-affinity

TABLE 2

Activated human platelets: procoagulant activity and functional binding sites

Activator	Prothrombin activation		Factor X activation	
	Rate	Sites	Rate	Sites
ADP (10 μM)	36	2 670	2	920
Thrombin (2 nM)	40	2 965	3	1 200
Collagen (10 μg/ml)	98	7 260	18	7 200
Collagen + thrombin	352	26 090	47	18 800
A23187 (1 μM)	793	58 780	94	37 600
Diamide (5 mM)	356	26 390	45	18 000
Lysed platelets	1 170	86 730	149	59 600

For calculations consult Table 1.

binding of factor X_a. The association constant of factor X_a alone for platelets and phospholipids is at least 3 orders of magnitude less than that of factor V_a, but factor X_a can be visualized to acquire high-affinity binding to a membrane surface due to its combined interaction with bound factor V_a and negatively charged phospholipids. A similar situation can be imagined for the factor X-activating complex, i.e. factor VIII_a and IX_a. In order to establish whether platelets, activated by various stimulators, show increased functional binding of both complexes the effect of various platelet activation procedures should be preferably compared at saturating concentrations of coagulation factors. This is particularly important for prothrombinase, to make it independent from release and activation of factor V. Under these conditions, the activity of various stimulated platelet preparations has been compared in prothrombin and factor X activation [77,92,98,104] (Table 2). Relative to control platelets, stimulation by thrombin hardly shows a rise in activity. This is consistent with binding data from the literature [89,101] showing that thrombin activation does not significantly change the number of membrane sites that bind the factor X_a–V_a complex. Also, ADP, PAF, serotonin, epinephrine and arachidonic acid are without effect, but collagen produces a substantial (3–7-fold) increase in the capacity of platelets to stimulate prothrombin and factor X activation. Platelets stimulated by the combined action of collagen and thrombin promote a 10-fold increase in prothrombin activation and a 20-fold increase in factor X activation. Therefore, the effect of collagen alone may in fact be brought about by a combination of collagen plus thrombin, since thrombin is rapidly formed in the prothrombinase assay and is also present in the assay system to measure factor X activation because factor VIII has to be activated by thrombin just before addition to the system. The most potent activation occurs with the non-physiological Ca-ionophore A23187, producing an activity increase in prothrombin and factor X activation which is twice as high as observed with collagen plus thrombin. Also diamide, an SH-oxidizing compound, stimulates platelets to become active in both procoagulant enzymatic reactions. In contrast to other activators, this occurs in the absence of release and aggregation. The highest increase in prothrombin and factor X activation is observed with completely lysed platelets, presumably representing a situation where the maximal amount of procoagulant phospholipid is exposed to the coagulation factors. To test the notion that the procoagulant surface of activated platelets also has a 'phospholipid-like' nature, platelets were first stimulated with collagen plus thrombin and then treated with *N. naja* phospholipase A_2 under conditions preventing significant cell lysis. Both prothrombin- and factor X-converting activities were almost completely abolished to values below those of unstimulated platelets. Since both activities were measured with saturating concentrations of coagulation factors, the increase in enzymatic activity upon platelet stimulation is proportional to the increase in functional binding sites at the platelet surface (Table 2). Thus, the highest state of activation by physiological stimulators, i.e. collagen plus thrombin, would represent some 26 000 binding sites for the complex of factors X_a and V_a and about 19 000 sites for the complex of factors IX_a and VIII_a. These numbers are sufficiently close to suggest that similar sites participate in prothrombin and factor X activation, also since increase in platelet prothrombinase activity resulting from a certain activation procedure is accompanied by a similar increase in factor X-converting activity. It should be noted, that the binding sites can be considered to be associated with the cell surface since less than 10% of the 'procoagulant effect' remained in the supernatant after centrifuging activated platelets at $7000 \times g$ for 5 min.

At first sight, it may look surprising that simultaneous (or sequential) platelet activation by two of the most potent stimulants is required to evoke maximal procoagulant activity. This situation, however, is not particularly unphysiological since combined triggering of platelets is likely to occur in situ. Upon vessel wall injury platelets will be activated by subendothelial collagen and traces of thrombin formed early in the hemostatic process; in fact, it can hardly be imagined that platelet activation in situ would occur with one single activator only. As required for the induction of platelet release and aggregation, it is essential that platelets are stirred during the activation procedure to evoke procoagulant activity [92]. Moreover, extracellular Ca^{2+} is required and no procoagulant activity is produced in the presence of calcium channel blockers dilthiazem and verapamil [105]. It is also of interest that platelets treated with prostacyclin or dibutyryl-cAMP lose their capability to become procoagulant when treated with collagen plus thrombin [106]. Aspirin, however, does not inhibit indicating that thromboxane A_2 formation is not an essential requirement for the generation of a procoagulant lipid surface. The two types of arterial wall collagens, i.e. collagen type I and type III, are equally effective in combination with thrombin. The effect of collagen can be completely abolished by a collagen-derived octapeptide [107], in that the activity of collagen-plus-thrombin-activated platelets is reduced to that of thrombin-activated platelets [105]. For the activation by collagen plus thrombin it is also essential that the active center of thrombin is not blocked. DIP–thrombin binds to platelets with the same affinity and number of binding sites as thrombin [108]. However, no procoagulant activity is produced above the level of collagen alone when collagen plus thrombin is replaced by collagen plus DIP-thrombin [105]. In combination with collagen, thrombin can be replaced, however, by γ-thrombin, trypsin or α-clostripain without significant loss in the extent of generating procoagulant activity. These enzymes have in common with thrombin that they split glycoprotein V at the platelet outer surface [4], suggesting that this event is a prerequisite (in combination with platelet binding to collagen) for the generation of a procoagulant surface. Indeed, when collagen plus thrombin is replaced by collagen plus enzymes with different substrate specificity, such as chymotrypsin, thermolysin and pronase, no procoagulant activity above that observed with collagen alone is generated.

4. Membrane phenomena in relation to platelet procoagulant activity

Although the platelet plasma membrane has many functions in common with plasma membranes of other cell types, it also performs a number of functions with regard to platelet hemostatic activities. An important part of this concerns its interaction with coagulation factors resulting in increased complex formation ensuring rapid generation of thrombin. It is very likely that membrane phospholipids actively participate in this process, while platelet activation by certain stimulants seems to improve the hemostatic performance of the plasma membrane. It is obvious that this phenomenon implies structural reorganization of membrane architecture, not only in its phospholipid complement but presumably also in its protein part since lipid organization in biological membranes is considered to be governed by membrane proteins. In this section, a number of membrane phenomena relevant for platelet procoagulant activities will be discussed.

(a) Intact versus lysed cells

Maximal exposure of procoagulant (i.e. negatively charged) phospholipid is obviously attained when platelets are completely lysed either by freezing and thawing or by sonication. This is reflected in maximal prothrombin- and factor X-converting activities of the platelet preparations (see Table 2). Moreover, when platelets are gradually disrupted by sonication at limited output of the sonifier, the loss of cytoplasmic lactate dehydrogenase to the supernatant runs in parallel with the increase in both procoagulant activities [104]. This strongly suggests that only limited amounts of negatively charged phospholipids at the outer surface of intact unstimulated platelets are available for interaction with coagulation factors, while disturbance of the membrane permeability barrier exposing the inner leaflet of the plasma membrane (as well as intracellular membranes) unmasks the majority of procoagulant phospholipid. The conspicuous difference in procoagulant activity between intact and lysed platelets is not at all specific for platelets. Table 3 shows a comparison of the capacity of intact and lysed blood cell preparations, as well as their phospholipid extracts, to promote prothrombinase activity under conditions where total phospholipid concentration is the same in each preparation. A dra-

TABLE 3

Activity of blood cells and their lipids in thrombin formation by factor X_a in the presence of factor V_a and calcium

	Rate of thrombin formation (nM/min)		
	Intact cells	Lysed cells	Phospholipid extract
Platelets	34	1170	1153
Erythrocytes	12	1137	1151
Leukocytes	8	910	1172
Endothelial	11	1056	1130

Phospholipid concentration is 1 μM in all cases, corresponding to 5×10^6 platelets/ml.

matic increase in the rate of thrombin formation is observed when the different blood cells are ruptured, and no significant differences are apparent between the different cells. Moreover, prothrombinase activity of lysed cells equals that of their lipid extracts suggesting that no components other than phospholipids are responsible for this effect. Both in platelets and in red cells, negatively charged phospholipids (phosphatidylserine and phosphatidylinositol) are almost absent from the outer leaflet of the plasma membrane [11–14,109,110]. This can easily explain the large difference in prothrombinase activity between intact and lysed cells. The similar behavior of leukocytes and endothelial cells strongly suggests that negatively charged phospholipids are predominantly confined to the cytoplasmic leaflet of the plasma membrane and to the subcellular organelles of these cells. Therefore, the asymmetric phospholipid distribution as observed for red cells and platelets may be uniformly present in all blood cells, and cells lining the vessel wall. Such a situation can be imagined to serve a physiological function in avoiding thrombosis and regulating hemostasis.

The relatively small activity of (unstimulated) intact cells may be real but might just as well result from minor cell lysis due to handling of the preparations in vitro. Considering that the prothrombinase activity in the presence of intact red cells, leukocytes and endothelial cells is some 100 times smaller than in the presence of the respective lysed cell preparations, activity of intact cells could be easily produced by 1% of the cell population being lysed. The activity of intact platelets is 3–4 times higher than that of other cell preparations. Since measurements of lactate dehydrogenase in the supernatant suggest cell lysis to be less than 1%, activity should be attributed to small amounts of phosphatidylserine already present at the exterior face of the plasma membrane. From a physiological point of view it can be imagined that the presence of procoagulant sites on unstimulated platelets would represent a situation with potential risk for undesired clotting. This raises the intriguing question of whether activity of unstimulated platelets, in as far as it cannot be explained by minor cell lysis, would originate from a minor fraction of platelets that has been activated in the circulation just prior to drawing the blood. Indeed, activated platelets in the circulation have been detected by measuring the extent of degranulation reflected in a decrease of buoyant density of the platelets, and increased levels of less dense platelets were shown to occur after cardiopulmonary bypass [111].

(b) Reorientation of membrane phospholipids

The importance of platelet lipids in the hemostatic properties of these cells has evoked an interest in possible alterations in exposure of phospholipids at the outer surface during platelet activation. Two inherent difficulties accompany the determination of the orientation of the membrane phospholipids in activated platelets. First, aggregation of platelets results in intimate platelet–platelet contact and may therefore reduce the amount of outer surface accessible for the probing agent. Second, fusion of granular membranes with the plasma membrane during the release reaction will increase the amount of phospholipids in the surface membrane or may even alter its phospholipid composition. This imposes certain limitations as to the accuracy with which the total amount of phospholipid exposed at the outer surface can be measured. Therefore, the best one can say is that the lipids which are available for a non-permeable probing agent at the outside of intact activated platelets are (at least temporarily) located at the outer surface, but the location of the lipids that do not react remains uncertain. The first indication for an alteration in phospholipid orientation in activated platelets was obtained by comparing the reaction of the non-permeable probe TNBS on thrombin-activated and control platelets [112]. In activated platelet preparations, some 25% of the phosphatidylethanolamine could be labeled being twice as much as observed with unactivated platelets. No labeling of phosphatidylserine could be detected, either in thrombin-activated or in control platelets. The main disadvantage of using probes such as TNBS is that the reaction is generally slow, incomplete, and limited to aminophospholipid. The use of phospholipases as tools to probe the phospholipid

TABLE 4

Composition of phospholipid fractions hydrolyzed by phospholipase A_2 and sphingomyelinase treatment of activated human platelets

	Unactivated	Activated by				
		Thrombin	Collagen	Collagen + thrombin	Diamide	A23187
PS	2.4	4.9	6.0	11.2	13.4	12.6
PC	31.0	39.3	41.4	33.9	39.0	29.5
PE	9.5	15.5	17.0	36.0	25.8	35.8
SM	57.1	40.2	35.6	18.7	21.7	22.0
Hydrolyzed fraction as % of total phospholipid	21	32	34	44	39	65

Values are expressed as percentage of the hydrolyzed fraction. PS, phosphatidylserine; PC, phosphatidylcholine; PE, phosphatidylethanolamine; SM, sphingomyelin.

orientation in biological membranes has the advantage over chemical reagents that a proper combination of them can in principle react with all phospholipid classes, and that reaction goes to completion. Although there are numerous pitfalls using phospholipases in sidedness studies [113,114], it appears possible to obtain detailed information on the outer surface orientation of phospholipids in a variety of activated platelets [98,115]. Table 4 shows the maximal attainable amount, as well as the composition, of the phospholipids that can be degraded by treatment of activated platelets with a mixture of sphingomyelinase and phospholipase A_2, in the absence of or prior to the onset of cell lysis [98]. With control platelets, some 21% of the total phospholipids can be hydrolyzed in the absence of cell lysis, representing the phospholipid fraction in the external leaflet of the plasma membrane. This fraction is mainly composed of choline-phospholipids, sphingomyelin and phosphatidylcholine, whereas the exposure of aminophospholipids (particularly phosphatidylserine) is limited. Activation of platelets by collagen or by thrombin prior to addition of phospholipases results in 32–35% of phospholipid hydrolysis. Relative to unactivated platelets, the surface-exposed fraction is somewhat less rich in sphingomyelin and this decrease is mainly compensated by an increase in phosphatidylethanolamine and phosphatidylcholine. It is difficult to ascertain whether or not phosphatidylserine is also increased in thrombin- or collagen-activated platelets, since for unknown reasons relatively large standard deviations are observed. Activation of platelets by a mixture of collagen plus thrombin, however, produces a quite different phospholipid pattern that is susceptible to exogenous phospholipases. The hydrolyzed phospholipid fraction shows a sharp increase in phosphatidylserine and phosphatidylethanolamine and a remarkable decrease in sphingomyelin. A very similar phenomenon is observed when platelets treated by diamide or by Ca-ionophore A23187 are subjected to treatment with phospholipases. Remarkably, some 65% of the phospholipids of ionophore-treated platelets can be degraded prior to the onset of cell lysis. As extensively discussed in ref. 98, the changes in phospholipid composition of the outer membrane leaflet of platelets activated by thrombin or collagen are mainly caused by the secretory event (release reaction), which involves fusion of granular membranes with the plasma membrane. On the other hand, the increased surface exposure of phosphatidylserine accompanied with a decreased exposure of sphingomyelin in platelets activated by collagen plus thrombin, diamide, or ionophore, presumably results from an induced transbilayer movement of phospholipids as a result of the activation procedure.

(c) Significance of altered phospholipid orientation

Since phosphatidylserine is the major negatively charged phospholipid in platelet membranes, its increased localization in the exterior half of the platelet plasma membrane can be expected to improve the procoagulant properties of platelets. From the data in Table 4, the percentage of total phosphatidylserine exposed at the exterior surface of platelets activated by various means can be calculated, and compared with the prothrombinase activity of the respective platelet preparations. As shown in Fig. 4, unstimulated platelets have little phosphatidylserine exposed at their outer surface, and this is reflected in the relatively poor capacity of resting platelets to stimulate the formation of thrombin by factors X_a and V_a in the presence of calcium. Depending on the activation procedure, platelets expose different amounts of phosphatidylserine at the outer surface, and the more phosphatidylserine they expose the higher is their capacity to stimulate prothrombinase activity. It should be realized, however, that the procoagulant activity of a membrane phospholipid surface is not solely dependent on the concentration of negatively charged phospholipid. The relationship is extremely complicated, and certainly depends on the nature of neutral phospholipids present in the membrane surface. It is obvious from Table 4 that an increase of phosphatidylserine in the outer leaflet is not the only result of platelet activation, but that this process is also accompanied by a drastic change in the phospholipid composition of this leaflet. Besides a rise in phosphatidylserine, there is also a considerable increase in phosphatidylethanolamine and a dramatic decrease in sphingomyelin, while phosphatidylcholine remains relatively constant. Reducing the content of sphingomyelin in the outer surface may indirectly contribute to the expression of procoagulant activity by negatively charged phospholipids. For example, when the prothrombinase activity of artificial lipid vesicles containing 10% of phosphatidylserine and 90% of choline-phospholipid is measured under the conditions used for platelets, the rate of

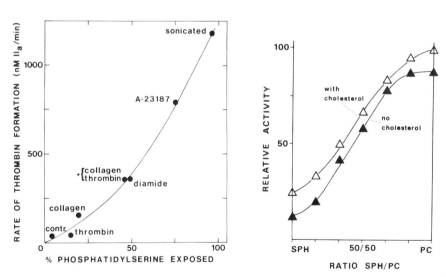

Fig. 4. Correlation between exposure of phosphatidylserine and prothrombinase activity of human platelets (contr., unstimulated platelet).

Fig. 5. Prothrombinase activity as function of the sphingomyelin:phosphatidylcholine ratio in phosphatidylserine-containing vesicles. Vesicle composition = 90 mole% (sphingomyelin (Sph) + phosphatidylcholine (PC)), 10 mole% phosphatidylserine, with or without 50 mole% cholesterol.

thrombin formation strongly depends on the ratio of sphingomyelin to phosphatidylcholine in these vesicles (Fig. 5). Vesicles which only contain sphingomyelin in addition to phosphatidylserine are much less active than vesicles in which sphingomyelin is replaced by phosphatidylcholine. Also, addition of cholesterol which is a naturally occurring lipid with a high affinity for sphingomyelin [116] does not influence this effect. Therefore, the relationship between platelet prothrombinase activity and surface-oriented phosphatidylserine as shown in Fig. 4 is an over-simplification, though demonstrating the relative importance of this effect. The decreased exposure of sphingomyelin can be expected to favor the expression of procoagulant activity by negatively charged phospholipids. In addition, the increased exposure of phosphatidylethanolamine might also have an influence on the procoagulant properties of the platelet outer surface [13]. Phosphatidylethanolamine by itself does not stimulate prothrombin or factor X activation, but can modulate the procoagulant activity of negatively charged phospholipids.

(d) Membranes of pathological platelets

The ability of platelets to alter their membrane phospholipid orientation upon platelet activation, can be expected to require the participation of other platelet (membrane) components or certain activation phenomena. In this respect, the behavior of a number of different pathological platelets is of interest, since most of these are known to be based on molecular or structural defects. In Table 5, prothrombinase activity of a number of pathological platelets is compared, before and after activation by collagen plus thrombin. Experiments were carried out using saturating amounts of coagulation factors in order to make the reaction independ-

TABLE 5

Prothrombinase activity of pathological platelets

	Platelet abnormality	Prothrombinase activity/10^6 platelets/ml (nM II_a/min)	
		Non-stimulated	Stimulated by collagen plus thrombin
Normal (n=13)	None	2–7	53–89
Thrombasthenia (n=5)	GP IIb–III deficient	3–9	42–78
Gray platelet (n=3)	α-Granule deficient	0.1–8	67–145
Hermansky–Pudlak (n=3)	δ-Bodies deficient	2–5	37–67
Bernard–Soulier (n=5)	GPIb (GPV) deficient	26–83	117–232

Activity given as range.

ent of release and activation of factor V. It is evident that platelets from storage pool deficiencies (i.e. gray platelet and Hermansky–Pudlak syndrome) exhibit a normal behavior with respect to prothrombinase activity. This can be taken to indicate that the release reaction is not a prerequisite for the exposure of a procoagulant lipid surface to occur at the exterior of the platelet membrane. This is consistent with the notion outlined earlier [98], that negatively charged phosphatidylserine is not brought to the outer surface as a result of the secretory event, which involves fusion between subcellular and plasma membranes. Since intracellular membranes of platelets do contain phosphatidylserine [117], this would imply that its location is restricted to the outer leaflet (i.e. cytoplasmic surface) of the granule membrane, which remains cytoplasmically oriented after the fusion process. Besides release, also platelet aggregation does not seem to be required for inducing a procoagulant surface. Platelets obtained from patients with Glanzmann's thrombasthenia fail to aggregate upon addition of collagen plus thrombin, but apart from normal release they exhibit a similar increase in prothrombinase activity as observed with normal platelets. Since these platelets show partial or complete deficiencies in membrane glycoproteins IIb and III [40,41], the involvement of these proteins in mediating transbilayer movement of phospholipids in platelet membranes can be excluded. On the other hand, platelets from patients with Bernard–Soulier syndrome exhibit a quite deviating behavior regarding their prothrombinase activity. In the unstimulated form, they are some 10 times more active than normal platelets. Stimulation by collagen plus thrombin produces some 3-fold increase in prothrombinase activity to reach levels that are somewhat higher than those obtained with activated normal platelets. Bernard–Soulier platelets have a characteristic deficiency of glycoprotein Ib [40,41], while deficiencies of glycoprotein V have also been reported [118]. In addition, they have an abnormally large size which may point to defects in cytoskeletal organization. It is also of interest that Bernard–Soulier platelets have been reported to display an abnormal phospholipid sidedness in their plasma membrane [119]. Without activation, the proportion of phosphatidylserine and phosphatidylethanolamine in the outer leaflet of the plasma membrane is increased at the expense of sphingomyelin. This situation markedly resembles the altered phospholipid orientation in activated normal platelets, and may in fact explain why unstimulated Bernard–Soulier platelets exhibit an increased prothrombinase activity. It remains to be established whether this is related to a genuine disturbance of membrane asymmetry, or to a partly activated state of the platelets induced during circulation due to an increased susceptibility towards activators.

(e) Possible mechanisms of phosphatidylserine exposure

Three distinct possibilities should be considered which can explain the increased availability of aminophospholipids at the exterior surface of activated platelets. First, aminophospholipids may be already present in considerable amounts at the outer surface of unstimulated platelets but they are segregated in distinct pools, e.g. shielded by interaction with certain membrane proteins, making them unavailable for chemical probes and phospholipases, as well as for interaction with coagulation factors. Non-reactivity of phospholipids at the outer surface towards phospholipases has been observed for mycoplasma hominis, but shielding was abolished after pretreatment with proteolytic enzymes [120]. However, proteolytic treatment of platelets does not increase the availability of phosphatidylserine for chemical probes [112]. Moreover, close to half of the plasma membrane phospholipids can be attacked by treatment of intact platelets with a suitable combination of phospholipases. This suggests but does not prove that, in analogy to erythrocytes, phosphatidylserine is virtually absent from the membrane exterior of resting platelets. Secondly, aminophospholipids might be brought to the cell surface during membrane fusion accompanying platelet release reaction. As discussed above, this mechanism may be operative for the increased exposure of phosphatidylethanolamine (e.g. after thrombin stimulation), but does not explain why phosphatidylserine appears to a significant extent at the outer surface when platelets are activated by a mixture of collagen and thrombin. Thirdly, the increased exposure of phosphatidylserine results from an increased transbilayer mobility of phospholipids. This may tend to a more random distribution of phospholipids and would therefore explain why increased availability of phosphatidylserine at the outer surface is accompanied by a decrease in sphingomyelin, since these two lipids have the most asymmetric orientation in resting platelets.

It is becoming increasingly obvious that flip-flop of phospholipids, the process whereby lipids move from one monolayer of the membrane to the other, can occur at significant rates when irregularities in the bilayer structure occur [121]. In artificial bilayer vesicles, transbilayer movement can be induced by introducing different physical properties between outer and inner monolayer, by insertion of bilayer-spanning proteins, and by triggering the formation of non-bilayer arrangements in the lipid bilayer. In addition, increased transbilayer movement of phospholipids in red cell membranes has been shown to occur when cytoskeletal organization becomes disturbed [122–124]. We have obtained some evidence that formation of non-bilayer structures as well as changes in cytoskeleton formation upon platelet activation might be involved in phospholipid flip-flop across the plasma membranes.

(i) Formation of non-bilayer structures

It has been known for many years that hydrated lipids can adopt a variety of phases in addition to the bilayer phase [125]. Also, certain lipids do not accommodate easily to the bilayer structure and tend to adopt non-bilayer arrangements within the bilayer [126]. These structures have been demonstrated using ^{31}P-NMR and freeze-fracture electron microscopy, and include cylindrical hexagonal phases as well as its limiting case, the inverted lipid micelle. In particular, lipids which are cone-shaped with the polar head group at the smaller end of the cone tend to form hexagonal structures with the polar head group inside. Examples of these are phosphatidylethanolamine, phosphatidic acid and (monoglucosyl)diglycerides. It

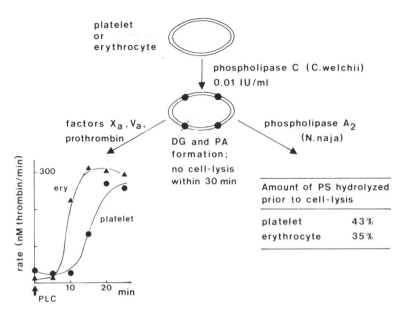

Fig. 6. Prothrombinase activity of platelets and erythrocytes and exposure of phosphatidylserine during treatment with *C. welchii* phospholipase C. DG, diacylglycerol; PA, phosphatidic acid; PS, phosphatidylserine.

has been shown both for red cells [127] and platelets [128], that introduction of diglycerides in the membrane by the action of exogenously added phospholipase C from *C. welchii* results in the formation of phosphatidic acid. This suggests a transbilayer movement of diglycerides to the inner aspect of the membrane where diglyceride kinase and ATP are available. Treatment of platelets with this phospholipase also elicits release and aggregation, and eventually leads to lysis of the cells [129]. However, using a particular combination of phospholipases, it could be demonstrated that before the onset of lysis substantial amounts of phosphatidylserine appear at the external surface [130]. This phenomenon is accompanied by a strongly increased ability of these platelets to promote thrombin formation in the presence of factors X_a, V_a, and calcium (Fig. 6). Remarkably, this behavior does not seem to be restricted to platelets. Treatment of red cells with this phospholipase C also leads to exposure of phosphatidylserine and these cells also acquire the property of stimulating prothrombinase activity. The amount of negatively charged phosphatidic acid formed during these incubations amounts to 2–4% (of total phospholipid) and this is too low to account for the observed prothrombinase activity. It is, however, of the same order as formed in activated platelets resulting from triggering of the phosphatidylinositol cycle [131,132]. The initial steps of this cycle are the conversion of phosphatidylinositol into diglyceride by an endogenous phospholipase C, followed by a phosphorylation catalyzed by diglyceride kinase to form phosphatidic acid. It is conceivable that triggering of the phosphatidylinositol cycle may, under certain conditions, produce threshold concentrations of diglyceride and phosphatidic acid, required to introduce non-bilayer arrangements in the membrane bilayer. These may perturb bilayer structure and form a locus for increased transbilayer mobility of phospholipids, leading to increased exposure of phosphatidylserine in the outer membrane leaflet.

(ii) Involvement of cytoskeletal proteins

There is increasing consensus in the literature that the membrane cytoskeleton plays a role in the maintenance of phospholipid asymmetry in biological membranes, particularly in the red cell membrane (see ref. 124 for a review). Therefore, loss of membrane phospholipid asymmetry can be suspected to be preceded or accompanied by alterations in the architecture of cytoskeletal proteins. The first

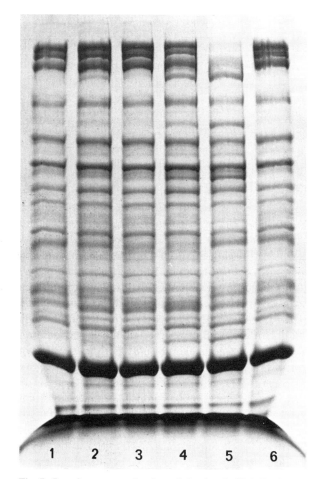

Fig. 7. Protein patterns of activated platelets in SDS–PAGE. Lane 1, unactivated platelet. Other lanes are from platelets activated by: 2, collagen; 3, thrombin; 4, collagen plus thrombin; 5, ionophore A23187; 6, ADP.

indication of the involvement of the cytoskeleton in phospholipid asymmetry was obtained from treatment of red cells with SH-oxidizing agents like diamide or tetrathionate [133]. Inner layer phospholipids became able to move to the outer leaflet upon oxidation of spectrin SH groups to disulfide bonds, which is paralleled by cross-linking of spectrin to form oligomers. As a result, an increased exposure of phosphatidylserine at the outer surface was demonstrated, while phosphatidylethanolamine even exhibited a random distribution over the two layers. Treatment of platelets with diamide also results in extensive polymerization of cytoskeletal proteins, particularly actin-binding protein (ABP), myosin and actin [134,135]. This process is also accompanied by increased exposure of aminophospholipids, formerly present in the internal leaflet of the membrane [98]. Apart from polymerization, hydrolysis of ABP in platelets is known to occur by endogenous calcium-dependent protease upon treatment of platelets with calcium ionophore A23187 in the presence of exogenous calcium chloride [136]. In this respect it is of interest that the extent of proteolysis of ABP upon platelet activation seems to correlate with the extent of exposure of phosphatidylserine at the platelet outer surface. As shown in Fig. 7, virtually complete hydrolysis of ABP is apparent when platelets plus exogenous $CaCl_2$ are treated with A23187, while partial degradation occurs upon platelet activation with a mixture of collagen and thrombin. Activation by collagen alone produces minor conversion of ABP, whereas thrombin activation is without effect on ABP hydrolysis. As shown above (Fig. 4), exposure of phosphatidylserine and concomitant platelet prothrombinase activity decrease in parallel with these series of platelet activation procedures. Moreover, when platelets are activated by collagen plus thrombin in the presence of calcium channel blockers dilthazem or verapamil no hydrolysis of ABP occurs, and, as mentioned before, no platelet prothrombinase activity is induced. This suggests that those platelet activation procedures which provoke transbilayer movement of phosphatidylserine require sufficient influx of calcium ions to activate calcium-dependent protease which subsequently degrades ABP.

It is interesting to note that ABP in platelets serves a similar function as spectrin in erythrocytes. Both proteins interact with F-actin, undergo reversible phosphorylation, and anti-spectrin antibodies cross-react with actin-binding proteins of different cells [137]. Spectrin has been shown to interact preferentially with negatively charged phospholipids like phosphatidylserine [138,139]. This interaction has been proposed to contribute to maintaining the cytoplasmic orientation of this lipid, since cross-linking of spectrin [133] or detachment from the membrane [140,141] allows phosphatidylserine to migrate to the outer leaflet. Whether or not induction of transmembrane movement of phospholipids upon degradation (or polymerization) of actin-binding protein occurs with a similar mechanism awaits further investigation.

References

1 Skaer, J. (1981) in: Platelets in Biology and Pathology (Gordon, J.L., Ed.) 2nd Vol., pp. 321–348, Elsevier, Amsterdam.

2 Behnke, O. (1970) Semin. Haematol. 3, 3–16.

3 White, J.G. and Gerrard, J.M. (1978) in: Platelets: A Multidisciplinary Approach (de Gaetano, G. and Garattini, S., Eds.) pp. 17–34, Raven, New York.

4 Berndt, M.C. and Phillips, D.R. (1981) in: Platelets in Biology and Pathology (Gordon, J.C., Ed.) 2nd Vol., pp. 44–75, Elsevier, Amsterdam.

5 Fox, J.E.B. and Phillips, D.R. (1983) Semin. Haematol. 20, 243–260.

6 Markey, F., Lindberg, V. and Eriksson, L. (1978) FEBS Lett. 88, 75–79.

7 Lind, S.E., Yin, H.L. and Stossel, T.P. (1982) J. Clin. Invest. 69, 1384–1387.

8 Sixma, J.J., Schiphorst, M.E. and Verhoeckx, C. (1982) Biochim. Biophys. Acta 704, 333–344.

9 Hartwig, J.H., Tyler, J. and Stossel, T.P. (1980) J. Cell. Biol. 87, 841–848.

10 Marcus, A.J., Ullman, H.L. and Safier, L.B. (1969) J. Lipid Res. 10, 108–114.

11 Perret, B., Chap, H. and Douste-Blazy, L. (1979) Biochim. Biophys. Acta 556, 434–446.

12 Chap, H., Zwaal, R.F.A. and van Deenen, L.L.M. (1977) Biochim. Biophys. Acta 467, 146–164.

13 Zwaal, R.F.A. (1978) Biochim. Biophys. Acta 515, 163–205.

14 Schick, P.K. (1979) Semin. Hematol. 16, 221–233.

15 White, J.G. (1972) Am. J. Pathol. 66, 295–312.

16 Käser-Glanzmann, R., Jakabova, M., George, J.N. and Lüscher, E.F. (1977) Biochim. Biophys. Acta 466, 429–440.

17 Käser-Glanzmann, R., Jakabova, M., George, J.N. and Lüscher, E.F. (1978) Biochim. Biophys. Acta 512, 1–12.

18 Gerrard, J.M., White, J.G. and Rao, G.H.R. (1976) Am. J. Pathol. 83, 283–298.

19 Holmsen, H. and Day, H.J. (1970) J. Lab. Clin. Med. 75, 840–852.

20 Broekman, M.J., Handin, R.I. and Cohen, P. (1974) Br. J. Haematol. 31, 51–63.

21 Broekman, M.J., Westmoreland, N.P. and Cohen, P. (1974) J. Cell. Biol. 60, 507–513.

22 Fukami, M.H. and Salganicoff, L. (1977) Thromb. Haemostas. 38, 963–970.

23 Kaplan, K.L. (1981) in: Platelets in Biology and Pathology (Gordon J.L., Ed.) 2nd Vol., pp. 77–90, Elsevier, Amsterdam.

24 Ross, R. and Vogel, A. (1978) Cell 14, 203–209.

25 Holmsen, H. (1972) Clin. Haematol. 1, 235–266.

26 Holmsen, H. (1977) Thromb. Haemostas. 38, 1030–1041.

27 Lüscher, E.F. and Massini, P. (1975) in: Biochemistry and Pharmacology of Platelets (Ciba Foundation Symp. 35) pp. 5–21, Elsevier/North-Holland, Amsterdam.

28 Salzman, E.W. (1972) New Engl. J. Med. 286, 358–363.

29 Bereziat, G. (1979) Agents Action, 9, 390–399.

30 Rodan, G.A. and Feinstein, M.G. (1976) Proc. Natl. Acad. Sci. (U.S.A.) 73, 1829–1833.

31 Bettex-Galland, M., Probst, E. and Behnke, O. (1972) J. Mol. Biol. 68, 533–535.

32 Weisenberg, R.C. (1972) Science 177, 1104–1105.

33 Papahadjopoulos, D. (1977) J. Coll. Interface Sci. 58, 459–470.

34 Baumgartner, H.R. (1977) Thromb. Haemostas. 37, 1–16.

35 Counts, R.B., Paskell, S.L. and Elgee, S.K. (1978) J. Clin. Invest. 62, 702–709.

36 Chiang, T.M. and Kang, A.H. (1982) J. Biol. Chem. 257, 7581–7586.

37 Kao, K.J., Pizzo, S.V. and McKee, P.A. (1979) J. Clin. Invest. 63, 656–664.

38 Sakariassen, K.S., Bolhuis, P.A. and Sixma, J.J. (1979) Nature (London) 279, 636–638.

39 Kao, K.J., Pizzo, S.V. and McKee, P.A. (1979) Proc. Natl. Acad. Sci. (U.S.A.) 76, 5317–5320.

40 Nurden, A.T. and Caen, J.P. (1976) Thromb. Haemostas. 35, 139–150.

41 Nurden, A.T. and Caen, J.P. (1977) Thromb. Haemostas. 39, 200–206.

42 Weiss, H.J., Tschopp, T.B. and Baumgartner, H.R. (1974) Am. J. Med. 57, 920–925.

43 Tschopp, T.B., Weiss, H.J. and Baumgartner, H.R. (1974) J. Lab. Clin. Med. 83, 296–300.

44 Born, G.V.R. (1970) J. Physiol. 209, 487–511.

45 Motamed, M., Michal, F. and Born, G.V.R. (1976) Biochem. J. 158, 655–657.
46 Kaplan, K.L., Broekman, M.J., Chernoff, A., Lesznik, G.R. and Drillings, M. (1979) Blood 53, 604–618.
47 Holmsen, H., Dangelmaier, C.A. and Holmsen, H.K. (1981) J. Biol. Chem. 256, 9393–9396.
48 Hamberg, M., Svensson, J. and Samuelson, B. (1975)
   Proc. Natl. Acad. Sci. (U.S.A.) 72, 2994–2998.
49 Smith, J.B. and Silver, M.J. (1973) Biochem. J. 131, 615–618.
50 Derksen, A. and Cohen, P. (1975) J. Biol. Chem. 250, 9342–9347.
51 Mauco, G., Chap, H., Simon, M.F. and Douste-Blazy, L. (1978) Biochimie 60, 653–661.
52 Rittenhouse-Simmons, S. (1979) J. Clin. Invest. 63, 580–587.
53 Bell, R.L. and Majerus, P.W. (1980) J. Biol. Chem. 255, 1790–1792.
54 Billah, M.M., Lapetina, E.G. and Cuatrecasas, P. (1980) J. Biol. Chem. 255, 10227–10231.
55 Roth, G.J. and Majerus, P.W. (1975) J. Clin. Invest. 56, 624–632.
56 Gerrard, J.M., Townsend, D., Stoddard, S., Witkop, C. and White, J.G. (1977) Am. J. Pathol. 86, 99–116.
57 Miller, O.V., Johnson, R.A. and Gorman, R.R. (1977) Prostaglandins 13, 599–605.
58 Moncada, S., Gryglewski, R.J., Bunting, S. and Vane, J.R. (1976) Prostaglandins 12, 715–737.
59 Gorman, R.R., Bunting, S. and Miller, O.V. (1977) Prostaglandins 13, 377–389.
60 Tateson, J.E., Moncada, S. and Vane, J.R. (1977) Prostaglandins 13, 389–397.
61 Weiss, H.J. (1980) Semin. Hematol. 17, 228–241.
62 Brinkhous, K.M., Read, M.S. and Mason, R.G. (1965) Lab. Invest. 14, 335–342.
63 Mustard, J.F., Packham, M.A., Kinlough-Rathbone, R.L., Perry, D.W. and Regoeczi, E. (1978) Blood 52, 453–466.
64 Mustard, J.F. and Packham, M.A. (1970) Pharmacol. Rev. 22, 97–187.
65 Jennings, L.K. and Phillips, D.R. (1982) J. Biol. Chem. 257, 10458–10466.
66 Hagen, I., Bjerrum, O.J. and Solum, N.O. (1979) Eur. J. Biochem. 99, 9–22.
67 Kunicki, R.J., Pidard, D., Rosa, J.P. and Nurden, A.T. (1981) Blood 58, 268–278.
68 Howard, L., Shulman, S., Sadamandan, S. and Karpatkin, S. (1982) J. Biol. Chem. 257, 8331–8336.
69 Bennett, J.S. and Vilaire, G. (1979) J. Clin. Invest. 64, 1392–1401.
70 Marguerie, G.A., Edgington, T.S. and Plow, E.F. (1980) J. Biol. Chem. 255, 154–161.
71 Lee, H., Nurden, A.T., Thomaidis, A. and Caen, J.P. (1981) Br. J. Haematol. 48, 47–57.
72 Walsh, P.N. (1972) Br. J. Haematol. 22, 237–254.
73 Walsh, P.N. (1972) Br. J. Haematol. 22, 393–405.
74 Walsh, P.N. and Griffin, J.H. (1981) Blood 57, 106–118.
75 Marcus, J.F. (1969) New Engl. J. Med. 280, 1213–1220.
76 Schiffman, S., Theodor, I. and Rapaport, S.I. (1969) Biochemistry 8, 1397–1405.
77 Bevers, E.M., Comfurius, P., Hemker, H.C. and Zwaal, R.F.A. (1982) Haemostasis 12, 268–274.
78 Chesney, C.M., Pifer, D.D. and Colman, R.W. (1983) Thromb. Res. 29, 75–84.
79 Breederveld, K., Giddings, J.C., ten Cate, J.W. and Bloom, A.L. (1975) Br. J. Haematol. 29, 405–412.
80 Chesney, C.M., Pifer, D.D. and Colman, R.W. (1981) Proc. Natl. Acad. Sci. (U.S.A.) 78, 5180–5184.
81 Hemker, H.C. and Kahn, M.J.P. (1967) Nature (London) 215, 1201–1202.
82 Walsh, P.N. (1978) Br. J. Haematol. 40, 311–331.
83 Shuman, M.A. and Majerus, P.W. (1977) J. Clin. Invest. 58, 1249–1258.
84 Suttie, J.W. and Jackson, C.M. (1977) Physiol. Rev. 57, 1–70.
85 Bloom, J.W., Nesheim, M.E. and Mann, K.G. (1979) Biochemistry 18, 4419–4425.
86 Pusey, M.L., Mayer, L.D., Wei, G.J., Bloomfield, V.A. and Nelsestuen, G.L. (1982) Biochemistry 21, 5262–5269.
87 Lajmanovich, A., Hudry-Clergeon, G., Freyssinet, J.M. and Marguerie, G. (1981) Biochim. Biophys. Acta 639, 132–136.
88 Tracy, P.B., Peterson, J.M., Nesheim, M.E., McDuffie, F.C. and Mann, K.G. (1979) J. Biol. Chem. 254, 10354–10361.

89 Kane, W.H., Lindhout, M.J., Jackson, C.M. and Majerus, P.W. (1980) J. Biol. Chem. 255, 1170–1174.
90 Tracy, P.B., Nesheim, M.E. and Mann, K.G. (1981) J. Biol. Chem. 256, 743–751.
91 Kane, W.H. and Majerus, P.W. (1982) J. Biol. Chem. 257, 3963–3969.
92 Rosing, J., van Rijn, J.L.M.L., Bevers, E.M., van Dieijen, G., Comfurius, P. and Zwaal, R.F.A. (1985) Blood 65, 319–332.
93 Nesheim, M.E., Taswell, J.B. and Mann, K.G. (1979) J. Biol. Chem. 254, 10952–10962.
94 Thiagarajan, P., Shapiro, S.S. and De Marco, L. (1980) J. Clin. Invest. 66, 397–405.
95 Dahlbäck, B., Nilsson, I.M. and Frohm, B. (1983) Blood 62, 218–225.
96 Weiss, H.J., Vicic, W.J., Lages, B.A. and Rogers, J. (1979) Am. J. Med. 67, 206–213.
97 Miletich, J.P., Kane, W.H., Hofmann, S.L., Stanford, N. and Majerus, P.W. (1979) Blood 54, 1015–1022.
98 Bevers, E.M., Comfurius, P. and Zwaal, R.F.A. (1983) Biochim. Biophys. Acta 736, 57–66.
99 Bevers, E.M., Comfurius, P. and Zwaal, R.F.A. (1982) Eur. J. Biochem. 122, 81–85.
100 Miletich, J.P., Jackson, C.M. and Majerus, P.W. (1977) Proc. Natl. Acad. Sci. (U.S.A.) 74, 4033–4036.
101 Miletich, J.P., Jackson, C.M. and Majerus, P.W. (1978) J. Biol. Chem. 253, 6908–6916.
102 Dahlbäck, B. and Stenflo, J. (1978) Biochemistry 17, 4938–4945.
103 Miletich, J.P., Majerus, D.W. and Majerus, P.W. (1978) J. Clin. Invest. 62, 824–831.
104 van Rijn, J., Rosing, J. and van Dieijen, G. (1983) Eur. J. Biochem. 133, 1–10.
105 Bevers, E.M., Karniguian, A., Legrand, Y.J. and Zwaal, R.F.A. (1985) Thromb. Res. 37, 365–370.
106 Zwaal, R.F.A., Comfurius, P., Hemker, H.C. and Bevers, E.M. (1984) Haemostasis, 14, 320–324.
107 Karniguian, A., Legrand, Y.J., Lefrancier, P. and Caen, J.P. (1983) Thromb. Res. 32, 593–604.
108 Tollefsen, D.M., Feagler, J.R. and Majerus, P.W. (1974) J. Biol. Chem. 249, 2646–2651.
109 Zwaal, R.F.A., Roelofsen, B., Comfurius, P. and van Deenen, L.L.M. (1975) Biochim. Biophys. Acta 406, 83–96.
110 Zwaal, R.F.A., Comfurius, P. and van Deenen, L.L.M. (1977) Nature (London) 268, 358–360.
111 van Oost, B., van Hien-Hagg, I.H., Timmermans, A.P.M. and Sixma, J.J. (1983) Blood 62, 433–438.
112 Schick, P.K., Kurica, K.B. and Chacko, G.K. (1976) J. Clin. Invest. 57, 1221–1226.
113 Op den Kamp, J.A.F. (1979) Annu. Rev. Biochem. 48, 47–71.
114 Zwaal, R.F.A. and Bevers, E.M. (1983) Subcell. Biochem. 9, 299–334.
115 Bevers, E.M., Comfurius, P., van Rijn, J.L.M.L., Hemker, H.C. and Zwaal, R.F.A. (1982) Eur. J. Biochem. 122, 429–436.
116 van Dijck, P.W.M. (1979) Biochim. Biophys. Acta 555, 89–101.
117 Barber, A.J. and Jamieson, G.A. (1970) J. Biol. Chem. 245, 6357–6365.
118 Nurden, A.T., Didry, B. and Rosa, J.P. (1983) Blood Cells 9, 333–358.
119 Perret, B., Levy-Toledano, S., Plantavid, M., Bredoux, R., Chap, H., Tobelem, G., Douste-Blazy, L. and Caen, J.P. (1983) Thromb. Res. 31, 529–537.
120 Rottem, S., Hasin, M. and Razin, S. (1973) Biochim. Biophys. Acta 323, 520–531.
121 van Deenen, L.L.M. (1981) FEBS Lett. 123, 3–15.
122 Franck, P.F.H., Roelofsen, B. and Op den Kamp, J.A.F. (1982) Biochim. Biophys. Acta 687, 105–108.
123 Franck, P.F.H., Chiu, D.T., Op den Kamp, J.A.F., Lubin, B., van Deenen, L.L.M. and Roelofsen, B. (1983) J. Biol. Chem. 257, 8435–8442.
124 Haest, C.W.M. (1982) Biochim. Biophys. Acta 694, 331–352.
125 Luzzatti, V. and Husson, F. (1962) J. Cell. Biol. 12, 207–219.
126 Cullis, P.R. and de Kruijff, B. (1979) Biochim. Biophys. Acta 559, 399–420.
127 Allan, B., Low, M.G., Finean, J.B. and Michell, R.H. (1975) Biochim. Biophys. Acta 413, 309–316.
128 Mauco, G., Chap, H., Simon, M.F. and Douste-Blazy, L. (1978) Biochimie 60, 653–661.
129 Chap, H. and Douste-Blazy, L. (1974) Eur. J. Biochem. 48, 351–356.
130 Comfurius, P., Bevers, E.M. and Zwaal, R.F.A. (1983) Biochem. Biophys. Res. Commun. 117, 803–808.

131 Lapetina, E.G. and Cuatrecasas, P. (1979) Biochim. Biophys. Acta 573, 394–402.
132 Bell, R.L. and Majerus, P.W. (1980) J. Biol. Chem. 255, 1790–1792.
133 Haest, C.W.M., Plasa, G., Kamp, B. and Deuticke, B. (1978) Biochim. Biophys. Acta 509, 21–32.
134 Davies, G.E. and Palek, J. (1982) Blood 59, 502–513.
135 Bosia, A., Spangenberg, P., Lösche, W., Arese, P. and Till, U. (1983) Thromb. Res. 30, 137–142.
136 McGowan, E.B., Yeo, K.T. and Detwiler, T.C. (1983) Arch. Biochem. Biophys. 227, 287–301.
137 Cohen, C.M. (1983) Semin. Haematol. 20, 141–158.
138 Marinetti, G.V. and Crain, R.C. (1978) J. Supramol. Struct. 8, 191–213.
139 Mombers, C., de Gier, J., Demel, R.A. and van Deenen, L.L.M. (1980) Biochim. Biophys. Acta 603, 52–62.
140 Lubin, B., Chiu, B., Bastacky, J., Roelofsen, B. and van Deenen, L.L.M. (1981) J. Clin. Invest. 67, 1643–1649.
141 Hill, J.S., Sawyer, W.J., Howlett, G.J. and Wiley, J.S. (1981) Biochem. J. 201, 259–266.
142 Rosing, J., Bevers, E.M., Comfurius, P., Hemker, H.C. van Dieijen, G., Weiss, H.J. and Zwaal, R.F.A. (1985) Blood 65, 1557–1561.

R.F.A. Zwaal and H.C. Hemker (Eds.), *Blood Coagulation*
© 1986 Elsevier Science Publishers B.V. (Biomedical Division)

CHAPTER 7

Fibrinogen, fibrin and factor XIII

AGNES HENSCHEN and JAN McDONAGH

*Max-Planck-Institut für Biochemie, D-8033 Martinsried bei München (F.R.G.),
and Beth Israel Hospital, 330 Brooklyn Avenue, Boston, MA 02215 (U.S.A.)*

1. Fibrinogen and fibrin

(a) Introduction

The importance of blood coagulation was recognized already several thousand years ago, and blood and blood flow were considered as essential for life. Hippocrates and Aristotle taught that all life processes take place in the blood, and one specific blood clot component which now can be identified as fibrin was indeed regarded as the symbol for one of the 4 elements, the 'water' or 'phlegm'. The amount of 'phlegm' in a patient's blood was of central medical diagnostic importance for about 2000 years.

100–150 years ago relatively pure preparations of the fibrous material from blood clots, now named fibrin, and its precursor from unclotted blood were analyzed by several scientists. Berzelius proposed the word protein first for fibrin. A soluble form of fibrin was named fibrinogen by Virchow.

(b) Occurrence and function

Fibrinogen is a blood plasma protein. It may be defined as the protein which induced by the action of the enzyme thrombin is converted into an insoluble gel or clot, called fibrin. Fibrinogen exists in free form in the blood, but thrombin is normally present as its inactive precursor prothrombin.

The fibrinogen–fibrin conversion proceeds in several steps. The first part of the reaction consists in the thrombin-catalyzed proteolytic cleavage of the fibrinogen molecule whereby a soluble fibrin monomer and low-molecular-weight peptides, called fibrinopeptides A and B, are formed. The second part of the reaction consists in a spontaneous polymerization of the monomers into the insoluble fibrin gel. The fibrin polymer may then be stabilized by a few covalent crosslinks, introduced by another enzyme, factor XIII_a.

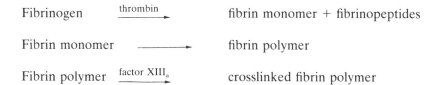

The fibrin gel, in non-crosslinked or crosslinked form, may be dissolved again and fibrinogen can become unclottable by proteolytic cleavage. Many proteases are able to degrade fibrinogen and fibrin; of special importance is the effect of plasmin, which is present in blood in the form of its inactive precursor plasminogen.

Blood plasma fibrinogen is synthesized in the parenchymal cells of the liver. Fibrinogen occurs, however, also in the platelets, and this form of the protein seems to be synthesized in the megakaryocytes of the bone marrow.

It is generally assumed that the most important biological function of fibrinogen is to clot and thereby form a barrier against blood leakage through a damaged blood vessel wall, the fibrin clot acting as a network retaining blood cells and certain plasma proteins. Fibrinogen and fibrin play, however, significant roles in many other physiological and pathological processes. The fibrin framework is believed to support fibroblast proliferation during wound healing. The function of fibrinogen is

TABLE 1

Identified and predicted functional sites in fibrinogen

Intrinsic sites
Thrombin cleavage
Polymerization
Crosslinking
Plasmin cleavage

Protein interaction or binding sites
Thrombin
Factor XIII
Plasmin(ogen)
Plasminogen activators
Fibronectin
α_2-Antiplasmin
Thrombospondin
Collagen
(Calcium and other metal ions)

Cell interaction or binding sites
Platelets
Erythrocytes
Monocytes
Macrophages
Endothelial cells
Fibroblasts
Staphylococci, Streptococci

---

also assumed to be related to tumor metastasis, and as it belongs to the group of acute-phase proteins it may be involved in the defence mechanisms.

The fibrin(ogen) molecules interact specifically with each other during coagulation and equally specifically with a large number of other proteins and cells during the execution of various functions. All these interactions must be governed by the structures of numerous functional sites. A tentative list of such sites is given in Table 1. Some of these sites have been well identified on the molecular level, others have so far been elusive.

Fibrinogen has even during the past few years been the subject of some reviews [1–4] and several international conferences devoted to fibrinogen have been published [5–9].

(c) Assay

A large number of assay methods for fibrinogen, fibrin and their degradation products have been described in the literature and a wide range of properties of these proteins have been utilized for the tests. The fibrinogen assay methods are in most cases based upon one of the following determination principles: coagulation time or velocity, and amount of coagulable protein or specifically precipitable protein or specifically immunoreactive protein. Problems may be encountered with most methods when the fibrinogen concentration is low or when fibrin(ogen) degradation products or certain abnormal plasma components are present.

In the classical coagulation time method of Clauss [10] large amounts of thrombin are added to diluted plasma; in this way the interference by various inhibitors is minimized. Instead of clotting time the velocity of clotting may be measured, e.g. photometrically [11].

The amount of coagulable protein is measured, after addition of a thrombic enzyme and separation of the fibrin clot, by quantitation of the protein in the clot. This is achieved by dissolving the clot and determining the tyrosine content colorimetrically according to Ratnoff and Menzie [12] or the ultraviolet absorption according to Blombäck [13].

The fact that fibrinogen will precipitate specifically from a solution when it is heated to 52–58°C for a few minutes was known already 100 years ago (quoted in [14]). The method is still regarded as useful. The precipitate may be quantitated nephelometrically or turbidimetrically [15].

A great variety of immunological fibrinogen assays have been developed, such as radial immunodiffusion, 'rocket' immunoelectrophoresis, latex agglutination, immunturbimetric measurement [16] and radioimmunoassay (see also under Section 1p, Antibodies).

For fibrin and fibrin(ogen) degradation products special assays are available. Fibrin and higher-molecular-mass degradation products can be selectively precipitated by means of the ethanol gelation [17] and the protamine sulfate precipitation [18] tests. In the staphylococcal clumping test fibrin(ogen) and degradation products will precipitate [19]. Highly specific radioimmunoassays may be employed to differentiate among fibrinogen and its various products (see under Section 1p, Antibodies). An extensive review of assay methods has appeared in 1977 [20].

(d) Purification

The concentration of fibrinogen in blood plasma is 2–4 g/l. It is a euglobulin and one of the least soluble plasma proteins. Purification methods have mainly been based on the low solubility, the isoelectric point or the affinity for immobilized fibrin.

Fibrinogen can be precipitated by many salts, amino acids and alcohols. It is particularly insoluble at lower temperature. In the now classical large-scale preparation method of Cohn et al. [21] fibrinogen is precipitated by cold ethanol. In the modification of Blombäck and Blombäck [14] the characteristically low solubility in the presence of glycine is utilized. Glycine alone was employed by Kazal et al. [22] and β-alanine by Straughn and Wagner [23]. Several procedures in which fibrinogen is precipitated by ammonium sulfate [24], low pH [25], polyethylene glycol [26] or freeze-thawing [27] have been described. In some instances fibrinogen subfractions with increased solubility could be isolated, the heterogeneity seeming to be due to proteolytic degradation [28–31].

Anion-exchange chromatography methods for fibrinogen purification are of special importance for the separation of fibrinogen subfractions which differ in charge [32]. By means of DEAE–cellulose [32,33] or –Sephacel [34] chromatography fibrinogens containing peptide chain variants could be isolated (see under Section 1n, Normal variants). A simple method for the purification of small amounts of fibrinogen has been developed; first the group of proteins of similar size as fibrinogen are fractionated out by gel filtration chromatography and then fibrinogen is isolated from this group by anion-exchange chromatography [35].

Fibrinogen may be highly selectively purified from plasma by means of affinity chromatography on immobilized fibrin, as described by Heene, Matthias and coworkers [36,37]. The column material is prepared by first coupling fibrinogen to cyanogen bromide-activated agarose, and then modifying the insolubilized fibrinogen by thrombin digestion or urea denaturation. The affinity of fibrinogen for this material is due to the same type of specific interaction as between fibrin molecules during polymerization (see under Section 1h, Polymerization). Subfractions with different molecular mass may be contained in the adsorbed fibrinogen [37,38]. A related method is being developed in which the affinity to Gly-Pro-Arg-Pro–agarose instead of fibrin–agarose is exploited [39], Gly-Pro-Arg corresponding to one of the fibrin polymerization sites.

Additional types of affinity chromatography for fibrinogen have been described. Here, ristocetin–agarose [49] and anti-fibrinogen-antibody–agarose [41] were employed as column material.

Many of the fibrinogen purification methods are connected with two types of problems, the contamination of the end product with proteins having affinity for fibrinogen and the heterogeneity of the end product. Plasma proteins with affinity for fibrinogen and which influence the quality of the preparation are: prothrombin, factor XIII, plasminogen and fibronectin. The activity of prothrombin may be removed by adsorption to barium sulfate [22], that of factor XIII by inactivation with a sulfhydryl-reactive reagent (see under Section 2, Factor XIII), that of plasminogen by affinity chromatography on lysine–agarose [42] and that of fibronectin by affinity chromatography on gelatine–agarose [43]. The heterogeneity of fibrinogen preparations is due to the fact that fibrin monomers and higher-molecular-mass degradation products of fibrin(ogen) often will be co-purified as their solubilities, charges or affinities may be related or because they have affinity for fibrinogen.

(e) Molecular shape and physicochemical properties

The molecular mass of fibrinogen has been calculated from sedimentation diffusion and light-scattering data to be 340 000 dalton, and this figure is in excellent agreement with the protein-chemical model (see under Section 1f, Covalent structure). Some physicochemical data for fibrinogen are summarized in Table 2 [44,45]. A large number of publications dealing with various types of light scattering, turbidity, neutron scattering, laser Raman spectroscopy and rheological measurements on fibrinogen and fibrin have appeared in recent years [46–54].

Much of the information about the shape of fibrinogen and about the molecular interactions during the fibrin polymerization comes from electron microscopic studies. Electron micrographs of fibrinogen, unidirectionally shadowed with platinum, were published by Hall and Slayter in 1959 [55]. These micrographs showed fibrinogen molecules to be composed of 3 discrete nodules, with the outer two larger than the central nodule. On the basis of these data, Hall and Slayter proposed the trinodular structure of fibrinogen [55]. Since then many new methods of sample preparation have been developed and results were obtained which disputed the trinodular model. However, these were later found to be artifactual, and at the present time a large number of micrographs of fibrinogen samples prepared in var-

TABLE 2

Physicochemical data for fibrinogen

Sedimentation coefficient ($S_{20, w}$)	7.9 S
Translational diffusion coefficient ($D_{20, w}$)	2.0×10^{-7} cm^2/sec
Rotary diffusion coefficient ($O_{20, w}$)	40 000/sec
Translational frictional coefficient ($f_{20, w}$)	2.0×10^{-7} g/sec
Frictional ratio (f/f_0)	2.34
Intrinsic viscosity ($[\eta]$)	25 cm^3/g
Partial specific volume ($\bar{v}$)	0.72 cm^3/g
Molecular volume (unhydrated)	3×10^5 Å^3
Hydration (g/g of protein)	5
Extinction coefficient ($E_1^{1\%}{}_{\text{cm, 280 nm}}$)	15
α-Helix content	33%
Isoelectric point	5.5

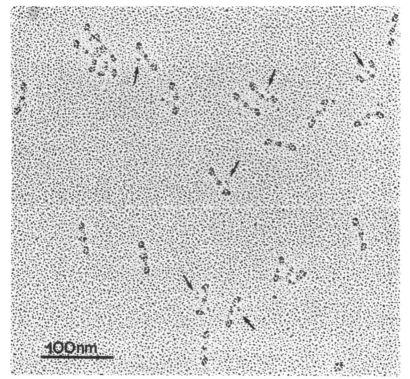

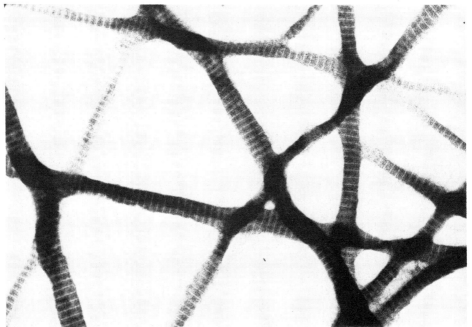

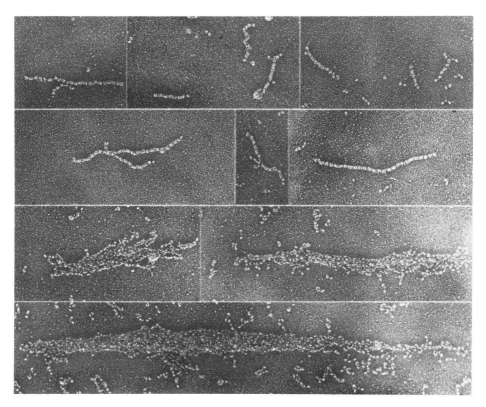

Fig. 1. Electron micrographs of fibrinogen and fibrin. (a) Human fibrinogen rotary shadow-cast with tungsten; magnification 50 000×; arrows indicate additional nodule. (b) Bovine fibrin fibers negatively stained with uranyl acetate; magnification 109 500×. (c) Polymerizing bovine fibrin rotary shadowed with platinum; increasing time after initiation of clotting from top to bottom panel. a was kindly provided by Dr. R. Gollwitzer and H. Wiedemann, Max-Planck-Institute for Biochemistry, Martinsried, and b and c by Dr. H. Slayter, Dana Farber Cancer Institute and Harvard Medical School, Boston, MA.

ious ways all confirm and refine the trinodular structure of fibrinogen [56–59].

Fig. 1a shows the structure of human fibrinogen which was rotary shadow-cast with tungsten. The two outer nodules appear to be somewhat variable in presentation, ranging from approximately spherical to elongated structures with two subdomains; they are connected to the central nodule by thin filaments. Fibrinogen has the following dimensions: length, 45 nm; diameter of the central nodule, 5 nm; diameter of the outer nodules, 6.5 nm in the least asymmetric presentation and 4.5 nm × 9 mm in the most asymmetric orientation; diameter of the connector filaments, 1 nm [57].

A number of observations have clearly shown that the structure seen in the electron microscope fits the structure derived from biochemical studies. Principal among these has been the use of antibodies or antibody fragments specific for the outer and central nodules, i.e. the D or E domains (see under Section 1f, Covalent structure), to label these domains in the electron microscope [60–62]. The two subdomains in the outer nodule are thought to correspond one to the C-terminal part of the β-chain and the other to the C-terminal part of the γ-chain. In some orientations of heavily shadowed fibrinogen there is an additional smaller nodule near the central one but not contiguous with it (Fig. 1a, at arrows). This additional nodule was only seen in fibrinogen samples which had not undergone any degradation; it was not visualized in fragment X preparations. The additional nodule has been interpreted as the carboxy-terminal α-chain segments looping over the outer nodules and coming together in the center [63]. Additional evidence in favor of this has come from scanning transmission electron microscopy, where extra mass, found in the region of the central nodule, was thought to represent these α-chain segments [64].

Proteolytically modified fibrinogen [58,59,65] and fibrinogen fragments [63,66] have also been analyzed by electron microscopy. Fragment X, i.e. fibrinogen which has lost the C-terminal parts of the Aα-chains, appears as a trinodular structure, with the central nodule being slightly smaller than in fibrinogen; fragment Y, a later degradation product, contains 2 nodules, and the end products D and E single nodules [63,66]. These observations are in agreement with the asymmetric plasmin cleavage pattern of fibrinogen (see Section 1j, Fibrinolysis).

Morphologic analysis of fibrin is more difficult but can provide useful information [55,56,67,68]. Fig. 1b is a typical example of fibrin fibers visualized by negative staining and showing a characteristic band pattern with a repeat unit of about 23 nm [55]. The band pattern reflects a half-staggered overlap arrangement of fibrin monomers (see Section 1h, Polymerization). Early and intermediate stages in fibrin formation can also be observed (Fig. 1c). Soon after initiation of clotting fibrin monomers and short protofibrils can be seen (top panel). As time increases, first longer protofibrils are seen (second panel) and then lateral association with thicker fiber formation (third and fourth panel). Fibrin-related ordered aggregates have been obtained from fibrinogen by protamine sulfate treatment [69] or other precipitation procedures [70]. Electron microscopy has also been used to demonstrate that the covalent crosslinking of γ-chains by factor XIII$_a$ occurs between molecules held end-to-end along the length of the protofibril [71] (see Section 1h, Polymerization).

Crystals of native [59] and of slightly degraded [58,59,65,67] fibrinogen have been grown and used for laser diffraction, X-ray crystallography as well as general electron microscopy studies.

The influence of strong magnetic fields on fibrinogen and polymerizing fibrin has been analyzed [72]. The molecules became oriented by the field and highly ordered polymers, similar to the ordinary polymers, were obtained.

The structural organization of fibrin(ogen) has also been studied by scanning microcolorimetry [73–75]. The results indicate that fibrinogen contains 12 domains, which can be located to central or terminal regions of the molecule and which differ in their thermal stability [73], and that the C-terminal regions of the α-chains (see below) interact with each other [75].

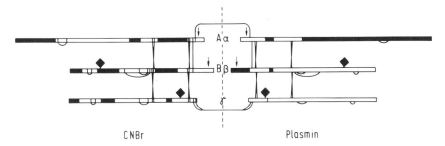

Fig. 2. Human fibrinogen, a model of the covalent structure. The chains have been aligned according to homology. The N-termini of the chains are in the center. The thin, connecting lines represent di-sulfide bonds, the arrows thrombin cleavage sites and the diamonds carbohydrate side chains. On the left-hand side the 5 disulfide knots formed by cyanogen bromide cleavage and on the right-hand side the plasmic fragments D and E are white.

(f) Covalent structure and protein-chemical properties

The overall covalent structure of fibrinogen is an assembly of 3 pairs of non-identical peptide chains connected by disulfide bridges (Fig. 2). Denoting the chains Aα, Bβ and γ (according to the recommendations of the International Committee on Haemostasis and Thrombosis in 1973) the structure may be described as (Aα, Bβ, γ)$_2$. On thrombin digestion fibrinopeptides A and B are released from the Aα- and Bβ-chain, respectively, and fibrin, with the structure (α, β, γ)$_2$ is formed. (In some literature, however, both fibrinogen and fibrin chains are named α, β and γ.)

$$(A\alpha, B\beta, \gamma)_2 \xrightarrow{\text{thrombin}} (\alpha, \beta, \gamma)_2 + 2A + 2B$$

Fibrinogen   Fibrin   Fibrinopeptides

The first clues to the structural organization of the fibrin(ogen) molecule came from the observations of Bettelheim and Bailey [76] and Lorand and Middlebrook [77] in 1952 and of Blombäck and Yamashina [78] in 1958 that fibrinogen and fibrin partly differed in their N-terminal amino acids. Tyrosine was found as N-terminal in both proteins, glycine in fibrin and various other amino acids in fibrinogen, depending on the species analyzed. From the yield and pattern of the N-terminal amino acids it was concluded that fibrin(ogen) contains 6 peptide chains which may be pairwise identical.

In 1962 the 3 types of peptide chains could be isolated for the first time by Henschen [79] and by Clegg and Bailey [80] after cleavage of the disulfide bridges by sulfite. Later research on the covalent structure proceeded mainly along three lines: isolation of the peptide chains, plasmin degradation products and cyanogen bromide fragments, in all cases attempts were gradually made to obtain the complete amino acid sequence information. All three approaches have been essential for our present-day understanding of the fibrinogen molecule.

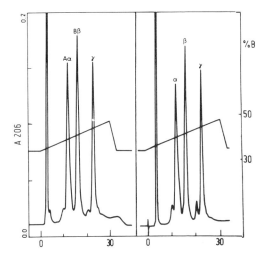

Fig. 3. Human fibrinogen and fibrin peptide chain isolation by reversed-phase high-performance liquid chromatography using a dilute trifluoroacetic acid–acetonitrile (% B) gradient.

(1) Amino acid sequence

The complete amino acid sequences of the 3 human fibrinogen chains have been elucidated. Most of the sequence information is a result of the strategy first to isolate the whole peptide chain and then to cleave it into fragments of a size which can be handled by the available sequencing methods. An obvious advantage of this strategy lies in the fact that fragments analyzed always can be definitely assigned to a certain peptide chain. For the purpose of this procedure the disulfide bridges of fibrin(ogen) were cleaved and modifed by *S*-carboxymethylation and the chains isolated in a pure form at that time by CM-cellulose chromatography in 8 M urea [81]. Nowadays, the corresponding separation would have been carried out by reversed-phase high-performance liquid chromatography [82], as shown in Fig. 3.

The first chain to be sequenced was the γ-chain. By cleaving the chain or parts of it with cyanogen bromide, trypsin, staphylococcal protease, hydroxylamine, *N*-bromosuccinimide and other enzymes or chemical reagents suitable fragments could be produced, and the analysis of these fragments led to the completion of the primary structure by Henschen and coworkers in 1977 [83]. The sequence of an N-terminal and C-terminal fragment had already been published by Blombäck et al. [84] and Sharp et al. [85], respectively. The sequence was completely confirmed by results from analysis of the complementary deoxyribonucleic acid (cDNA) coding for the γ-chain in 1983 [86,87]. The human γ-chain contains 411 amino acid residues and the sequence is shown in Fig. 4 (bottom panel) and the composition in Table 3.

The charge heterogeneity of human fibrinogen was early related to the existence of γ-chain variants [88]. These two [32,33] or three [34] γ-chain forms were later separated and characterized. It was demonstrated that the difference resides in the

```
  1  A D S G E G D F L A E G G G V R⁺G P R V V E R H Q S A C K D S D W P F C S D E D
 41  W N Y K C P S G C R M K G L I D E V N Q D F T N R I N K L K N S L F E Y Q K N N
 81  K D S H S L T T N I M E I L R G D F S S A N N R D N T Y N R V S E D L R S R I E
121  V L K R K V I E K V Q H I Q L L Q K N V R A Q L V D M K R L E V D I D I K I R S
161  C R G S C S R A L A R E V D L K D Y E D Q Q K Q L E Q V I A K D L L P S R D R Q
201  H L P L I K M K P V P D L V P G N F K S Q L Q K V P P E W K A L T D M P Q M R M
241  E L E R P G G N E I T R G G S T S Y G T G S E T E S P R N P S S A G S W N S G S
281  S G P G S T G N R N P G S S G T G G T A T W K P G S S G P G S T G S W N S G S S
321  G T G S T G N Q N P G S P R P G S T G T W N P G S S E R G S A G H W T S E S S V
361  S G S T G Q W H S E S G S F R P D S P G S G N A R P N N P D W G T F E E V S G N
401  V S P G T R R E Y H T E K L V T S K G D K E L R T G K E K V T S G S T T T T R R
441  S C S K T V T K T V I G P D G H K E V T K E V V T S E D G S D C P E A M D L G T
481  L S G I G T L D G F R H R H P D E A A F F D T A S T G K T F P G F F S P M L G E
521  F V S E T E S R G S E S G I F T N T K E S S S H H P G I A E F P S R G K S S S Y
561  S K Q F T S S T S Y N R G D S T F E S K S Y K M A D E A G S E A D H E G T H S T
601  K R G H A K S R P V


  1  Z G V N D N E E G F F S A R⁺G H R P L D K K R E E A P S L R P A P P P I S G G G
 41  Y R A R P A K A A A T Q K K V E R K A P D A G G C L H A D P D L G V L C P T G C
 81  Q L Q E A L L Q Q E R P I R N S V D E L N N N V E A V S Q T S S S S F Q Y M Y L
121  L K D L W Q K R Q K Q V K D N E N V V N E Y S S E L E K H Q L Y I D E T V N S N
161  I P T N L R V L R S I L E N L R S K I Q K L E S D V S A Q M E Y C R T P C T V S
201  C N I P V V S G K E C E E I I R K G G E T S E M Y L I Q P D S S V K P Y R V Y C
241  D M N T E N G G W T V I Q N R Q D G S V D F G R K W D P Y K Q G F G N V A T N T
281  D G K N Y C G L P G E Y W L G N D K I S Q L T R M G P T E L L I E M E D W K G D
321  K V K A H Y G G F T V Q N E A N K Y Q I S V N K Y R G T A G N A L M D G A S Q L
361  M G E N⁺R T M T I H N G M F F S T Y D R D N D G W L T S D P R K Q C S K E D G G
401  G W W Y N R C H A A N P N G R Y Y W G G Q Y T W D M A K H G T D D G V V W M N W
441  K G S W Y S M R K M S M K I R P F F P Q Q


  1  Y V A T R D N C C I L D E R F G S Y C P T T C G I A D F L S T Y Q T K V D K D L
 41  Q S L E D I L H Q V E N⁺K T S E V K Q L I K A I Q L T Y N P D E S S K P N M I D
 81  A A T L K S R K M L E E I M K Y E A S I L T H D S S I R Y L Q E I Y N S N N Q K
121  I V N L K E K V A Q L E A Q C Q E P C K D T V Q I H D I T G K D C Q D I A N K G
161  A K Q S G L Y F I K P L K A N Q Q F L V Y C E I D G S G N G W T V F Q K R L D G
201  S V D F K K N W I Q Y K E G F G H L S P T G T T E F W L G N E K I H L I S T Q S
241  A I P Y A L R V E L E D W N G R T S T A D Y A M F K V G P E A D K Y R L T Y A Y
281  F A G G D A G D A F D G F D F G D D P S D K F F T S H N G M Q F S T W D N D N D
321  K F E G N C A E Q D G S G W W M N K C H A G H L N G V Y Y Q G G T Y S K A S T P
361  N G Y D N G I I W A T W K T R W Y S M K K T T M K I I P F N R L T I G E G Q Q H
401  H L G G A K Q A G D V
```

Fig. 4. Human fibrinogen Aα-chain (top), Bβ-chain (middle) and γ-chain (bottom) amino acid sequences. Arrows indicate thrombin cleavage sites and + carbohydrate side chains. For one letter code see Table 3. Z denotes pyroglutamic acid.

C-terminus of the chain and this region of the most high-molecular-mass variant which is denoted as the γ'-chain, has subsequently been sequenced on the protein [33] as well as the cDNA [89] level. As shown in Fig. 5 the last 4 residues in the γ-chain main variant are replaced by 20 residues in the γ'-variant. The extended sequence has been explained as due to alternative processing during chain synthesis, giving rise to a read-through into an intron sequence and different mRNAs for

TABLE 3

Amino acid and carbohydrate composition of human fibrinogen and its peptide chains: residues/mole, and calculated molecular weights

		Fibrinogen	Aα-Chain	Bβ-Chain	γ-Chain
Amino acids					
Asp	D	190	35	28	32
Asn	N	168	29	32	23
Thr	T	196	48	22	28
Ser	S	284	86	31	25
Glu	E	192	44	30	22
Gln	Q	136	18	26	24
Pro	P	138	35	23	11
Gly	G	292	69	42	35
Ala	A	142	22	23	26
Cys	C	58	8	11	10
Val	V	134	28	25	14
Met	M	66	10	15	8
Ile	I	116	17	16	25
Leu	L	166	29	28	26
Tyr	Y	100	9	21	20
Phe	F	94	19	10	18
Lys	K	208	39	31	34
His	H	64	15	7	10
Arg	R	154	40	27	10
Trp	W	66	10	13	10
Sum		2 964	610	461	411
Carbohydrates					
N-Acetylglucosamine	GlcNAc	16	–	4	4
Galactose	Gal	8	–	2	2
Mannose	Man	12	–	3	3
N-Acetylneuraminic acid	NeuAc	4–8	–	1–2	1–2
Molecular mass		338 162	66 161	54 375	48 545

the γ- and γ'-chain [33,89]. The presence of a different type of γ-chain variants [81] with lower molecular mass has remained unexplained.

The analysis of the next chain, the Bβ-chain, proceeded very similarly to that of the γ-chain. The 461-residue sequence was published by Henschen and co-workers in 1977 [90]. A long N-terminal segment of the chain was sequenced by

```
γ -chain 401   H L G G A K Q A G D V
γ'-chain 401   H L G G A K Q V R P E H P A E T E Y D S L Y P E D D L
```

Fig. 5. Human fibrinogen γ-chain and γ'-chain C-terminal amino acid sequences. The numbers indicate the positions of the first residues.

Hessel et al. [91]. The human Bβ-chain was analyzed on the protein level once more in 1979 [92] and on the cDNA level in 1983 [87,93] with minor disagreements in the results. Sequence and composition are shown in Fig. 4 (middle panel) and Table 3, respectively.

The Aα-chain, finally, was sequenced first in its N-terminal part by Blombäck et al. [94] and in one intermediate and the C-terminal part by Doolittle and co-workers [95,96]. The rest of the partly very difficult sequencing was carried out in parallel in the laboratories of Doolittle and Henschen, the complete primary structure with 610 amino acid residues appearing in print in 1979 [97,98]. Most of the Aα-chain was sequenced protein-chemically once more [99]. The entire cDNA of the chain has been analyzed, and only minor differences between the two types of sequences were found, except for an unexpected 15-residue C-terminal extension in the cDNA coding for the Aα-chain [87,100] (see also under Section 1g, Genes). Sequence and composition are shown in Fig. 4 (top panel) and Table 3, respectively.

The size and solubility heterogeneity of human fibrinogen has since some time been related to Aα-chain degradation [28–31,101], shorter or longer segments from the most C-terminal part of the Aα-chain missing in lower-molecular-mass or higher-solubility preparations. It has been noticed that Aα-chains lacking the most C-terminal 27 amino acid residues will separate from the full-length Aα-chains during CM-cellulose peptide chain isolation [96,102].

A complete primary structure is only available for the human protein. However, a few additional fibrinogen peptide chains have been sequenced. In bovine fibrinogen the total Bβ-chain [103–106] and almost half of the Aα-chain [103,105,107] have been analyzed, most of it on the cDNA level. In rat fibrinogen the Aα- and γ-chains [108–110] are known, and in lamprey fibrinogen the sequence of the γ-chain [111] has been determined, in both species mainly by cDNA analysis. Rat γ-chain occurs in two forms [110], just as the corresponding human chain, although the biosynthetic mechanism for their formation is slightly different [89,110].

(2) Disulfide bridges

The 6 peptide chains in fibrinogen are held together by 29 disulfide bridges [112]. No free sulfhydryl groups are present in the molecule [112]. The half-cystine residues are located in 3 clusters along each chain, i.e. one N-terminal cluster, one intermediate and one C-terminal. The disulfide bridge pattern was mainly elucidated by cleaving native fibrinogen with cyanogen bromide after the methionine residues and isolating cystine-containing fragments, so-called disulfide knots [113–116]. It turned out that the 29 disulfide bonds are also clustered, and that they are contained in 5 disulfide knots, denoted FCB 1–5 (*fibrinogen–cyanogen bromide fragment*), according to their order of appearance on gel filtration chromatography, or NDSK, IDSK, αCDSK, βCDSK and γCDSK (N, I and C for *N*-terminal, *i*ntermediate and *C*-terminal, respectively; DSK for *di*sulfide *k*not), according to their position within the molecule. Some of their characteristics are listed in Table 4. The chain segments contained are indicated in Fig. 2 (left side, white segments).

TABLE 4

Disulfide knots in human fibrinogen

Designations	FCB 1 NDSK	FCB 2 IDSK	FCB 3 αCDSK	FCB 4 βCDSK	FCB 5 γCDSK
Position	N-terminal	Intermediate	C-terminal	C-terminal	C-terminal
Number per molecule	1	2	2	2	2
Chains involved	Aα, Bβ, γ	Aα, Bβ, γ	Aα	Bβ	γ
Number of peptides	2 × 3	5	1	1	2
Number of sulfur bridges	11	6	1	1	1
Number of residues	2 × (51 + 118 + 78) = 494	(60 + 34 + 18 + 63 + 170) = 345	236	53	(43 + 26) = 69
Disulfide bridges	Aα28–Aα28[a] Aα36–Bβ65 Aα45– γ23 Aα49–Bβ76 Bβ80– γ19 γ8– γ9[a] γ9– γ9[a]	Aα161– γ139 Aα165–Bβ193 Bβ197– γ135 Bβ201–Bβ286 Bβ211–Bβ240 γ153– γ182	Aα442–Aα472	Bβ394–Bβ407	γ326–γ339

[a] Opposite half of the molecule.

The 5 disulfide knots can be separated from each other and from additional fragments by the combination of gel filtration chromatographies and counter-current distribution [115,116]. In order to find the unique half-cystine partners it is, however, necessary to isolate peptide fragments which only contain 2 half-cystines, and as several disulfide bonds are contained in the two largest disulfide knots, subfragmentation and isolation of simpler knots had to be undertaken to complete the disulfide assignment [114–117]. The positions of the half-cystine residues involved in each disulfide bond are given in Table 4. The arrangement of the disulfide bridges is to a large extent supported by data from other types of fragments than those obtained by cyanogen bromide cleavage, e.g. plasmic fragments (see under Section 1j, Fibrinolysis).

The largest disulfide knot, NDSK, encompasses the N-terminal regions of all peptide chains [113]. Like fibrinogen itself it is dimeric [114]. Out of its 11 disulfide bonds, three connect the two halves of the fibrinogen molecule [114], one bond between the Aα-chains and two between the γ-chains. Those between the γ-chains link these chains in an antiparallel fashion [117]. Three bridges connect all 3 chains in a ring-like structure [114].

The second-largest disulfide knot, IDSK, contains the middle part of the 3 peptide chains [116]. Here, like in NDSK, 3 bridges arrange the chains in a ring-like structure [116]. Remaining disulfides are found in intra-chain bonds. The 3 smallest disulfide knots are located in the C-terminal region, one in each peptide chain [115,118], i.e. all bonds are of the intra-chain type.

The disulfide bridges in fibrinogen are all remarkably stable, strongly denaturing conditions being needed to cleave them chemically [81,112]. It has, however, been possible to split 5 of the 29 bonds selectively under native conditions by means of the thioredoxin system, the susceptible bonds being those three between the two halves of the molecule and those at the C-termini of the two Aα-chains [119].

(3) Posttranslational modifications

Three types of modified amino acid side chains have been found in fibrinogen, i.e. those carrying carbohydrate, those with phosphate and those with sulfate.

Carbohydrate	(+)		
Aα-chain	N	269	S P R N P S S A G
Aα-chain	N	400	V S G N V S P G T
Bβ-chain	N	364	M G E N$^+$R T M T I
γ-chain	N	52	Q V E N$^+$K T S E V
Phosphate	(o)		
Aα-chain	S	3	A D S^{o}G E G D L
Aα-chain	S	345	N P G S^{o}S E R G S

Fig. 6. Human fibrinogen potential carbohydrate- and phosphate-carrying amino acid sequences. The numbers indicate the positions of modified amino acid residues.

Of the two common amino sugars, glucosamine and galactosamine, fibrinogen contains only the first mentioned [81], which implies that the carbohydrate side chains are of the N-glycosidic type. Scanning the amino acid sequences for attachment sites, i.e. for the sequence Asn-Xaa-Thr or -Ser, 4 potential sites are found, as shown in Fig. 6 (upper panel). However, only the Bβ- [120] and γ-chains [84] carry indeed carbohydrate, the neighbouring proline residues in the Aα-chain sequences might prevent glycosylation of this chain. The compositions of the sugar moieties are given in Table 3 (lower part). The structures of the side chains have been determined by nuclear magnetic resonance measurements and by sequential exoglycosidase digestion analyses [121–123]. They are of the biantennary type. The carbohydrate moieties are heterogeneous as regards the terminal neuraminic (sialic) acid residues, and both disialylated and monosialylated species have been found, but asialo side chains are not present in normal fibrinogen [124,125]. The structure is presented in Fig. 7.

Human fibrinogen has been shown to contain phosphate linked to serine, but not threonine, residues in the Aα-chain [126,127]. In normal fibrinogen this chain is the exclusive phosphate carrier [127]. The modified serines are located close to the N-terminus in fibrinopeptide A [126] and in the middle of the chain in position 345 [127], respectively. The sequences around the modified residues are shown in Fig. 6 (lower panel). The two sites are only partially phosphorylated, approximately 20% of position 3 and 34% of position 345 occurring in the modified form in adult fibrinogen [126,127]. However, newly synthesized fibrinogen seems to be fully phosphorylated [128,129]. Several kinase preparations have been demonstrated to incorporate phosphate into plasma fibrinogen, preferentially into the non-fibrinopeptide part of the Aα-chain [130,131].

Sulfate in the form of tyrosine-O-sulfate has been detected in human fibrin, the content being about 2.3 moles/mole of protein [132]. The location of the modified tyrosine residues in human fibrinogen is unknown. In several animal fibrinogens tyrosine-O-sulfate is found in the fibrinopeptides B, but this is not the case with the human peptide, which is devoid of tyrosine [126].

(4) Primary structure-based model building

It is generally assumed that the primary structure data, including the amino acid sequences, the disulfide bridges and the posttranslationally modified side chains, must contain the complete information for all higher-order structures, and obviously all constructed models must be in agreement with the facts of the primary structure, as outlined in Fig. 2. In this sense the sequences of fibrinogen have been

```
+NeuAc(α2→6)Gal(β1→4)GlcNAc(β1→2)Man(α1→3)
                                                >Man(β1→4)GlcNAc(β1→4)GlcNAc(β1→N)Asn
+NeuAc(α2→6)Gal(β1→4)GlcNAc(β1→2)Man(α1→6)
```

Fig. 7. Human fibrinogen carbohydrate side chain structure. For abbreviations see Table 3. ± indicates the partial absence of one of the N-acetyl neuraminic acid residues.

used to predict the secondary structure of the γ-chain [133] and a three-dimensional coiled-coil structure of the peptide chain regions between the disulfide rings of the N-terminal and intermediate disulfide knots [134,135].

(g) Genes, biosynthesis and turnover

(1) Gene location and coding sequences

Plasma fibrinogen is synthesized by the hepatic parenchymal cells. It has been demonstrated that the 3 peptide chains, Aα, Bβ and γ, are synthesized separately from 3 different mRNAs, i.e. they are not formed by cleavage of a single precursor peptide chain [136–139]. The location of the human fibrinogen genes on the long arm of chromosome 4 was first reported when it was observed that a certain genetically abnormal fibrinogen variant cosegregated with the variants of the MNSs blood group [140], these blood group genes being known as located on chromosome 4. The finding was confirmed by analyzing human–rodent somatic cell hybrids containing rearranged chromosomes and by in situ hybridization of fibrinogen cDNA to chromosomes of mitotic spreads [141–143]. The exact location was found to be the distal third of the long arm, band q23–q32 [143].

Each peptide chain gene occurs as a single copy, and the 3 human genes are closely linked in the 5'-3' direction in the order γ–Aα–Bβ [143]. The γ- and Aα-chain genes are oriented in tandem and transcribed towards the Bβ-chain gene, and the Bβ-chain gene is transcribed from the opposite DNA strand towards the Aα- and γ-chain genes, according to Kant et al. [143].

Genomic DNA sequences have been determined for the human Bβ- [93] and γ-chains [144] and for the rat Aα- [109] and γ-chains [110]. The number of introns in the regions coding for the mature peptide chains were 3, 7 and 8 for the Aα-, Bβ- and γ-chain genes, respectively. Of these intervening sequences only two in each chain occur in the homologous positions in all 3 chains [109]. The γ-chain variants are formed from a single gene by alternative mRNA splicing at the last intron of the γ-chain [89,110,144,145]. (For cDNA sequences see under Section 1f, Covalent structure).

Fibrinogen synthesis has recently been shown to take place also in the megakaryocytes [146,147]. The platelet fibrinogen, which is synthesized in the megakaryocytes, contains only the 411-residue γ-chain, the elongated γ'-form is absent [148–150].

(2) Assembly and modification

The peptide chains of fibrinogen are all synthesized in a precursor form [128,136,137,139,151], and according to Chung and coworkers the cDNA sequences indicate the presence of signal peptides of 16 or 19 amino acid residues for the human pre-Aα-chain [100], 16, 27 or 30 residues for the pre-Bβ-chain [93] and 26 residues for the pre-γ-chain [86,144]. All these N-terminal extensions have the characteristics of leader sequences involved in the translocation from the cytosolic to the cisternal side of the rough endoplasmatic reticulum. They have been suggested to be important in chain assembly [137], and are lost before fibrinogen leaves the hepatocyte. The Aα-chain has an additional C-terminal 15-residue extension, as demonstrated by cDNA analysis, which is removed during assembly, secretion or early during circulation in blood plasma [100,107].

The time course of the synthesis seems not identical for the 3 chains, as judged from incorporation of radioactive label [151,152]. According to Yu et al. [151] fibrinogen assembly commences already at the stage when nascent, incomplete Bβ-chains still are attached at the polysomes, by combination between the Bβ-chains and preformed Aα- or γ-chains from an intracellular pool; later the Bβ–Aα and Bβ–γ complexes are completed by the missing chain. Within the rough endoplasmatic reticulum nascent fibrinogen is already fully disulfide-linked in dimeric form [128]. No mechanism has so far been found which convincingly explains the fact that in heterozygous cases of dysfibrinogenemia, when two different genes for one of the chains must be present, only symmetrically normal and symmetrically abnormal molecules, but no hybrids, can be detected in the blood plasma [153].

The time course of glycosylation was investigated by Nickerson and Fuller [154]; the γ-chain was demonstrated to receive its core carbohydrate as an early cotranslational event and the Bβ-chain at the time of polypeptide termination or shortly after the release into the rough endoplasmatic reticulum. Phosphorylation and sulfation occur somewhat later during the secretory stage [128].

(3) Regulation and turnover

Fibrinogen is normally synthesized at a rate of about 30 mg/kg and day. The synthesis is stimulated during acute-phase reaction, by defibrination and fibrin(ogen) degradation products and by certain hormones. Using non-specific traumatic agents, like turpentine, the synthesis can be increased 10-fold in laboratory animals [147,155].

Acute-phase reaction, defibrination and fibrinogen degradation may all have the formation of the degradation products of the D and E type (see Section 1j, Fibrinolysis) in common, and it seems likely that these breakdown products have an effect on leukocytes or monocytes [156,157] from the blood and macrophages [158] from the liver, i.e. Kupffer cells, which then produce factor(s) which stimulate the hepatocytes to synthesize more fibrinogen. Treatment with defined degradation products increased the synthesis [156,159–161]. Glucocorticoids had a stimulatory effect on cell cultures, but no effect when administered to animals [162]. Interleukin-1 may also stimulate the synthesis [163]. The hepatocyte-stimulating factor seems to control the synthesis at the level of gene transcription, i.e. by increasing the amount of specific mRNA, and not at the level of translation or secretion [157,161].

The normal catabolic pathways for fibrinogen are only partially known. Fibrinogen has been reported to have a half-life of 4.1 days, corresponding to a fractional catabolic rate of 24% of the plasma pool per day [164]. The blood clearance has been determined as being highly different for the various plasmic degradation products [165]. Asialo-fibrinogen and normal fibrinogen differed only modestly in

Designation	Sequence
AP	A D S⁰G E G D F L A E G G G V R
A	A D S G E G D F L A E G G G V R
AY	D S G E G D F L A E G G G V R
B-Arg	Z G V N D N E E G F F S A
B	Z G V N D N E E G F F S A R

Fig. 8. Human fibrinopeptide amino acid sequences. B-Arg, des-Arg-fibrinopeptide B; Z, pyroglu-tamic acid; S⁰, phosphorylated serine.

half-life time, indicating that fibrinogen is not removed from circulation by means of the liver asialo–glycoprotein receptor [166].

(h) Fibrinogen–fibrin conversion

(1) Fibrinopeptide release and interaction with thrombin
When the fibrinogen–fibrin transition is initiated by thrombin cleavage only 1–2% of the molecular mass is removed. In each molecule of fibrinogen 2 molecules of each fibrinopeptide A and B may be released by proteolysis from the amino-terminal ends of the Aα- and Bβ-chains, respectively (see Figs. 2 and 4). The removal of fibrinopeptides A is, however, sufficient for clotting to occur.

The human fibrinopeptides were first isolated and sequenced by Blombäck and coworkers in 1966 [126]. The peptides are present in the clot supernatant liquid in several forms, as shown in Fig. 8. Fibrinopeptide A occurs in 3 variants, i.e. a phosphorylated variant (AP) which accounts for about 20% of the total A-peptide, a main variant (A) accounting for 70%, and an N-terminally shorter variant (AY) accounting for 10% [126,167]. The missing N-terminal amino acid residue in peptide AY compared to A may be explained as caused by an aminopeptidase in blood. Fibrinopeptide B is present in fibrinogen in only one form. However, upon release it rapidly loses its carboxy-terminal arginine, due to the action of a carboxy-peptidase which occurs in blood and contaminates most fibrinogen preparations, and the des-Arg form (B-Arg) is obtained. Two molecules of an additional peptide, Gly-Pro-Arg, are split off by thrombin from the amino termini of the fibrin α-chains in fibrin(ogen) which has been denatured by cyanogen bromide cleavage into disulfide knots and other peptides [113] or by mercaptan cleavage into free peptide chains [81].

Many methods have been developed for the isolation, identification and/or quantification of fibrinopeptides. Older procedures were based on colorimetry, electrophoresis [81, 126] or ion-exchange chromatography [see ref. 168]. Nowadays, mainly immunoassays and HPLC analyses are employed. Radioimmunoassays for fibrinopeptides have been extensively applied in many types of coagulation-related research. The great advantage of the methods lies obviously in their high sensitivity and selectivity even in solutions containing many other peptides. Different antisera have to be used for the analyses of fibrinopeptide A [169–174], fibrinopeptide B [175–177] and des-Arg fibrinopeptide B [176]. Fibrinogen and certain degradation products interfere, as they cross-react, if not removed beforehand by precipitation [169] or adsorption [170]. Sensitive enzyme-linked immunoassays have also been developed [178,179].

Recently, HPLC-based procedures for fibrinopeptide analysis have been published [167,168,180–183]. Using reversed-phase HPLC columns all fibrinopeptide variants and their common degradation products can be isolated, identified as defined peptides and quantified simultaneously in pre-purified systems. It is noteworthy that in most of the structurally elucidated cases of genetically determined fibrinogen abnormality HPLC-fibrinopeptide analysis has been of decisive importance [168]. (For HPLC patterns, see under Section 10, Abnormal variants).

Thrombin is a trypsin-like enzyme, but cleaves higher-molecular-mass substrates, like fibrinogen, with a remarkably high degree of proteolytic specificity [81,113,184,185]. Under conditions where trypsin would split 120–130 out of a total of 181 different arginyl and lysyl bonds in denatured human fibrinogen [186], thrombin will only split 3 arginyl bonds, i.e. those at positions 16 and 19 in the $A\alpha$-chain and 14 in the $B\beta$-chain.

The thrombin-catalyzed cleavages of the various peptide bonds proceed with different rates in native as well as in denatured fibrinogen. The relative order of the cleavages has been investigated by means of N-terminal amino acid analysis [187–189], radioimmunoassay of the free fibrinopeptides [175,189,190] and HPLC-fibrinopeptide analysis [168,191–193,195–197]. Fibrinopeptide A always appeared with the highest initial release rate and fibrinopeptide B was delayed [168,175, 187–196]; the tripeptide Gly-Pro-Arg is, as already mentioned, only split off from denatured fibrin(ogen) and appeared later than the fibrinopeptides [81,197]. Typical curves for the time course of fibrinopeptide release are shown in Fig. 9.

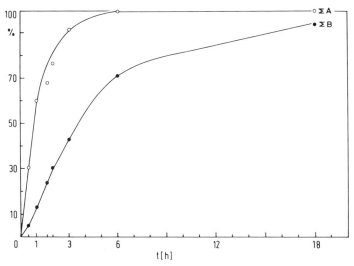

Fig. 9. Human fibrinopeptide kinetics of release as determined by HPLC analyses.

Much research work has been devoted to interpret the significance of the differences between the fibrinopeptides as regards liberation kinetics. In principle, two explanations have been proposed. According to one of them the peptides are released sequentially [188–190,196], i.e. prior release of A-peptide is essential for release of B-peptide; in other words, thrombin recognizes only the N-terminal region of the Aα-chain and splits off A-peptide, which initiates polymerization (see below) and conformational change, which then leads to the recognition by thrombin of the N-terminal region of the Bβ-chain and B-peptide removal. According to the other explanation the peptides are released independently of each other and the N-terminal regions of the Aα- and the Bβ-chain compete for the active site of thrombin [191,194], i.e. B-peptide is liberated at a lower rate, as the N-terminal part of the Bβ-chain is a poorer substrate for thrombin than that of the Aα-chain.

In favor of the first-mentioned explanation speak the facts that polymerization inhibition by addition of urea [189] or the peptide Gly-Pro-Arg-Pro [190] (see below) will slow down B-peptide liberation, and also certain calculations of kinetic data [196]. However, the accessibility of the thrombin cleavage sites both in the Aα- and in the Bβ-chain of native fibrinogen to the interaction with specific antibodies [198,199], and perhaps also the fact that trypsin will cleave off both fibrinopeptides, B-peptide even at a higher rate [175], indicate at least that the two cleavage sites are freely available on the surface of fibrinogen. As an appropriate compromise it has been suggested that a mechanism, characterized by independent, competitive cleavage, most accurately describes the early stages of the thrombin–fibrinogen reaction, and that another mechanism, characterized by polymerization-dependent, sequential cleavage, describes the later stages [194].

The influence of the phosphorylation of serine in position 3 of fibrinopeptide A on the release kinetics has been studied, with the result that at higher fibrinogen concentrations A and AP are cleaved off at the same rate [168,192], but at lower substrate concentrations AP seems to be cleaved off slightly faster than A [194].

The interaction between thrombin and fibrinogen is not limited to the specific proteolytic fibrinopeptide liberation. Thrombin also binds in a specific and saturable way to fibrin [200–205]. The maximum molar ratio between thrombin and fibrin seemed to be 0.5 [200], and the binding was independent of the state of the active site in thrombin [200,204,205]. Thrombin could be desorbed by calcium ions [202] or released by proteolytic clot lysis [203].

Several thrombin-like snake venom enzymes have been isolated [206] and characterized as regards their specificity towards fibrinogen. Of special interest have been those enzymes which selectively remove either fibrinopeptide A or B, but not both. Batroxobin from *Bothrops atrox* or *moojeni*, often called reptilase, and ancrod from *Agkistrodon rhodostoma*, also called arvin, will exclusively cleave off the A-peptide [175,187,206]. An enzyme from *Agkistrodon contortrix contortrix* will preferentially release the B-peptide, but slowly also the A-peptide, the reaction being more specific for the B-peptide at lower temperatures [175,206–208]. These snake venom enzymes provide the opportunity to study the A- and B-peptide-specific effects on the properties of fibrin(ogen) [175,187,207,208].

192

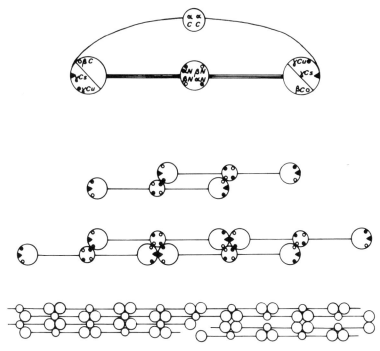

Fig. 10. Schematic representation of the localization of binding sites in fibrin(ogen), and of various fibrin polymerization stages.

(2) Polymerization

Fibrin polymerization is a highly ordered process in which the monomers interact with each other in a most specific way. The interacting regions of the molecules are called polymerization sites, contact sites or binding sites. The models for the polymerization process are to a large extent based on the electron microscopic trinodular structure of fibrinogen and band pattern of fibrin (see Section 1e, Molecular shape). The polymerization process has been investigated with a great variety of methods. In many types of experiments fragments of fibrin(ogen) have been employed in order to establish the functional properties of the various regions of the molecule. Both fragments obtained by proteolytic degradation with plasmin (see Section 1j, Fibrinolysis), i.e. fragments X, Y, D and E, and fragments formed by cyanogen bromide cleavage, i.e. disulfide knots, have been tested. Small, synthetic peptide analogues of certain regions have also provided useful information.

Several types of functional sites participate at the fibrin polymerization process. Certain sites are present both in fibrinogen and fibrin, others are only exposed or activated on fibrinopeptide release. Some kinds of interaction are symmetrical or homotypic, i.e. the corresponding regions of two molecules are in contact, and other interactions are unsymmetrical or heterotypic, i.e. the regions of the two molecules making contact are different from each other [209].

According to the present-day concept a number of consecutive stages may be discerned in the polymerization process as outlined in Fig. 10. On release of fibrinopeptide A from the N-terminal end of the Aα-chain an essential polymerization site is activated. This site may be called A-site [188], or GPR-site [4] or αN-site. It is located on the central nodule, i.e. the E-domain. The αN-site interacts with a preformed, complementary site in the C-terminal region of the γ-chain of another molecule. The latter site is denoted as a-site [188] or γCu-site (u for unsymmetrical), and is located on an outer nodule, i.e. a D-domain. A dimer with a half-staggered overlap between the participating units is formed, as indicated in Fig. 10. The contacts between the molecules have therefore been called DE-stag contacts [210].

Additional interaction between a D- and an E-domain may arise as a result of fibrinopeptide B release from the N-terminal part of the Bβ-chain within the central nodule, the new site being called B-site [188], or GHR-site [4] or βN-site. Its preformed complementary site is assumed to reside in the β-chain within the outer nodule, and is called the b-site [188] or βC-site. The βN–βC interaction may have a different function than the αN–γC interaction.

When more fibrin monomer units are added to the growing polymer, a new type of contact is established (see Fig. 10). This contact is situated between two adjacent outer nodules, and is therefore called the DD-long contact [210]. As the most C-terminal segments of the γ-chains with the γ-chain cross-linking sites (see below) should be of special importance for this contact, the corresponding site may be denoted γCs (s for symmetrical). The polymer is now composed of two rows of end-to-end linked monomer units where the units in one row are arranged in a half-staggered overlap with respect to the units in the other row. This type of polymer is called a protofibril.

Protofibrils combine to form straight or branching fibrin fibers by lateral association. The interacting regions are less well defined than the previous, but have provisionally been denoted DD-lat contacts [210] and DE-lat contacts [209], depending on the assumed configuration (see Fig. 10). The βN–βC interaction seems to be relevant to lateral association.

Finally, it may be predicted that important polymerization sites are present in the C-terminal region of the α-chain. These αC-sites are at least partially active and give rise to symmetrical contacts in fibrinogen in form of the small additional nodule near the central one. Their fate during fibrin polymerization is largely unknown, but the difference in properties between polymers obtained from complete fibrin molecules and from those lacking the C-terminal α-chain regions, i.e. X-type fragments, indicates their functional significance.

The polymerization-related interactions between fibrinogen, fibrin and various fibrin(ogen) fragments have been studied with ultracentrifugation, gel chromatography, light scattering, gel electrophoresis, coagulation measurement, equilibrium dialysis, affinity chromatography, amino acid or carbohydrate modification and several other methods.

Ultracentrifugation experiments were performed with soluble fibrinogen–fibrin complexes [211,212]. The complexes were found to be specific but unstable.

The fibrin-solubilizing effect of fibrinogen was also analyzed by gel chromatography [213–216]. When fibrinogen was activated with small amounts of thrombin stable oligomers in form of half-activated fibrinogen–fibrin complexes were observed [214,216]. Higher temperature, i.e. 37°C, favored desaggregation of fibrinogen–fibrin complexes [215].

Light-scattering [48–52] data indicated a correlation between B-peptide release and lateral association in some studies [48], but failed to indicate this in other studies [49]. It provided evidence for the polymerization-inhibiting effect of fragment D [217] and for the significance of the C-terminal region of the α-chain, when the polymerization rates of undegraded and slightly degraded fibrin monomers were compared [218].

Polyacrylamide gel electrophoresis [219] and crossed immunoelectrophoresis in agarose [220] were employed to demonstrate the complex formation between fragment DD, i.e. crosslinked D-fragments (see below), and fragments E of various sizes.

The inhibitory effect on fibrin monomer polymerization has been one of the most useful parameters for testing polymerization sites [221–225]. It could be shown that X-fragment is more inhibitory than fibrinogen and Y- and D-fragments [221]. Comparing D-fragments of various sizes the polymerization site of the γ-chain could in some laboratories be precisely localized to the 40 most C-terminal amino acid residues [222–224]; conflicting results were, however, obtained in other laboratories [225]. In a direct coagulation test fibrinogen devoid of the first 42 amino acid residues of the Bβ-chain was compared with undegraded fibrinogen; the pronounced delay in polymerization of the degraded sample points to the importance of the β-chain N-terminus in fibrin polymer formation [226].

Synthetic di-, tri- and tetra-peptides, identical with or related to the first few amino acid residues of the amino terminal in the fibrin α- and β-chains, and first described by Laudano and Doolittle, have found extensive use as probes for the functional sites involved in the polymerization process [4,227–229], e.g. in polymerization inhibition tests [227–229] and in binding experiments, using equilibrium dialysis [227]. Peptides similar to the N-terminus of the α-chain, i.e. starting with the sequence Gly-Pro-Arg, were shown to be efficient inhibitors of polymerization, provided sufficiently high concentrations were used. They strongly bound to fibrinogen or D-fragments in which the C-terminal end of the γ-chain still was preserved, thus providing evidence for the C-terminal polymerization site of the γ-chain. Peptides similar to the N-terminus of the β-chain, i.e. beginning with the sequence Gly-His-Arg, did not inhibit clot formation, but bound to fibrinogen and D-fragments of all sizes. The effects of the peptides were calcium ion concentration dependent [227,228]. Photoaffinity label-containing peptides, similar to the α-chain N-terminus, displayed potent inhibitory effects in monomer reaggregation tests [229].

The procedure of affinity chromatography on solid-phase-bound fibrin(ogen) was originally reported by Heene and Matthias [36,37,230,231]. It has gradually been developed into a most versatile and informative method for analyzing the various interactions between fibrinogen, fibrin types, many fibrin(ogen) fragment types [36,37,39,230–237], and also other proteins (see Section 11, Interaction with other proteins). Fibrinogen or soluble fragments were covalently linked to activated agarose, and then if required modified by cleavage with thrombin, reptilase, mercaptoethanol or other agents. Fibrinogen-derived samples to be tested were reacted with the solid-phase-bound material under physiological conditions; adsorbed material was desorbed with solvents containing high salt concentrations, denaturing agents and/or having an acidic pH.

The results obtained strongly supported the concept of the complementary binding sites, i.e. sites of the type which can be exposed or activated by fibrinopeptide release and sites of the preformed type. The former type was shown to be present in isolated form in the thrombin- or reptilase-treated N-terminal disulfide knot and in activated, but not extensively degraded fragment E [232,235]. The latter type of site was found in isolated form in D-fragment with C-terminally undegraded or only slightly degraded γ-chain component [234–236] and especially in the cross-linked D-fragment, i.e. DD [235]. Recently it has been reported that a tetrapeptide analogue of the fibrin α-chain N-terminus, Gly-Pro-Arg-Pro, when attached to agarose, also can be employed for affinity chromatography of fibrinogen [39].

Chemical modification of certain amino acid residues has been used in the studies of the polymerization sites. However, only in a few cases has it been feasible to achieve sufficiently specific and selective effects, so that the modification could be assumed to have changed the properties of single amino acid residues with preserved nearly-native molecular structure.

Alkylation of approximately 18 histidine residues by reaction with iodoacetate or iodoacetamide interfered with polymerization; histidines from both the D- and the E-region were affected [238]. Modification of about 16 tryptophan residues by oxidation with hydrogen peroxide did not influence the fibrin monomer polymerization, but further oxidation of 7 more residues destroyed the clotting activity; similarly oxidized fragment D lost its polymerization-inhibitory effect [239].

On photooxidation of fibrinogen in the presence of rose bengal and on reaction with diethyl pyrocarbonate histidine residues, primarily in the Bβ-chain, were modified; the reaction was accompanied by decreased susceptibility to thrombic cleavage [240]. However, on photooxidation in the presence of methylene blue, which also led to histidine modification, at least the initial fibrinopeptide release rate was normal, but the polymerization was strongly affected [241]. Photooxidation of the N-terminal disulfide knot from fibrin reduced its overall ability to bind to fibrinogen–agarose, so that a binding and a non-binding fraction could be separated, in the dysfunctional fraction the histidine residue in position 2 of the fibrin β-chain was demonstrated to be selectively destroyed, indicating the essential function of this histidine residue in fibrin polymerization [241].

The influence of the carbohydrate side chains on the fibrinogen–fibrin conversion has been investigated by comparing biosynthetically non-glycosylated fibrinogen with ordinary fibrinogen as regards their incorporation into fibrin clots; no differences were found [242]. Desialylation of fibrinogen by neuraminidase treatment increased the polymerization rate [166,243], which may be regarded as a result of decreasing the acidic charges in fibrin(ogen), in a related way to the effects of decrease in negative charges on fibrinopeptide release or protamine sulfate treatment [69].

The gel structure of fibrin has been evaluated by measuring the permeation of liquid or particles through it; many factors, such as fibrin type and concentration, enzyme concentration, calcium concentration, were found to influence the fibrin network [50,244]. The mechanical properties of a fibrin gel [54] could be modified by allowing the tetrapeptide analogues of the fibrin α- and β-chain N-termini, Gly-Pro-Arg-Pro and Gly-His-Arg-Pro, to diffuse into it, and the clot would eventually liquefy [245]. Effects of calcium ions on the changes in fibrin(ogen) domain structure during clotting were measured calorimetrically [246].

A large number of different antibodies which can discriminate among various products of fibrinogen have been produced (see Section 1p, Antibodies). In this context it is of special interest that antibodies have been described which will differentiate between fibrinogen and fibrin [247–251], some of them by recognizing the amino terminus of the fibrin α-chain [250] or β-chain [248,249], and another by recognizing fibrinopeptide A in the linked form [251]. Antibodies specific for a polymerization site [252] and a crosslinking site [253] in the α-chain and such which are specific for the crosslinking of the γ-chain region [254] have also been reported (see Section i, Crosslinking).

(i) Crosslinking

After fibrinogen has been converted to fibrin, the polymerized product may be crosslinked by the introduction of isopeptide bonds. The reaction is catalyzed by coagulation factor XIII_a, a plasma transglutaminase, which is calcium ion-dependent and has an active center sulfhydryl group (see Section 2, Factor XIII). The isopeptide bonds are formed between the ϵ-amino groups of a few, selected lysine residues and the γ-carbamoyl groups of some specific glutamine residues.

Crosslinking sites are present only in the γ- and α-chains. Lysine in γ-chain position 406 is connected to glutamine in γ-chain position 398 of the neighboring fibrin molecule, and the corresponding lysine of the second molecule is connected in the same way to the glutamine of the first molecule, so that the C-termini of the γ-chain are linked in antiparallel [85,255]. As it seems, only fibrin molecules within the same row of the protofibril in end-to-end contact will crosslink their D-domains (see Section 1h, Polymerization). The isopeptide bond formation in the γ-chain is fast. The higher-molecular-mass γ-chain variants crosslink to the same extent as the 411-residue γ-chain [33,34].

The crosslinking sites in the Aα-chains have not been as well identified, but it has been assumed that the participating glutamines are those in positions 328 and 366, i.e. in the middle part of the chain, and the lysines may be those in positions 508, 556 and/or 562, i.e. in the C-terminal region of the chain [97,253,256–258]. Several α-chains are gradually crossconnected. The reaction in the α-chain is considerably slower than in the γ-chain. (For further details concerning crosslinking and interactions between fibrin(ogen) and factor XIII see Section 2, Factor XIII.)

(j) Fibrinolysis

When fibrinogen and fibrin are degraded by common proteolytic enzymes fibrinogen is rendered unclottable and the fibrin clot is dissolved. Of special medical and biochemical interest are the degradations caused by plasmin and leukocyte proteinases (cf. Ch. 8).

(1) Degradation by and interaction with plasmin

Plasmin is a trypsin-like enzyme, which is present in plasma as an inactive precursor, plasminogen. Plasmin cleaves fibrinogen at lysyl and arginyl bonds, i.e. with the same peptide bond specificity as trypsin and thrombin. In native fibrinogen plasmin will split about 34 out of the 181 different arginyl and lysyl bonds. However, these bonds are split at highly different rates, so that series of characteristic fragments are formed.

Early detailed examinations of degradation products were made by Nussenzweig et al. in 1961 [259]. Since then much research has been devoted to the interpretation of the fibrinolytic pathway. The results have been of greatest importance for the understanding of the fibrinogen structure and function [260–262]. To begin with, gel electrophoresis was the most common analytical method, but gradually many fibrinolysis products have been isolated and characterized in terms of N-terminal sequence [95,96,118,219,223,263–268]. As special purification method affinity chromatography on fibrin–agarose [231,234–236] or lysine–agarose [42] has often proven useful. In recent years, HPLC-based methods have been introduced [224,225,269,270].

A general scheme for the plasminolytic degradation has gradually emerged. First the C-terminal two thirds of the Aα-chain and a short N-terminal segment of the Bβ-chain are removed and fragment X is formed. This large fragment is cleaved asymmetrically, giving rise to one each of fragments Y and D. Finally, fragment Y is divided into one more fragment D and one fragment E.

Fibrinogen ⟶ fragment X + peptides from Aα- and Bβ-chains

Fragment X ⟶ fragment Y + fragment D + small peptides

Fragment Y ⟶ fragment D + fragment E + small peptides

The regions of fibrinogen contained in fragments D and E are indicated in Fig. 2 and first characterizations of the plasmic fragments are listed in Table 5. It should, however, be noted that each fragment designation represents a whole family of fragments, which differ from each other in their peptide chain components, as often several cleavages will give rise to similar-size fragments.

TABLE 5

Main plasmic fragments of human fibrinogen

Designation	X	Y	D	E
Structure	Dimeric symmetric	Dimeric non-symmetric	Monometric	Dimeric symmetric
Number per molecule	1	1	2	1
Number of peptides	2×3	3+3	3	2×3
Mass (approx.)	250 000	155 000	90 000	50 000

All the so far identified plasmic cleavage sites and their relative positions within human fibrinogen are indicated in Fig. 11 [102]. The first point of attack is near to the C-terminus of the Aα-chain, i.e. after position 583, and a 27-amino acid residue fragment is released [96]. This cleavage occurs partially already in the circulating fibrinogen and partially during preparation [101], and on ion-exchange chromatography of the peptide chains the Aα-chain eluting late contains the complete chain, but the material eluting earlier contains the shorter chain [96,101,102]. These two Aα-chains show up as a characteristic doublet on SDS–gel electrophoresis.

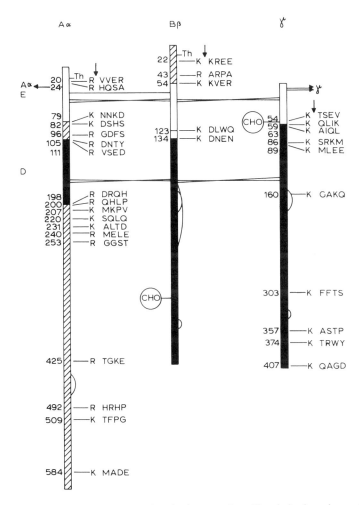

Fig. 11. Human fibrinogen plasmic cleavage sites. The chains have been aligned with the N-termini at the top. The thin, connecting lines represent disulfide bridges. The arrows point to the cleavages in the indicated sequences, the numbers give the positions of the new N-terminal residues. Fragment E is white and D black. Th, thrombin cleavage site; CHO, carbohydrate side chain.

Further early cleavages in the $A\alpha$-chain are those after positions 206 and 230. Hereby a 40 000-molecular-mass fragment is liberated [263] and fragment X is formed. This large $A\alpha$-chain fragment is quickly degraded into fragments of half the size [95,263,266]. There is strong evidence that all these early clips partly already take place in plasma, leading to fibrinogens with higher solubility and lower molecular mass, i.e. 305 000 and 270 000 [28–31,101,218,266]. In parallel with these early splits in the $A\alpha$-chain, the $B\beta$-chain N-terminus is attacked and the first 21, 42, 53 or 54 amino acid residues, including fibrinopeptide B, are removed [269,271]. At this stage fibrinogen is progressively losing its clottability [30,31,218].

Next set of cleavages occur in the regions between D- and E-fragments in all 3 chains, and fragments Y, D and slightly later E are produced. Earlier, less degraded, and later, more degraded, variants of the fragments have been characterized [219,234–236,264,265,267,269,270]. The first formed fragment E has intact $A\alpha$- and γ-chain N-termini, but is missing the 54 most N-terminal residues in the $B\beta$-chain; the C-termini of the peptide chain components are in positions 78 or 81, 122 and 62 for $A\alpha$-, $B\beta$- and γ-chain, respectively [219,265]. In the most degraded form of fragment E the N-terminal 19 residues of the $A\alpha$-chain, including fibrinopeptide A, have been removed, together with a few C-terminal residues in the $A\alpha$- and γ-chain components [219].

The immunological and chemical relationship between fragment E and the N-terminal disulfide knot had been discovered already at an early stage of the investigations [260,261]. Fibrinogen-derived E-fragments were shown to be devoid of active polymerization sites, but early and intermediate fibrin-derived E-fragments would bind to crosslinked fibrin–agarose [219,235].

Early fragment D encompasses the positions 105–197 of the $A\alpha$-chain [234, 264,265]. Subsequently, a few N-terminal residues of the $A\alpha$- and γ-chain components, and, depending on the presence or absence of calcium ions, C-terminal segments of the γ-chain disappear. The $A\alpha$-chain component of intermediate and late fragment D starts at position 111, the γ-chain component at positions 86 and 89, respectively [234,264,265].

Examining the protective effect of calcium ions in plasmin degradation Haverkate, Nieuwenhuizen and coworkers [222,272] observed that the γ-chain component of fragment D obtained in the presence of 2 mM calcium ions has a size indicating that the C-terminus of the chain is included, but the γ-chain component obtained in the presence of metal ion chelators, such as EGTA, has lost approximately 100 amino acid residues from its C-terminal region. The calcium ion-protected peptide bond was tentatively localized to position 302 [273]. The two D-fragment species were called D cate (for *ca*lcium *te*rminal) and D EGTA [272]. D cate, but not D EGTA, could be shown to bind 1 mole of calcium/mole of peptide [222]. The stabilizing effect of calcium and certain other divalent cations has been confirmed by several investigations [274–276] (see also Section 1l, Interactions).

It had been noted that early and late D-fragments differed in their ability to bind to fibrin monomer–agarose and to inhibit fibrin polymerization [234,235,264]. As late D-fragments were devoid of these activities, it was concluded that a polymerization site is located in the C-terminal region of the γ-chain. More recently an intermediate D-fragment, Dint, was described, which binds calcium ions, but lacks anticlotting properties [222]. The finding was interpreted as that the calcium binding site was more distant from the γ-chain C-terminus than the polymerization site. First attempts to isolate the segment of the γ-chain responsible for polymerization inhibition and, thus, containing the polymerization site seemed succesful, and segments corresponding to amino acid residues 374–411 [223] or 374–396 [224] inhibited polymerization efficiently. However, segments 303–356, 357–373 and 374–405 were found to be devoid of inhibitory activity in another investigation [225], and it was suggested that the polymerization site would correspond to a more extended region of the γ-chain C-terminus.

Fibrin and especially crosslinked fibrin are, to some extent, degraded in a different way from fibrinogen [277–284]. The main end products are not the fragments D and E, but a non-covalent complex, DD–E or D-dimer E, as N-terminal polymerization site(s) are activated in fibrin E-fragment, which has an especially high affinity for the site(s) in crosslinked D-fragment [279–280]. Higher-molecular-mass intermediate complexes of the types DY–YD, DXD–YY and YXD–DXY have been characterized [280,281]. It was demonstrated that increased α-chain crosslinking, but not γ-chain crosslinking, made the fibrin clot more resistant to plasmin [277]. Also crosslinked products of the DD–E type are more susceptible to further degradation in the presence of a calcium ion chelator, EDTA, and late fragments D, devoid of affinity for fibrin fragment E, are released [278].

It may be sumarized that in native fibrin(ogen) about twice as many lysyl as arginyl bonds are split by plasmin, and that about half the number of cleavages occur in the Aα-chain. Most of the cleavage sites are found in a few hydrophilic clusters (see Fig. 11). The information about fibrinogen structure and functional sites gained by studying plasmic fragments is in excellent agreement with that obtained by analyzing chemical fragments and electron microscopy data [60–66].

A large number of antibodies against various plasmic fragments have been described. These antibodies have found extensive application mainly in clinical investigations [285–296], but also as probes for degradation-related surface exposure in fibrin(ogen) [297,298]. Antibodies against D-dimer [254,285–291] and against the N-terminus of the Bβ-chain, i.e. positions 1–42 or 15–42 [269,270,292,293], have attracted considerable interest as markers for fibrinolysis in patients. An additional useful antibody is the one directed against the C-terminal region of the Aα-chain [294].

Fibrinogen and fibrin bind Glu and Lys plasminogen and plasmin, mediated by the lysine-binding sites of the enzyme [299–305]. Limited degradation created additional binding sites [304], and certain regions within both fragments D and E seemed essential for binding [303]. Plasminogen and plasmin were found to bind in higher amounts to non-crosslinked than to crosslinked fibrin [302]. Furthermore plasminogen was observed to enhance fibrin polymerization [299].

(2) Degradation by other enzymes

Fibrinogen and fibrin can be degraded by a large number of other proteinases than plasmin. A few of these enzymes have clinical relevance, some others are of interest as the degradation products are endowed with special biochemical properties. To the group with medical importance belong enzymes from polymorphonuclear neutrophil (PMN) leukocytes, i.e. leukocyte elastase [306–309] and cathepsin G [306], from monocytes–macrophages [310] and those contained in certain animal venoms.

The cleavage pattern obtained with leukocyte elastase has been shown to resemble that with plasmin, in the way that X-, D- and E-like fragments were obtained, that calcium ions would protect against the most extensive degradation, and that certain fragments would possess anticlotting properties [306–309]. Little is, however, known about the positions of the cleavage sites.

Many snake venoms have been demonstrated to contain fibrinolytic enzymes [226,311–314]. Only in rare cases have the cleavage sites been identified [226]. Powerful fibrinolytic enzymes have also been found in a leech [315] and a caterpillar [316].

A protease from Pseudomonas has the unique property to degrade fibrinogen into a crystalizing form [58,59,67].

(k) Biologically active fragments

Several well-defined low-molecular-mass fibrinogen fragments have been reported to display biological activity. Fibrinopeptides A and B showed an effect in experimental allergic encephalomyelitis and in carrageenan-induced inflammatory rat paw edema [317]. A pentapeptide, corresponding to positions 123–127 of the Bβ-chain, was isolated from a patient and demonstrated to inhibit lymphocyte E-rosette formation [318].

Another pentapeptide from the Bβ-chain, this time positions 43–47, induced vasodilation, prostacyclin release and an increase in cyclic AMP; it also inhibited angiotensin-converting enzyme, released histamine, and increased microvascular permeability and coronary blood flow [319,320]. A 14-residue peptide from the Bβ-chain, positions 30–43, increased also vascular permeability and coronary blood flow, and furthermore, it induced leukocyte emigration [321]. One more fragment, the 11-residue peptide from the Aα-chain, positions 220–230, was demonstrated to increase vascular permeability and release histamine; it also inhibited thymidine uptake in kidney cell culture [320].

It should be mentioned in this context that a putative cell attachment site sequence, Arg-Gly-Asp, occurs twice in the Aα-fibrinogen, i.e. positions 95–97 and 572–574; the C-terminal localization could possibly be implicated in platelet binding [322].

(l) Interactions with other proteins and metal ions

Fibrin(ogen) interacts in specific and unspecific ways with a large number of proteins, cells and metal ions (Table 1). Many of the specific interactions are of physiological importance, those related to thrombin and plasmin(ogen) having been mentioned above (see Section 1h, Fibrinogen–fibrin conversion and 1j, Fibrinolysis) and those related to factor XIII and the crosslinking with several proteins being described below (see Section 2, Factor XIII).

Fibrin binds certain types of plasminogen activators and may enhance the conversion of plasminogen to plasmin, especially when both plasminogen and activator are bound to fibrin [301,323–333]. Tissue-type plasminogen activator shows a specific affinity for fibrin, but not for fibrinogen. The affinity has been suggested to be due to the so-called finger domain, which is present in this activator, but not in urokinase or streptokinase [324]. Most recently, however, it could be shown that tissue plasminogen activator devoid of the finger domain also binds strongly to fibrin [325]. Single-chain urokinase-type plasminogen activator, i.e. prourokinase, has a higher affinity for fibrin than the activated two-chain form of the enzyme [328–329]. Cyanogen-bromide-cleaved and plasmin-digested fibrin enhance the plasminogen activation by tissue-type and urokinase-type activators [301,327,331] and by streptokinase [332,333].

The α_2-plasmin inhibitor interacts in several ways with fibrin. It may be crosslinked to fibrin (see Section 2, Factor XIII), and it inhibits the binding of plasminogen to fibrin [334]. Two forms of the inhibitor, which differ in fibrin-binding properties, have been described [335].

The affinity of fibronectin for fibrin(ogen) has been well documented [43, 336–340]. The fibrin-binding regions of fibronectin contain large numbers of the so-called finger domains, which were first described for this protein [336] and later also discovered in a plasminogen activator [324]. Fibronectin has been demonstrated to be incorporated into and crosslinked with fibrin clots (see below). The possible inhibitory effect on clot formation, the enhancing effect on fibrin monomer solubility and the influence on gel structure have been discussed [337–339]. Fibronectin or its fragments may mediate the binding of fibrin to various cells, such as macrophages [340].

Fibrin(ogen) may furthermore bind certain types of collagen [341], serum amyloid P component [342], various unrelated immunoglobulins and other plasma proteins [343,344]. Some plasma proteins affect fibrin polymerization [343,344]. The physiological significance is often unknown. Several autoantibodies against fibrin(ogen) or fibrinolytic degradation products have been described [345], some of which influence the fibrinogen function. Hepatitis B surface antigen binds to fibrinogen [346].

Physiologically less relevant, but still quite specific interactions have been demonstrated to occur between fibrin(ogen) and concanavalin A [347] or protamine sulfate [69].

Calcium ions influence many properties, functions and reactions of fibrinogen,

```
                                      x   y   z  -y  -x  -z
Calmodulin                     + E X + + X X + + X D + O + O G - + I O + + E X + + X X + + X

γ -chain     301   D K↓F F T S H N G M Q F S T W D N D N D K F E G N C A E Q D G S G W W M
Bβ-chain     364   N⁺R T M T I H N G M F F S T Y D R D N D G - W L T S - D P R K Q C S K E
```

Fig. 12. Homology between calcium-binding sequence in calmodulin and suggested calcium-binding sequence in human fibrinogen γ- and Bβ-chain. x – –z, calcium ligands in calmodulin; X, hydrophobic residue; O, oxygen-containing ligand residue; –, deletion; +, arbitrary residue; N⁺, asparagine residue with carbohydrate side chain; arrow, calcium-protected peptide bond. Underlined are residues in agreement with calmodulin 'test sequence'.

e.g. those related to fibrinopeptide release [348], fibrin polymerization, crosslinking, fibrinolytic degradation [222,272,274–276] and conformation [246,275]. The fibrinogen molecule contains 3 calcium-binding sites [222,348,349], one in each D-domain [222,272,274,275] and one in the E-domain [349]. The difference in calcium ion-binding properties between D-fragments of certain sizes [222,272], the position of the calcium ion-protected peptide bond in the γ-chain and the structural similarity between C-terminal sequences in the γ- and Bβ-chains and the calcium-binding sequence in calmodulin and related proteins [273,350], as shown in Fig. 12, provided strong evidence for the localization of the calcium-binding site. The interpretation was recently supported by results of terbium ion-binding studies [351].

Fibrinogen can be precipitated by many different metal ions. However, a specific interaction seems to exist with zinc ions, which bind to D-fragments, but not at the calcium-binding site [352], and which reduce the thrombin clotting time [353]. Several other divalent metal ions increase both the fibrin polymerization and the fibrinogen precipitation rate [354].

(m) Interactions with cells and their constituents

Fibrin(ogen) interacts in a specific and physiologically important manner with a large number of cells, primarily those of the blood and the blood vessel wall. The cell constituents responsible have so far not been identified for most cells.

Much research work has been devoted to the interaction between fibrinogen and platelets, especially with the purpose to elucidate the properties of the fibrinogen receptors and the relationship with the aggregation state of the platelets [355–359]. In fibrinogen, C-terminal regions of both the γ-chain [357–359] and the Aα-chain [356,359] can bind to the platelets. In the γ-chain the residues 400–411 have been identified as being of primary importance [357,358]. On the platelet side, the membrane glycoproteins IIb and IIIa are involved in the binding [355–359]. The platelet protein thrombospondin, which is secreted from the platelet during coagulation, also binds to fibrinogen, is incorporated into fibrin clots and may crosslink to fibrin [360–361].   The enhancing effect of increased fibrinogen concentration on erythrocyte aggregation and sedimentation was utilized for diagnostic purposes already several thousand years ago (see Section 1a, Introduction). Recent investigations demonstrate the importance of fibrinogen concentration and erythrocyte aggregation for blood viscosity and flow and for erythrocyte adhesion [362–364].

Studies of the interactions between fibrin(ogen) and endothelial cells have been conducted. In some reports the binding of fibrinogen to these cells is described as specific [365], in other reports as unspecific [366]. Fibrinogen has been shown to induce endothelial cell migration [365], and fibrin seems to stimulate the formation of capillary-like tubes from endothelial cells [367], as well as influence the shape of the cells in the culture [368]. Fibrin(ogen) may form an endoendothelial lining of the blood vessels [369].

A number of reports dealing with the interaction between fibrin(ogen) and monocytes [370], macrophages [371,372], fibroblasts [372,373] and melanoma cells [374] have also appeared. The binding region within fibrin(ogen) has been indicated to be the α-chain for monocytes [370], the amino terminus of the α-chain for macrophages [371] and the E-domain for fibroblasts [373].

The interaction of fibrinogen with many different types of bacteria has recently been reported. The interactions seem to be of pronounced pathophysiological importance, as the bacterial surface may get masked by fibrinogen binding. Several strains of *Staphylococcus aureus* both bind and are clumped by fibrinogen [358,375], others only bind [376]. The fibrinogen sites for the staphylococcal clumping reaction are localized at the carboxy termini of the γ-chains, positions 397–411 [358,375]. Many types of Streptococcus bind fibrinogen [376–380], and the fibrinogen site seems to be present in the Aα- and Bβ-chains [376], the bacterial site is related to the M protein, as extracted M protein will bind to and even precipitate fibrinogen [378–380].

(n) Normal variants

Human fibrinogen occurs in a great number of different molecular forms, as there are several sites or sections of the molecule which exist in a number of different forms and the regional variants may be combined in various ways. The hetero-

Aα-chain	S/T	47	K C P S/T G C R
Aα-chain	T/A	296	S S G T/A G G T
Aα-chain	T/A	312	P G S T/A G S W
Bβ-chain	P/A	162	S N I P/A T N L
Bβ-chain	N/D	296	W L G N/D D K I
Bβ-chain	R/K	448	Y S M R/K K M S
γ -chain	K/I	88	K S R K/I M L E

Fig. 13. Human fibrinogen amino acid sequences containing tentatively identified microheterogeneous positions. The numbers indicate these positions.

geneity of fibrinogen is evident already from the variations in solubility properties [28–31], ion-exchange chromatographic behavior of total fibrinogen [32–34,88] and of its peptide chain components [81,96,381], as well as the gel-electrophoretic behavior of the peptide chains [124,382,383].

Heterogeneity in the Aα-chain is related to various degrees of C-terminal, probably mainly fibrinolytic degradation [28–31,96,101,102,218] and to the phosphorylation state of the serine residues in positions 3 [126,129] and 345 [127]. Variants of the Bβ-chain are due to its carbohydrate side chain, i.e. the presence of one or two neuraminic acid groups [121–125,381]. The γ-chain may differ in its C-terminal region depending on the type of mRNA involved at the synthesis [32–34,88,89,110,144,145] and in its carbohydrate side chain depending on the presence of one or two neuraminic acid groups [121–125,381] (see also under Sections 1d, f, g and j). All fibrinogen forms which may arise from the above-mentioned regional variations are expected to exist in all normal human beings.

A different category of human fibrinogen variants is made up of those caused by genetic polymorphism in the population. The so far tentatively identified sites for microheterogeneity are listed in Fig. 13. Only for the 3 types of Aα-chain variants have both forms been observed on the protein-chemical level [99,114]. The DNA sequence of the Aα-chain predicted Ser in position 47,Thr in 296, but Thr [87] or Ala [100] in position 312. For the site in position 162 of the Bβ-chain only the Pro-containing protein sequence was reported [90,92], but both DNA sequences corresponding to Pro and such corresponding to Ala were detected [93]. For the Bβ-chain sites in positions 296 and 448, the protein sequences [90,92] and one of the DNA sequences [93] indicated Asn and Arg, respectively, the other DNA sequence [87] Asp and Lys, respectively. For the site in the γ-chain, both the protein [83] and the cDNA sequence [144] showed Lys, but the gene sequence predicted Ile [144].

It is clear that further research is needed for the unambiguous interpretation of the results summarized in Fig. 13 as due to polymorphism. A truly polymorphic site has, however, been identified by restriction fragment length analysis in a non-transcribed region of the Aα-chain locus [142].

Human platelet or megakaryocyte-synthesized fibrinogen seems to be identical with plasma fibrinogen, synthesized in the liver [146–150], except for the absence of the higher-molecular-mass γ-chain variant [148–150]. However, more evidence for the identity is required.

The existence of a fetal form of fibrinogen has already been discussed in the literature for a long time, as fibrinogen isolated from cord blood seems to differ in many of its properties from fibrinogen isolated from adult blood. Thus, cord plasma fibrinogen has often been described as characterized by delayed fibrin aggregation and a distinct fibrin clot appearance [384–388]. It has been firmly established that fetal fibrinogen contains at least twice as much phosphate as adult fibrinogen [127,389]; the phosphorylation degree is higher in the fetal form both in fibrinopeptide A and in the interior of the Aα-chain [127] (see Fig. 6). It seems that fetal fibrinogen contains more neuraminic acid than adult fibrinogen and that enzymatic removal of the excess will normalize the clotting time [385–388]. Fetal fibrinogen has been fingerprinted and most of its Aα-chain has been sequenced, but the results were in complete agreement with those for adult fibrinogen [99].

(o) Abnormal variants

(1) Acquired abnormalities

Acquired functional abnormalities of fibrinogen are associated with certain diseases, primarily those of the liver, such as cirrhosis, hepatitis, liver cell tumor [385,388,390,391]. The fibrinogen molecule may be defective in several ways, but the most common and best characterized abnormality is related to a delay in fibrin polymerization, which is caused by an increase in carbohydrate content, especially neuraminic acid. The relative excess in neuraminic acid is correlated with the thrombin time prolongation, and on treatment with neuraminidase both the number of neuraminic acid residues and the thrombin time were normalized in a similar manner as described for fetal fibrinogen [385,388,390,391].

The additional neuraminic acid residues are only present in the Bβ- and γ-chains, and are most likely accommodated by extra branches of the carbohydrate side chains [390], i.e. in the form of triantennary sugar moieties. The effect of the abnormally high neuraminic acid content on fibrin polymerization may be explained as due to the additional negative charges of the acidic residues.

A different type of fibrinogen with increased carbohydrate content is found in diabetic subjects [392] and may be obtained by incubation of fibrinogen with glucose [393]. The glucose is bound in a rearranged form to the ϵ-amino groups of lysine and possibly to α-amino groups, and seems not to be of major importance for the fibrinogen function [392,393].

(2) Genetically determined abnormalities

Several types of inherited fibrinogen disorders have been described: the fibrinogen synthesized may be dysfunctional, resulting in a dysfibrinogenemia, and the synthesis itself may be deficient, resulting in a hypo- or afibrinogenemia.

The inherited fibrinogen dysfunctions are assumed to be due to mutations which lead to the synthesis of structurally abnormal variants. These variants differ usually only in a single amino acid residue from the normal fibrinogen, and provide thus the unique means to correlate the details of the structure to the function. Various laboratory tests and clinical observations have led to the detection of dysfibrinogenemias in over 130 families, and the number is rapidly increasing. Several detailed reviews have appeared during the last years [3,168,385,394–397].

Until recently the number of structurally elucidated cases of dysfibrinogenemia was small, because of the great problems related to identifying a single substituted amino acid residue in a molecule containing 2×1482 residues, most substitutions being expressed heterozygously. However, functional tests and protein-chemical analyses have been employed to find clues to the localization of the structural error. The most commonly observed functional defect is the prolonged coagulation

TABLE 6

Classification of genetically abnormal fibrinogens according to the number and type of fibrinopeptide released

Group	Homozygote				Heterozygote			
	FPA		FPB		FPA		FPB	
	Abnormal	Normal	Abnormal	Normal	Abnormal	Normal	Abnormal	Normal
IA	–	–	–	2	–	1	–	2
IB	–	2	–	–	–	2	–	1
IIA	2	–	2	2	1	1	–	2
IIB	–	2	2	–	–	2	1	1
III	–	2	–	2	–	2	–	2

TABLE 7

Structurally elucidated, genetically abnormal fibrinogens

Group		FPA abn	FPA norm	FPB abn	FPB norm	Rep. clott.	Add. thr. clott.	Error	Gene expr.
IA	Metz	–	–	–	2	–	++	Aα16 R→C	ho
	Amsterdam I	–	1	–	2	+	+	Aα16 R→C	he
	Bergamo I *	–	1	–	2			Aα16 R→C	he
	Frankfurt II	–	1	–	2			Aα16 R→C	he
	Frankfurt III	–	1	–	2	+	+	Aα16 R→C	he
	Paris	–	1	–	2			Aα16 R→C	he
	Stony Brook	–	1	–	2	+	+	Aα16 R→C	he
	Schwarzach	–	1	–	2			Aα16 R→C	he
	Zürich I	–	1	–	2	+	+	Aα16 R→C	he
IB	New York I *	–	2	–	1			Bβ9–72 Del.	he

TABLE 7 (continued)

Group	FPA abn	FPA norm.	FPB abn.	FPB norm.	Rep. clott.	Add. thr. clott.	Error	Gene expr.
IIA								
Bicêtre	2	–	–	2	–	++	Aα16 R→H	ho
Bicêtre	1	1	–	2	+	+	Aα16 R→H	he
Amiens *	1	1	–	2			Aα16 R→H	he
Bern II *	1	1	–	2			Aα16 R→H	he
Chapel Hill II	1	1	–	2	+	+	Aα16 R→H	he
Clermond-Ferrand *	1	1	–	2			Aα16 R→H	he
Leitchfield	1	1	–	2			Aα16 R→H	he
Louisville	1	1	–	2	+	+	Aα16 R→H	he
Manchester	1	1	–	2			Aα16 R→H	he
New Albany	1	1	–	2			Aα16 R→H	he
Petoskey *	1	1	–	2			Aα16 R→H	he
Sydney I	1	1	–	2			Aα16 R→H	he
Sydney II	1	1	–	2			Aα16 R→H	he
White Marsh *			–	2			Aα16 R→H	
Lille *			–	2			Aα 7 D→H	
Rouen	1	1	–	2	++	–	Aα12 G→V	he
III								
Detroit *	–	2	–	2			Aα19 R→S	ho, he
München I	–	2	–	2	++	–	Aα19 R→N	he
Pontoise	–	2	–	2			Bβ335A→T	he
Bergamo II	–	2	–	2			γ275R→H	he
Essen	–	2	–	2			γ275R→H	he
Haifa	–	2	–	2			γ275R→H	he
Milano I	–	2	–	2	++	–	γ330D→V	he

Abn., abnormal; norm., normal; rep. clott., reptilase clotting; add. thr. clott., additional thrombin clotting; expr., expression; ho, homozygous; he, heterozygous; del., deletion.

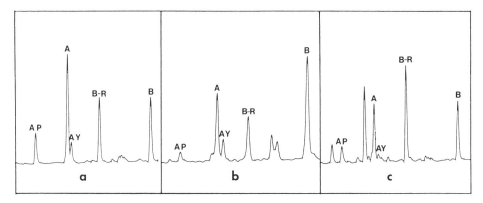

Fig. 14. Human fibrinopeptides from normal and genetically abnormal fibrinogen separated by reversed-phase high-performance liquid chromatography using an ammonium acetate, pH 6–acetonitrile gradient and detection at 220 nm. a, normal fibrinogen; b, abnormal fibrinogen from group IA (Aα 16R→C); c, abnormal fibrinogen from group IIA (Aα16R→H).

time. The delay may either be due to incomplete or slow release of fibrinopeptides A and/or B, or due to impaired fibrin polymerization in the absence of a release defect.

The development of HPLC-based methods for quantitative and qualitative fibrinopeptide analysis [167,168,182] has made it possible to classify the genetically abnormal fibrinogens in a convenient way [168,396,397]. Thus, by determining the yields and types of fibrinopeptides released by an excess of thrombin after an excess of time the 3 main groups shown in Table 6 may be discerned. Group I is characterized by the absence of fibrinopeptide release, group II by the release of an abnormal fibrinopeptide and group III by normal release. Groups I and II can be subdivided into A and B depending on the type of fibrinopeptide showing abnormal behavior. Different patterns are obtained in homozygous and in heterozygous cases. Typical HPLC patterns for fibrinopeptides derived from normal fibrinogen and from heterozygous cases belonging to groups IA and IIA are presented in Fig. 14.

The 32 cases of structurally elucidated genetically determined fibrinogen abnormality are listed in Table 7, and the corresponding sequences surrounding the substituted amino acid residues are compiled in Fig. 15. All variants, except those marked with *, have been elucidated by Henschen and coworkers. Detailed references to most of the variants have been published [3,168].

All 9 variants in group IA have the same amino acid substitution, i.e. Aα 16 Arg→Cys [168,385,396–400]. When the C-terminal Arg residue in the fibrinopeptide A sequence is replaced by Cys, no cleavage occurs, but when Cys is derivatized by S-aminoethylation thrombin will cleave after the Lys analogue formed and a modified peptide may be identified [400]. In the single homozygous case, the fibrinogen variant clotted after release of only fibrinopeptide B [398].

A single variant belonging to group IB has hitherto been identified. A large N-terminal deletion corresponding to the second exon of the Bβ-chain explains the absence of fibrinopeptide B release [401].

In group IIA 13 of the 15 cases are characterized by the substitution Aα 16 Arg→His [153,168,193,197,385,402,403], i.e. this is the most common type of structurally elucidated genetic fibrinogen variant. Surprisingly, thrombin cleaves quantitatively and selectively, though much more slowly after His replacing Arg at the C-terminus of the A-peptide sequence. The modified A-peptide has a distinct HPLC retention time (see Fig. 14).

In group III the amino acid substitutions are localized in the fibrin part of fibrinogen, in 2 cases close to the N-terminus of the α-chain [35,168,396,399,404] and in 5 cases in the C-terminal part of the β- or γ-chain [405,406]. The substitution in the Bβ-chain induces a new carbohydrate attachment site, which indeed is fully glycosylated [405]. The substitutions in the γ-chain are associated with impaired calcium ion interaction [406]. It may be expected that inherited, dysfunctional fibrinogen variants corresponding to all the various properties and functional sites will be discovered some time in the future.

Much less is known about the other categories of fibrinogen-related disorders and the causes of hypo- and afibrinogenemia have in most cases not yet been discovered [394,395,407–409]. However, one family has been described in which the low plasma fibrinogen level was due to disturbed secretion of fibrinogen from the hepatocytes, and massive deposits of fibrin(ogen) could be demonstrated in the liver [408], i.e. the family suffered from a liver storage disease. In two afibrinogenemic patients no gross defects in the fibrinogen genes could be detected [409].

(p) Antibodies

Antibodies directed against fibrin(ogen) or specific regions of it have, obviously, found wide application in very many types of fibrinogen-related research. Recently, the preparation and properties of a number of the highly specific mono-

```
Aα-chain    D   7    A D S G E G D F L A E G G G V R↓G P R V V
            G  12                N              V         C     S
            R  16                                         H     N
            R  19


Bβ-chain    G   9 -  L 72 Deletion

            A 335    F T V Q N E A N K Y Q I
                             N⁺ T

γ-chain     R 275    P E A D K Y R L T Y A Y
                                 H

            D 330    G N C A E Q D G S G W W
                               V
```

Fig. 15. Human fibrinogen structurally elucidated genetically abnormal variants. The top line in each sequence represents the normal sequence, the amino acid substitutions are shown below. The numbers indicate the positions of the substitutions.

clonal antibodies have been reported. Only a few examples for the use of antibodies can be given here.

General antifibrinogen antibodies have been employed as immunosorbents or immunoprecipitants during fibrinogen purification [41,137,138,151,156], for detection of fibrinogen in gel electrophoresis [291], histologic sections [408] or for quantification of fibrinogen and degradation products in plasma [16,20,290].

Antibodies against fibrinopeptide A [169–174,178,179,189,198], fibrinopeptide B [175–177,189,191], Bβ 1–42 or 15–42 or similar [199,248,249,269,270,283,292,293] have been used extensively both for studying patients and fibrinopeptide release-related biochemical mechanisms. Certain antibodies can differentiate between fibrinogen and fibrin [247–251] or can recognize polymerization or crosslinking sites in the α-chain [252,253] or the crosslinking site in the γ-chain [254,285–290].

Also antibodies against fibrin(ogen) degradation products D, E and the C-terminal region of the Aα-chain have been of great value both for clinical and biochemical investigations [60–62,155,220,294–298,305], such as electron microscopic localization [60–62] or surface exposure during degradation [297,298] (for Bβ 1–42, see above). A number of autoantibodies with various specificities have been discovered in healthy subjects as well as in patients [345].

It may be mentioned in this context that not only antibodies [297] but also chemical reagents [410,411] have been employed to analyze the surface of the fibrinogen molecule and its solvent exposure.

(q) Evolutionary aspects

Speculations around the evolution of fibrinogen started when especially Blombäck and coworkers were able to demonstrate that fibrins from several animal species have the same N-terminal amino acids [78], but the corresponding fibrinopeptides differ enormously in sequence [42], in fact show more inter-species variation than any other protein [413].

The evolutionary origin of the 3 peptide chains has also been discussed for a long time, and the fact that two of the chains, i.e. Aα and Bβ, release fibrinopeptides during coagulation was taken as an indication of their common ancestry. However, when the two first peptide chain sequences, i.e. those of γ and Bβ, became available [83,90], a striking and unexpected degree of homology between these chains was observed [414]. Identical residues were found in about 30% of the positions (depending on alignment and gaps), the degree of identity being higher in the C-terminal two thirds of the chains [105,273,397]. The alignment of the chains offered an explanation for the absence of a γ-chain fibrinopeptide C, as the γ-chain is 'too short' at the N-terminus [105]. When later the Aα-chain sequence was completed [97,98], it turned out that this chain is much less similar to the two other chains, only approximately 10% of the positions containing identical residues as the Bβ- or γ-chain [105,273,397], but the N-terminal regions being somewhat more homologous. The internal, 13-residue repeat in the middle of the Aα-chain has 66% of the positions in agreement with an 'average' sequence [97,273,397].

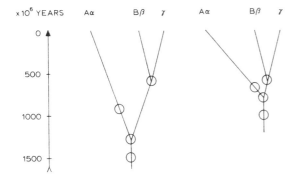

Fig. 16. Evolution of the 3 fibrinogen chains.

The recently reported animal fibrinogen chains may also be compared with their human counterparts. Human and rat [109] Aα-chains show 53% identity, human and bovine [106] Bβ-chains 82%, human and rat [110] γ-chains 83%, and finally human and lamprey [111] γ-chains 50%.

Because of the pronounced homologies among the 3 chains, it may be assumed that they all have a common evolutionary ancestor, and that they arose by gene duplications and subsequently have diverged due to separate mutations [103,273,397,415]. The 3 fibrinogen chains, also the Bβ and γ, must have diverged during evolution before the appearance of vertebrates, as even the most primitive vertebrates [111] possess 3 different peptide chains. The Aα-chain should have diverged from a Bβ–γ-common ancestor earlier, as it is less similar. The evolutionary time course may have been as outlined in Fig. 16. The two variants of the scheme illustrate how similar (left side) and quite dissimilar (right side) amino acid exchange rates (symbolized by the relative slopes) relate to an earlier (left side) or later (right side) time point for the gene duplication event (marked as a ring). Assuming the Aα-chain to evolve faster than the other chains, it might have diverged from the common ancestor only 800 million years ago (right side of Fig. 16).

The internal repeats in the Aα-chain would have arisen by partial gene duplications (ring in Fig. 16) after the divergence of this chain from the others [87,100,109]. The ring on the common Aα–Bβ–γ line symbolizes that the chains were elongated by means of gene duplication before they diverged from each other, as deduced from the sequence identities arount the half-Cys residues involved in the triple connections of the chains [273,397].

Fibrinogen, especially the γ-chain, has been suggested to be related to κ-casein [133,273] and to β-thromboglobulin [416].

It seems worthwhile noting that the amino acid substitutions of the genetically abnormal, dysfunctional human fibrinogens are always found in positions which are evolutionary strictly non-variant. This fact may serve to illustrate the difference between 'allowed' and 'not allowed' structure in relation to appropriate and non-appropriate function [168,397,405,406].

2. Factor XIII

(a) Occurrence and function

Factor XIII_a (plasma transglutaminase, fibrinoligase, fibrin-stabilizing factor) belongs to a group of calcium ion-dependent enzymes designated as endo-γ-glutamine: ϵ-lysine transferases. The enzymes are more commonly referred to as transglutaminases, although this name is not strictly appropriate. The Enzyme Commission nomenclature recommends glutaminyl-peptide γ-glutamyltransferase (EC 2.3.2.13). The function of these enzymes is catalysis of isopeptide bond formation between the γ-carbamoyl group of peptide-bound glutamine and the ϵ-amino group of lysine. By this mechanism, two polypeptides can be covalently joined together.

Factor XIII is essential for normal hemostasis, as evidenced by the bleeding problems of patients who are either congenitally deficient or who have acquired inhibitors. Factor XIII may also have a more general role in the various processes involving cell proliferation, including wound healing and tissue repair, tumor growth and metastasis, and atherosclerosis. In addition, factor XIII has also certain unique biochemical properties. The zymogen exists in two molecular forms, one of which is found intracellularly in platelets, megakaryocytes, monocytes, placenta, uterus and prostate tissue and is a dimer of two identical A chains $(A_2)^*$. The extracellular zymogen is found only in plasma; it has two A subunits and two B subunits (denoted A_2B_2). Activation of factor XIII to XIII_a is a multi-step process that results in exposure of an active center cysteine. Cysteine enzymes are principally intracellular, and plasma factor XIII_a is the only sulfhydryl enzyme known to function extracellularly. Factor XIII_a is also the only enzyme in the blood coagulation mechanism which is not a serine proteinase.

(b) Purification and assay

Factor XIII can be isolated from plasma, platelet lysate, and placental extract entirely in zymogenic form. Normal plasma does not have any transglutaminase activity, and there is evidence that in vivo both the intracellular and extracellular forms of factor XIII normally exist as zymogens. However, activation can readily occur during purification, particularly of A_2. In order to prevent activation, purification should be done with EDTA present in all buffers and in the absence of reducing agents.

The concentration of A_2B_2 in human plasma is 30 μg/ml, i.e. 0.0004% of the total protein [417]. It can be purified from plasma by procedures involving differential precipitation, removal of fibrinogen, and ion-exchange chromatorgraphy on

---

* The following nomenclature is used: A_2, intracellular zymogen; A_2B_2, extracellular zymogen; A'_2 and A'_2B_2, thrombin-activated zymogens; A_2 and A_2B_2, Ca^{2+}-activated zymogens; $A_2\star$, active enzymes, also called factor XIII_a. A and B refer to the separated polypeptide subunits.

DEAE-cellulose [418–421]. Precipitation is usually carried out from citrated plasma at pH 7.0–7.5 with ammonium sulfate, and fibrinogen is removed by denaturation at 56°C [418,419]. The final factor XIII precipitate is chromatographed on DEAE–cellulose. A_2B_2 is 2000–4000 times purified after elution from the ion-exchange column, and the yield is 20–30%. Further purification may be achieved by a second chromatography on DEAE–cellulose, HPLC or agarose gel filtration. Purified A_2B_2 can be stored at 4°C in buffer containing EDTA. When factor XIII is purified from fresh or fresh frozen human plasma, essentially all of the factor XIII protein isolated is in the tetrameric A_2B_2 complex.

Intracellular factor XIII, free of contamination by the plasma component, can be prepared from washed platelets by ammonium sulfate precipitation, followed by DEAE-cellulose chromatography and affinity chromatography on organomercurial agarose [422]. Rapid fractionation results in isolation of all the factor XIII in the zymogenic form. A_2 can also be purified from placental concentrate [417].

Although A and B are held together non-covalently in the plasma zymogen, they do not readily dissociate. Isolation of B protein from A_2B_2 can be achieved electrophoretically in SDS buffer [423]. B protein can also be isolated if the zymogen is first activated. In the absence of reducing agent A_2^* tends to precipitate, leaving the supernatant enriched in B.

Factor XIII will covalently bind to organomercurial agarose through free sulfhydryls in A. B protein has no free SH groups and is bound to the matrix only through its non-covalent association with A. B can be eluted in denaturing buffers or in non-denaturing buffers if the complex is first activated [422].

Quantitative assays to measure factor XIII activity have been developed by Lorand and colleagues [419] and are based on the normal function of the enzyme, which is covalent bond formation between lysine and peptide-bound glutamine (Fig. 17). In the most widely used assays, a labeled lysine analogue such as monodansylcadaverine or radiolabeled (^{14}C or ^{3}H) putrescine is incorporated into a protein acceptor such as casein, and increased fluorescence or radioactivity of the protein is a measure of factor XIII activity. These assays can also be used to quantitate factor XIII in plasma. However, in order to prevent clot formation when thrombin and calcium ions are added to activate factor XIII, fibrinogen is first heat-precipitated [419] or the tetrapeptide fibrin polymerization inhibitor, Gly-Pro-Arg-Pro, is added to the assay mixture [424]. The assays can detect about 1% of the normal plasma factor XIII level or 0.15 µg/ml A protein. Totally synthetic assays using thiol esters, such as β-phenylpropionylthiocholine, and dansylcadaverine have primarily been used for kinetic studies with purified enzyme [419]. The active center can be titrated with iodoacetamide.

Factor XIII activity can be measured by in situ activity staining of gels following non-denaturing agarose electrophoresis [419]. The gels are overlayed with a staining solution containing thrombin, calcium ions, dansylcadaverine and casein, which results in formation of a fluorescent band proportional to the amount of A protein in the gel. An additional method is based on quantitation of the amount of γ–γ dimer formation in fibrin crosslinking [425]. In this assay, factor XIII is added to

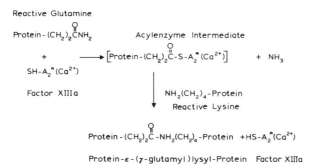

Fig. 17. Diagrammatic representation of the covalent crosslinking of two substrate proteins by factor XIII$_a$.

fibrinogen, and the mixture is clotted with thrombin and calcium ions. Clots are dissolved and analyzed by SDS gel electrophoresis under reducing conditions.

A and B proteins can also be measured immunochemically by radioimmunoassay or electroimmunoassay [417,426]. Not all antibodies react equally well with the various conformational forms of A protein. With radioimmunoassays and dansylcadaverine activity assays, the specific activity of factor XIII$_a$ has been found to be 1.5–1.7 units/μg A protein, where 1.0 unit is defined as the incorporation of 1.0 μmole dansylcadaverine/30 min in a standard assay [417].

(c) Biosynthesis

All of the intracellular forms of factor XIII are immunochemically identical and are generally thought to be synthesized by the cells in which the zymogens are found. Platelet factor XIII was identified by immunofluorescence in megakaryocytes and in platelets [427]. Platelet A$_2$ is not adsorbed from plasma [428]. These observations indicate, therefore, that megakaryocytes are the site of synthesis of A$_2$ in platelets. A$_2$ in monocytes and in a promonocyte tumor cell line has been shown by metabolic labeling and immunoprecipitation to be synthesized by these cells. A$_2$ is found in the cytoplasm of megakaryocytes, platelets, and monocytes [427,429,430]. It is not present in platelet granules and is not a constituent of the platelet release reaction [429]. Placental tissue is a rich source of A$_2$, but biosynthesis has not been studied in this tissue.

Until recently, little was known concerning the biosynthesis of plasma factor XIII, but the liver has been implicated as the source since some, but not all, patients with chronic liver disease have decreased factor XIII [431,432]. Recently, synthesis of plasma factor XIII has been demonstrated in a human hepatoma cell line by metabolic labeling (Fig. 18) [433]. Mechanisms for regulating the biosynthesis have not yet been determined, although transfusion studies in factor XIII-deficient patients (see below) indicate a regulatory effect of A on the concentration of B in plasma.

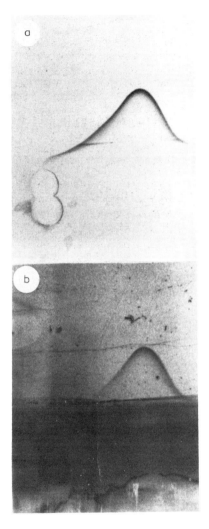

Fig. 18. Metabolic labeling of factor XIII synthesized by human liver cell line (Hep G2). Crossed immunoelectrophoresis with monospecific antiserum to B protein demonstrates that the immunoprecipitation arc of culture medium intrinsically labeled with [^{35}S]methionine (b) is identical to the immunoprecipitation arc of A_2B_2 (a).

(d) Physicochemical properties

The physicochemical characteristics of factor XIII proteins are shown in Table 8. The data are consistent with a tetrameric A_2B_2 structure for the extracellular zymogen, and a dimeric A_2 complex for the intracellular zymogen. Intracellular factor XIII has the characteristics of a globular protein composed of two identical A subunits held together non-covalently. On SDS gel electrophoresis the migra-

TABLE 8

Physicochemical data for factor XIII

	A_2B_2	A_2	A	B
Molecular mass	309 000	154 000	74 000	88 000
Sedimentation coefficient ($S_{20, w}$)	9.9 S	7.3 S		3.7 S
Frictional ratio (f/f_{min})	1.8	1.4		1.8
Stokes' radius (R_s)	82 Å	50 Å		59 Å
Extinction coefficient ($E_1^{1\%}{}_{cm, 280 nm}$)	14			
Isoelectric point	5.2			

TABLE 9

Amino acid and carbohydrate composition of human factor XIII A and B proteins: residues/mole (amino acids) and % (carbohydrate), respectively

	A	B
Amino acids		
Asp	80	72
Thr	40	64
Ser	46	72
Glu	75	96
Pro	32	56
Gly	51	74
Ala	37	27
Cys	6	32
Val	57	36
Met	14	10
Ile	29	28
Leu	45	52
Tyr	25	39
Phe	28	27
Lys	37	53
His	14	24
Arg	40	38
Trp	5	4
Sum	661	804
Carbohydrates		
N-Acetylhexosamine	0.2	1.6
Hexoses	1.2	1.9
Fucose	–	0.2
N-Acetylneuraminic acid	0.2	1.2

tion of A is the same under reducing and non-reducing conditions. The molecular mass of the A protein has been reported to be about 73 600 by sedimentation equilibrium [423]; for A_2 the molecular mass estimates are about 153 600 [434]. Electron microscopy of rotary-shadowed samples shows that the A protein is approximately spherical with a diameter of 5 nm. It is usually seen as a dimer, but sometimes as a monomer [435]. These observations confirm that A_2 consists of two identical globular subunits that self-associate in dimers. The molecular mass of the B chain is 87 800 by sedimentation equilibrium [423]. In electron microscopy, it appears as a long, thin, flexible strand with a length of 30 nm and a width of 2 nm [435].

Summation of the subunit molecular masses gives a value of 320 600 for the plasma zymogen, in good agreement with the values determined by sedimentation equilibrium for A_2B_2 [423]. The two A subunits are held together by strong non-covalent interactions, and there are interactions between A and B. However, the B subunits do not appear to be bound to each other. The tetrameric structure of the plasma zymogen has also been demonstrated by chemical crosslinking experiments with dimethylsuberimidate [434]. By combining the appearance of the subunits in the electron microscope with other physical data, a model of A_2B_2 can be constructed, consisting of the two globular domains of the A chains with the flexible B strands wound around them, i.e. B is more exposed to the surface than A in the zymogen. The model also explains why A_2B_2 behaves anomalously in sucrose density gradient centrifugation, i.e. corresponding to a molecular mass of 160 000, and why its gel filtration characteristics are different from fibrinogen, even though the molecular weights of the two proteins are nearly the same.

(e) Protein characterization

Table 9 shows the amino acid and carbohydrate compositions reported for factor XIII proteins. The A chains of A_2 and A_2B_2 are immunochemically identical [426], and have the same amino acid and carbohydrate compositions [422,423,436]. The B chain is immunochemically and structurally distinct [422,423]. The B protein contains about 5% carbohydrate and the A protein about 1% [436]. The heterogeneity in B, observed in isoelectric focusing, is due in part to sialic acid [419,436]. A protein has 6 free sulfhydryls, one of which is in the active center, and no disulfide bridges; in contrast, B protein contains 16 intrachain disulfide bonds and no free sulfhydryls [434]. This distribution of disulfides results in aberrant migration of B on non-reduced SDS gels in the Weber–Osborn system, where B has a faster migration than A [423]. However, in the Laemmli SDS gel system, B migrates more slowly than A, as would be expected from the molecular weights (Fig. 19). The amino terminal residues are N-acetyl-serine for A and glutamic acid for B [437].

A large cyanogen bromide fragment ($M_r \sim 48 000$) of B chain has been isolated. This fragment, which contains disulfide bonds and about 50% of the B chain carbohydrate, retains the ability to complex with A. Reduced and alkylated B will also bind to A_2, but denatured B will not [438].

The activation peptide, active center, and principal calcium ion-binding sites are located in the A protein [419,421]. The active center cysteine is buried in the zymogen and cannot be alkylated with iodoacetamide. However, it is readily alkylated in the active enzyme, and this results in loss of enzymatic activity [439]. Fluorescence polarization experiments indicate that the thrombin-binding site is contained

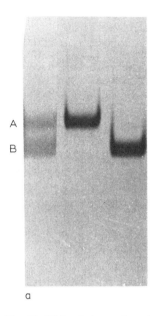 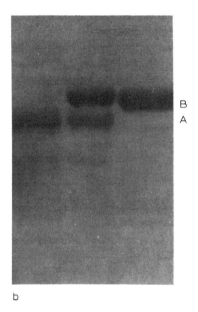

a   b

Fig. 19. SDS gel electrophoresis of factor XIII, A_2B_2, on 7% polyacrylamide gels. a, Weber–Osborn system with non-reducing buffer; b, Laemmli system with reducing buffer. The 3 lanes correspond to isolated A and B protein and their mixture.

in the activation peptide, since A_2 did not bind thrombin [440]. The activation peptide, cleaved from the amino-terminal end of A by thrombin, has been sequenced for human and bovine factor XIII (Fig. 20) [437]. The two peptides show a high degree of identity. The sequence around the active center of human factor XIII has been determined to be -Gly-Gln-Cys-Trp- [442], which is identical to the active center sequence in guinea pig liver transglutaminase [443] and similar to that in papain [444]. The amino-terminal sequence of the B chain is Glu-Glx-Lys-Pro [437]. Additional primary structure data have not been reported.

(f) Zymogen activation

Expression of activity of factor XIII and other transglutaminases requires calcium ions. However, factor XIII is unique in that it is present in plasma, platelets

```
    1              10                 20
Ac  S E T S R T A F G G R R A V P P N N S N

               30                 40
    A A E D D L P T V E L Q G V P R↓G V B L Z Z
```

Fig. 20. Amino acid sequence of the amino-terminal activation peptide of human factor XIII A protein. The bovine activation peptide is homologous, with 5 substitutions (Ser_3, Gly_5, Ile_{14}, Thr_{18}, Pro_{26}) and insertion of Leu following Gly_{33} in the human sequence. Arrow shows thrombin cleavage site.

and monocytes entirely in zymogenic form, while other tissue transglutaminases appear to be present as enzymes. Complete activation of A_2 or A_2B_2 can be achieved in vitro by exposure of the zymogens to thrombin and calcium ions, and this is also presumed to be the principal mechanism for in vivo activation. Thrombin cleaves the human A chain between Arg in position 36 and Gly in 37 (Fig. 20) to release the amino-terminal activation peptide. This cleavage does not result in full exposure of the active center, and only a small amount of activity is expressed. Complete exposure of the active center is then induced by calcium ions [439]. High concentrations of these ions alone, without activation peptide cleavage, can also result in some activity [419].

A model for the general mechanism of plasma factor XIII activation is summarized in Fig. 21. It indicates that at least 4 conformationally distinct chemical states can be defined. State I is the metal-free zymogen which is fully maintained in vitro only in the presence of a chelating agent. Calcium ions can bind both to the intact zymogen and to the thrombin-cleaved intermediate [440]. Binding to zymogen produces state II and to the thrombin intermediate, state III. In a purified system, the K_d for calcium ions–A_2B_2 complex is 2.5 mM [445]. The calcium concentration in plasma is 2.5 mM, the free ion concentration being about 1.3 mM. Hence, both state I and state II should exist in normal plasma, with about 30–50% of the molecules being in state II. Any event, such as endothelial cell injury or death or platelet degranulation, which could raise the calcium ion concentrations in the microenvironment of incipient coagulation would also shift the equilibrium toward state II. In vitro, the conformational effects of calcium ions can be reversed by EDTA. State III is the conformational state induced by thrombin cleavage of the zymogen in the absence of calcium ions, and state IV is the fully active enzyme.

The dots in Fig. 21 represent non-covalent interactions between A and B and indicate that these are altered during activation. During the activation of the plasma zymogen, B becomes fully dissociated from A. That this occurs physiologically is demonstrated by the observation that B protein can be entirely recovered in serum

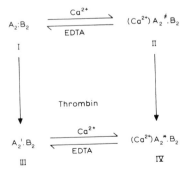

Fig. 21. Proposed mechanism for activation of extracellular factor XIII. Intracellular zymogen can be activated similarly except that B subunit is not present. Dots indicate non-covalent interactions.

after clotting normal plasma [417]. B protein will combine with A_2 in purified systems to generate A_2B_2, but it will not recombine with A_2^* [434]. These studies have led to the assumption that release of B occurs concomitantly with activation. However, under physiological conditions, it is more likely that B is released when A'_2 or A_2^* binds to substrate.

The specific function of B protein in A_2B_2 is uncertain, although its presence in the extracellular complex and not the intracellular one implies that an additional protective or regulatory function is necessary in the plasma environment. The basic activation steps for A_2 are the same as for A_2B_2 except that A_2 activation is more rapid and maximum activation can occur at a lower calcium ion concentration [434]. In a purified system with thrombin cleavage of activation peptide, the calcium ion concentration needed for generation of optimal activity from A_2B_2 is about 20 mM and from A_2, 2 mM [418,434].

The high calcium ion concentration needed for maximal activation of A_2B_2 in purified systems could not be obtained in plasma. However, in the presence of physiological concentrations of fibrinogen, the calcium ion concentration required is lowered to about 1.5 mM [446]. This effect is mediated through the middle region of the $A\alpha$-chain of fibrinogen (residues 242–424), which presumably contains a factor XIII-binding domain [447]. It has also been observed that fibrinogen or reptilase fibrin significantly enhances the cleavage rate of factor XIII activation peptide by thrombin [448]. The mechanisms for these interactions are not known.

(g) Enzyme action

The reaction catalyzed by factor XIII_a is the formation of a covalent bond between the γ-carbamoyl group of a peptide-bound glutamine and the ϵ-amino group of lysine (Fig. 17). This reaction occurs via intermediary acylation and deacylation steps in which glutamine functions as the electron acceptor (or acyl donor) and lysine as the electron donor (or acyl acceptor). In the absence of amine substrate, hydrolysis of the glutamine substrate will occur. Factor XIII_a, like all transglutaminases, requires calcium ions for expression of enzyme activity. The catalytically active species is a metal–enzyme complex formed between calcium ions and A_2^*. Zn^{2+} inhibits enzyme activity ($K_i \sim 10^{-7}$ M) [418]. However, divalent metal ions can substitute for calcium ions ($Sr^{2+} > Ba^{2+} > Mg^{2+}$) [439].

The enzymatic action of factor XIII_a requires formation of a trimolecular macromolecule complex between the enzyme and two protein substrates. The active center cysteine of the calcium ion A_2^* complex reacts with the γ-carbamoyl of peptide-bound glutamine which results in formation of a γ-glutamyl–S-ester intermediate complex and aminolysis. It is postulated that the enzyme–substrate complex is conformationally altered so that a functional site for interaction of a lysine ϵ-amino group with the active center is then formed [449]. The amino group reacts with the acylenzyme thioester bond, and formation of an ϵ-(γ-glutamyl)-lysyl bond occurs.

Factor XIII_a demonstrates a high degree of substrate specificity, so that only a

Glutamine sites		
Fibrinogen Aα-chain	Q 328	S T G N <u>Q</u> N P G S P
Fibronectin	Q 3	Z A <u>Q</u> - Q V Q P
α₂-Plasmin inhibitor	Q 2	N <u>Q</u> E Q V S P
β-Casein	Q 167	L S L S <u>Q</u> S K V L P
Fibrinogen Aα-chain	Q 366	G S T G <u>Q</u> W H S E S
Fibrinogen γ-chain	Q 398	I G E G <u>Q</u> Q H H L G
Lysine sites		
Fibrinogen Aα-chain	K 508	A S T G <u>K</u> T F P G F
Fibrinogen Aα-chain	K 556	P S R G <u>K</u> S S S Y S
Fibrinogen Aα-chain	K 562	S S Y S <u>K</u> Q F T S S
Fibrinogen γ-chain	K 406	L G G A <u>K</u> Q A G D V

Fig. 22. Sequences around reactive glutamine and lysine sites in factor XIII$_a$ substrates. The numbers indicate these positions.

few glutamine and lysine residues can participate in the crosslinking reaction. Although the determinants of this specificity are not entirely clear, secondary interactions between the extended active site and the glutamine substrate are thought to be critical. The active center of factor XIII$_a$ is thought to be located in a hydrophobic pocket, and the extended active site contains about 10 amino acids [449]. Hydrophobic interaction between the active site and amino acids around the reactive glutamine is important. Examination of the linear sequences around known glutamine crosslinking sites shows some evidence for homology (Fig. 22). Glutamine 167 in β-casein has been found to be highly reactive with factor XIII$_a$ [450]. Synthetic peptides modelled after the linear sequence around Gln 167 have been used to study the determinants of specificity. A tridecapeptide corresponding to the sequence around Gln 398 in the γ-chain of fibrinogen was found to be a poor substrate for factor XIII$_a$ [450]. These studies all indicate that important determinants of specificity are provided by the tertiary structure of the substrate.

Little information is available concerning specificity of the lysine substrates, and specific reactive lysines have been identified only in the γ- and perhaps in the α-chains of fibrin (Fig. 22). Studies with small synthetic peptides have shown that introduction of a hydrophobic residue on the amino-terminal side of the reactive lysine significantly enhances the reactivity [449]. It has been proposed that the glutamine substrate contributes to the specificity for the lysine substrate [449].

(h) Substrates of factor XIII$_a$

Proteins are designated as substrates for factor XIII$_a$ if they can specifically incorporate a lysine analogue such as putrescine or dansylcadaverine in a concentration- and time-dependent manner or if formation of a crosslinked complex can be demonstrated, usually by reduced SDS gel electrophoresis. Covalent complex formation has been observed for all of the plasma proteins which are considered

TABLE 10

Crosslinked complexes formed by factor XIII$_a$

Fibrin-fibrin
Fibrin-fibrinogen
Fibrin-α_2-plasmin inhibitor
Fibrin-fibronectin
Fibrin-von Willebrand factor
Fibrin-actin
Fibrin-thrombospondin
Fibronectin-collagen
Fibronectin-myosin
von Willebrand factor-collagen
Actin-myosin

---

to be physiologically relevant substrates. These are listed in Table 10. Although a specific protein could be a substrate by virtue of either a reactive glutamine or lysine, the plasma proteins designated thus far all contribute reactive glutamines or both lysines and glutamines. These proteins also have several other features in common. Most of them are large, sticky proteins. They are both plasma constituents and platelet α-granule components, secreted by activated platelets. They all participate in assembly of a macromolecular protein complex on a surface, whether the surface be platelet or other cell membrane, fibrin polymer, or subendothelium.

(1) Fibrinogen and fibrin

Fibrin is the most well characterized crosslinking substrate with the most obvious physiologic significance. It was earlier observed that the fibrin clot formed from plasma in the presence of EDTA was more soluble than that formed without EDTA, which led to the discovery of factor XIII and also gave rise to the name fibrin-stabilizing factor [451]. In this regard, factor XIII differs from other coagulation factors, many of which were discovered through observations on patients with unexplained bleeding disorders.

The crosslinking of fibrin is an orderly process that results in the formation of γ-chain dimers and α-chain polymers. These can readily be observed by reduced SDS gel electrophoresis (Fig. 23). There is one reactive glutamine (Gln 398) and one reactive lysine (Lys 406) at the carboxy-terminal end of each γ-chain (see Fig. 4). Gln 398 in one γ-chain forms a crosslink with Lys 406 in a second γ-chain, and Lys 406 in the first γ-chain and Gln 398 in the second one form another crosslink [85,255]. Crosslinking of γ-chains is intermolecular and results in a product composed of one γ-chain from each of two fibrin molecules, held together by two crosslinking bonds and oriented in antiparallel [85,255].

Crosslinking of fibrin γ-chains is very rapid and occurs at low enzyme concentration. It occurs at the stage of protofibril formation in the fibrin assembly process (see Section 2 h (2), Polymerization). Electron microscopy and gel electrophoresis have shown that crosslinks form linearly, along the length of the protofibril, re-

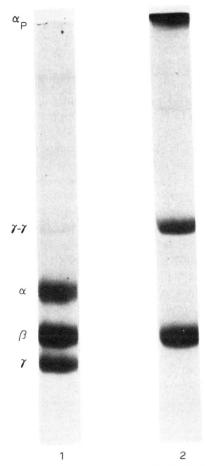

Fig. 23. Analysis of fibrin crosslinking by SDS gel electrophoresis under reducing conditions. Gel 1 has been allowed to crosslink for 1 min and contains predominantly the α-, β- and γ-chains of non-crosslinked fibrin plus a trace of γ-dimer. Gel 2 is completely crosslinked and contains high-molecular-weight α-polymer, γ-dimer, and β-chain.

sulting in the monomer units in each strand of the protofibril being covalently joined together. However, the two strands of the protofibril are not crosslinked to each other [71]. γ-Chain crosslinking alone does not make the fibrin gel insoluble in dilute acid; this requires the crosslinking of α-chains [452].

α-Chain crosslinking is slower, requires a higher factor XIII_a concentration, and is more complicated than γ-dimer formation. The crosslinked polymer contains 5 or more α-chains per polymeric unit. Spatial organization of the polymer has not been determined. However, the reactive glutamine and lysine residues are in the carboxy-terminal half of the α-chain, which is hydrophilic and not disulfide bonded to the rest of the molecule. Glutamine residues that may participate in α-polymer formation are at positions 328 and 366 [95,97,256]. The reactive lysines have been tentatively assigned to positions 508 and 556 or 562 [258]. There is an additional glutamine, i.e. residue 237, that incorporates lysine analogues, but which seems not to be involved in α-polymer formation [95,97]; however, it may participate in the crosslinking of α-chains to other proteins [257].

α-Polymer is difficult to solubilize, and it conveys this insolubility to crosslinked fibrin. In crosslinked fibrin, the average number of crosslinks is 4–6/fibrin monomer unit. Plasmin hydrolysis of crosslinked fibrin differs from non-crosslinked fibrin in that fragment D contains the γ-chain crosslinks, which results in the appearance of dimeric D as a terminal digestion fragment [453]. Crosslinking of α-chains also increases resistance of the fibrin gel to plasmin [454]. High-molecular-mass, early cleavage fragments of α-polymer can also be observed; but these are lost as plasmin digestion proceeds, due to the large number of plasmin cleavage sites in the α-chain [291].

Both γ-dimer and α-polymer form readily in fibrin. There is no apparent difference in the crosslinking of fibrin formed through cleavage of fibrinopeptide A only or fibrin from which both fibrinopeptides A and B have been cleaved. However, fibrinogen is a relatively poor substrate. It can be crosslinked to form γ-dimers and α-polymers, but the rates are much slower. With high factor XIII_a concentration fibrinogen can be covalently crosslinked to form a gel [455]. It is generally assumed that the principal difference between fibrinogen and fibrin as crosslinking substrates resides in the orderly arrangement of fibrin monomers in the protofibril so that α-chains are appropriately aligned for crosslinking. Soluble fibrinogen–fibrin oligomers can also be easily crosslinked; fibrinogen in high concentration inhibits fibrin crosslinking [455]. Binding of factor XIII to fibrin monomer and activation at the site of polymerization may be an additional mechanism for concentrating factor XIII activity and thus enhancing the rate of crosslinking.

(2) α_2-Plasmin inhibitor

α_2-Plasmin inhibitor is the primary, fast acting inhibitor of plasmin activity in plasma. It can complex with plasmin both in solution and when it is crosslinked to fibrin. Plasmin inhibition is more efficient when the inhibitor is crosslinked to fibrin and a trimolecular fibrin–α_2-plasmin inhibitor–plasmin complex is formed. Covalent crosslinking occurs through a reactive glutamine (residue 2) in α_2-plasmin inhibitor and a reactive lysine residue in the α-chain of fibrin, which has not yet been defined [456]. The average molar ratio of α_2-plasmin inhibitor to fibrin monomer in the fibrin gel from blood plasma is 1:45.

Crosslinking of α_2-plasmin inhibitor to the fibrin gel is a principal mechanism for increasing the resistance of crosslinked fibrin to plasmin degradation [457]. Patients who are congenitally deficient in α_2-plasmin inhibitor have significant bleeding problems due to uncontrolled plasmin activity [457].

(3) Fibronectin, von Willebrand factor and thrombospondin

After fibrin monomer, fibronectin is the next most abundant protein in the normal fibrin gel and constitutes approximately 4% of the total protein in it [458].

Under normal circumstances, the fibronectin in the gel is covalently crosslinked to the α-chain of fibrin [459]. This crosslinking reaction occurs principally through a glutamine at the amino terminus of fibronectin (residue 3) and a lysine in the fibrin α-chain [460]. A consequence of fibronectin–fibrin crosslinking is that the initial rate of α-polymer formation is decreased. If the crosslinking reactions are allowed to proceed, all the fibronectin and α-chains become crosslinked into high-molecular-mass heteropolymers. Crosslinking of fibronectin to itself can occur if the fibronectin dimer is first reduced [458]. Rapid crosslinking of fibronectin to α-chain requires a higher factor XIII_a concentration than is needed for α-polymer formation.

The α-granule protein, thrombospondin, is a substrate for factor XIII_a [461]. In vitro, in purified systems, thrombospondin readily crosslinks to itself to form high-molecular-weight polymers. Under certain conditions, it also appears to crosslink to fibrin.

Plasma von Willebrand factor is also a substrate for factor XIII_a and can be crosslinked to fibrin during gel formation [462]. Reduced, monomeric, but not polymeric von Willebrand factor, will crosslink to itself. It crosslinks to fibrin through the α-chain and decreases the initial rate of α-polymer formation. This crosslinking reaction will occur in plasma when the clotting time is prolonged and can result in covalent crosslinking of 80% of the plasma von Willebrand factor to fibrin.

(4) Collagen

Factor XIII_a will crosslink fibronectin to collagen types I, II, III, and V but not type IV collagen [463]. There is also evidence that von Willebrand factor can be crosslinked to collagen. Direct crosslinking of fibrin to collagen has not been substantiated. Both fibronectin and von Willebrand factor could serve as covalent bridges between fibrin and collagen in a wound site, but direct evidence for such crosslinked complexes has not yet been obtained. It is also possible that other structural proteins in the subendothelial matrix may be substrates for factor XIII_a.

(5) Platelet membrane and contractile proteins

$A_2{}^*$ binds to thrombin-activated platelets [464]. There is evidence for crosslinking between platelet actin and fibrin, actin and myosin, and myosin and fibronectin. Tropomyosin also incorporates lysine analogues and is thought to be a substrate for factor XIII_a [465]. Actin crosslinking is inhibited by ATP. Since platelet factor XIII is readily activated when the cytosolic calcium ion concentration is raised, as would occur during platelet activation, it has been proposed that crosslinking of the platelet contractile system by platelet factor XIII_a may be a mechanism for irreversibly stabilizing an activated platelet aggregate. Covalent crosslinking of the membrane glycoproteins IIb and III has also been observed [465]. It is not known whether crosslinking substrates secreted from platelet α-granules or distributed in the plasma environment can be crosslinked to platelet membrane proteins.

(i) Physiological consequences of factor XIII activity

The concentration of factor XIII in normal plasma is approximately 90 nM. Radioimmunoassay data indicate that the molar concentration of the A and B proteins are equal and that the A_2B_2 tetramer accounts for all of the A and B proteins in normal plasma [417]. However, there is a molar excess of B to A in the plasma of patients who are heterozygous for factor XIII deficiency, and homozygous deficient patients have decreased but measurable B protein and no detectable A protein in their plasma [417].

The crosslinking of fibrin is a principal catalytic function of factor XIII_a in blood coagulation. Analysis of fibrin clots obtained at surgery has shown clearly that the fibrin crosslinking pattern observed in vitro also occurs in vivo. Clots formed in vivo contain crosslinked γ-dimers and α-polymers [257]. In vivo crosslinking of other proteins to fibrin has not been assessed.

An important consequence of fibrin crosslinking is that equilibrium is shifted in favor of gel formation and therefore less fibrin monomer is required for formation of a stable hemostatic plug. Polymerization of fibrin monomers is readily reversible in the absence of factor XIII activity; but once crosslinking has occurred, depolymerization is effectively inhibited. Crosslinking of α-chains alters the fibrin gel so that mechanical stability and resistance to plasmin degradation are increased [209]. In purified systems containing crosslinked or non-crosslinked fibrin, the initial stage of plasmin cleavage at α-polymer sites is slowed down, indicating that α-chain is a better plasmin substrate than α-polymer [454]. The crosslinking of $α_2$-plasmin inhibitor to fibrin is also a critical reaction for inhibiting plasmin degradation of the gel [456,457]. In summary, it is apparent that the net effect in vivo of factor XIII_a on fibrin is to promote the formation and maintenance of a fibrin network, both by enhancing and stabilizing the network and by protecting it from mechanical and enzymatic disruption.

The hemostatic significance of fibrin crosslinking and $α_2$-plasmin inhibitor–fibrin crosslinking is also substantiated by observations of the hemorrhagic disorders in patients who are deficient in factor XIII or $α_2$-plasmin inhibitor. The plasma concentration of factor XIII is greatly in excess of that needed for fibrin crosslinking, and there is also a high intracellular concentration in platelets and monocytes. The availability and distribution of factor XIII, have led to suggestions that factor XIII has important roles in platelet reactions and wound healing.

There is also evidence for factor XIII function in wound healing and tissue repair. Crosslinking of fibronectin to fibrin promotes fibroblast adhesion and spreading [466]. Fibroblast proliferation also occurs more readily on crosslinked plasma clots than on non-crosslinked clots.

Placenta is a rich source of intracellular factor XIII. A specific physiologic function for placental factor XIII has not been established. However, in all reported cases of homozygously factor XIII-deficient women who became pregnant, spontaneous abortion occurred unless the patient was treated during the pregnancy [467]. The incidence of spontaneous abortion also appears to be higher than normal in women who are heterozygous for factor XIII. What role placental factor XIII may play is unknown, but crosslinking reactions may be necessary for placental adherence or to prevent uterine or placental hemorrhage.

(j) Factor XIII deficiency

The gene loci for factor XIII A and B proteins are located on autosomal chromosomes. The gene for A is linked to the HLA locus on chromosome 6 [468]. Both A and B are genetically polymorphic, as indicated by electrophoretic analyses [468]. Pedigree analyses of families with congenital factor XIII deficiency also show autosomal transmission of factor XIII genes and indicate that phenotypic expression of a hemorrhagic disorder is recessive. Heterozygotes do not generally have bleeding problems, but they can be identified by laboratory analysis [467]. About 200 cases have been recorded in various countries around the world [469]. There is a high incidence of consanguinity in families with factor XIII deficiency [467].

Congenital factor XIII deficiency is characterized biochemically by very low or undetectable levels of A in plasma, measured either functionally as factor XIII activity or immunochemically as A protein [417]. Immunochemical analysis of B shows that homozygous deficient patients have about 50% of the normal plasma B level [426]. A patient totally deficient in B has also been observed. Assays for A in the platelets of one deficient patient showed that A was also absent in the platelets [428]. In the deficiency state, there is no crosslinking of the patient's fibrin, although the fibrin will crosslink normally if exogenous factor XIII is added. Infusion of deficient patients with placental factor XIII concentrate (Fibrogammin, Behringwerke) results in rapid in vivo complex formation between the infused A_2 and the patient's plasma B protein. There is an immediate, expected rise in factor XIII activity in the patient's plasma which slowly decreases. In addition there is a delayed increase in the plasma concentration of B, which appears to reach a maximum about 5 days after transfusion. The increase is a function of the amount of A_2 infused.

These observations indicate that addition of A_2 into the circulation of deficient patients has a specific effect on circulating B protein, which could be due to increased biosynthesis or secretion of B or to decreased degradation of B when it is complexed with A. This effect also complicates determination of the half-life of plasma factor XIII in deficient patients. However, in transfused patients who receive only A_2 concentrate, the half-life of A in the tetrameric zymogen complex has been found to be approximately 8.5 days [470].

Heterozygous members of factor XIII-deficient kindreds have decreased plasma levels of A and B, with A being approximately 50–60% and B 80% of normal.

Factor XIII deficiency is characterized clinically by a moderate to severe hemorrhagic diathesis. The reason for this variation is not obvious since all the patients have less than 1% plasma factor XIII. One possibility is that some patients have platelet factor XIII while others do not. Delayed, repeat bleeding from superficial wounds is highly characteristic of factor XIII deficiency. Hemorrhage in factor XIII

230

deficiency can be treated with plasma, cryoprecipitate, or factor XIII concentrates. Antibody inhibitors to factor XIII have been reported in a few patients, and antibodies to fibrin crosslinking sites have also been described [470].

*References**

1 Henschen, A. (1981) Hämostaseologie 1, 30–40.
2 Doolittle, R.F. (1981) in: Haemostasis and Thrombosis (Bloom, A.L. and Thomas, D.P., Eds.) pp. 163–191, Churchill Livingstone, London.
3 Beck, E.A. and Furlan, M. (1984) Variants of Human Fibrinogen, pp. 1–328, Huber, Bern.
4 Doolittle, R.F. (1984) Annu. Rev. Biochem. 53, 195–229.
5 Henschen, A., Graeff, H. and Lottspeich, F. (1982) Fibrinogen – Recent Biochemical and Medical Aspects, Vol. 1, pp. 1–400, de Gruyter, Berlin.
6 Haverkate, F., Henschen, A., Nieuwenhuizen, W. and Straub, P.W. (1983) Fibrinogen – Structure, Functional Aspects and Metabolism, Vol. 2, pp. 1–343, de Gruyter, Berlin.
7 Mosesson, M.W. and Doolittle, R.F. (1983) Molecular Biology of Fibrinogen and Fibrin, Ann. N.Y. Acad. Sci. 408, 1–672.
8 Henschen, A., Hessel, B., McDonagh, J. and Saldeen, T. (1985) Fibrinogen – Structural Variants and Interactions, Vol. 3, pp. 1–418, de Gruyter, Berlin.
9 Lane, D.A., Henschen, A. and Jasani, M.K. (1986) Fibrinogen, Fibrin Formation and Fibrinolysis, Vol. 4, pp. 1–396, de Gruyter, Berlin.
10 Clauss, A. (1957) Acta Haematol. 17, 237–246.
11 Becker, U., Bartl, K. and Wahlefeld, A.W. (1984) Thromb. Res. 35, 475–484.
12 Ratnoff, O.D. and Menzie, C. (1951) J. Lab. Clin. Med. 37, 316–320.
13 Blombäck, B. (1958) Ark. Kem. 12, 99–113.
14 Blombäck, B. and Blombäck, M. (1956) Ark. Kem. 10, 415–443.
15 Desvignes, P. and Bonnet, P. (1981) Clin. Chim. Acta 110, 9–17.
16 Harmoinen, A., Uppa, H., Lehtinen, M., Jokela, H. and Koivula, T. (1983) Clin. Lab. Haematol. 5, 101–107.
17 Godal, H.C. and Abildgaard, U. (1966) Scand. J. Haematol. 3, 342–350.
18 Gurewich, V. and Lipinski, B. (1976) Am. J. Clin. Pathol. 65, 397–401.
19 Drewinko, B., Surgeon, J., Cobb, P., Callahan, L., Schmidt, D., Bollinger, P. and Trujillo, J.M. (1985) Am. J. Clin. Pathol. 84, 58–66.
20 Shaw, S.T. (1977) CRC Crit. Rev. Clin. Lab. Sci. 8, 145–192.
21 Cohn, E.J., Strong, L.E., Hughes, W.L., Mulford, D.J., Ashworth, J.N., Melin, M. and Taylor, H.L. (1946) J. Am. Chem. Soc. 68, 459–475.
22 Kazal, L.A., Amsel, S., Miller, O.P. and Tocantins, L.M. (1963) Proc. Soc. Exp. Biol. Med. 113, 989–994.
23 Straughn, W. and Wagner, R.H. (1966) Thromb. Diath. Haemorrh. 16, 198–206.
24 Laki, K. (1951) Arch. Biochem. Biophys. 32, 317–324.
25 Hafter, R., von Hugo, R. and Graeff, H. (1978) Hoppe-Seyler's Z. Physiol. Chem. 359, 759–763.
26 Longas, M.O., Newman, J. and Johnson, A.J. (1980) Int. J. Biochem. 11, 559–564.
27 Ware, A.G., Guest, M.M. and Seegers, W.H. (1947) Arch. Biochem. Biophys. 13, 231–236.
28 Galanakis, D.K., Mosesson, M.W. and Stathakis, N.E. (1978) J. Lab. Clin. Med. 92, 376–386.
29 Phillips, H.M. (1981) Can. J. Biochem. 59, 332–342.
30 Galanakis, D.K. and Mosesson, M.W. (1983) Thromb. Res. 31, 403–413.
31 Holm, B., Nilsen, D.W.T., Kierulf, P. and Godal, H.C. (1985) Thromb. Res. 37, 165–176.
32 Stathakis, N.E., Mosesson, M.W., Galanakis, D.K. and Menache, D. (1978) Thromb. Res. 13, 467–475.
33 Wolfenstein-Todel, C. and Mosesson, M.W. (1981) Biochemistry 20, 6146–6149.

---

* The list covers primarily recent literature, in which references to earlier work may be found.

34 Francis, C.W., Keele, E.M. and Marder, V.J. (1984) Biochim. Biophys. Acta 797, 328–335.
35 Henschen, A. and Southan, C. (1980) in: Fibrinolyse, Thrombose, Hämostase (Deutsch, E. and Lechner, K., Eds.) pp. 290–293, Schattauer, Stuttgart.
36 Heene, D.L. and Matthias, F.R. (1973) Thromb. Res. 2, 137–154.
37 Matthias, F.R., Hocke, G. and Lasch, H.G. (1975) Thromb. Res. 7, 861–870.
38 Stemberger, A. and Hörmann, H. (1975) Hoppe-Seyler's Z. Physiol. Chem. 356, 341–348.
39 Kuyas, C., Haeberli, A. and Straub, P.W. (1985) Thromb. Haemostas. 54, 40 (abstr.).
40 Suzuki, K., Nishioka, J. and Hashimoto, S. (1980) Thromb. Res. 18, 707–715.
41 Vila, V., Reganon, E. and Aznar, J. (1978) Clin. Chim. Acta 87, 245–252.
42 Rupp, C., Sievi, R. and Furlan, M. (1982) Thromb. Res. 27, 117–121.
43 Engvall, E., Ruoslahti, E. and Miller, E.J. (1978) J. Exp. Med. 147, 1584–1595.
44 Scheraga, H.A. and Laskowski Jr., M. (1957) Adv. Prot. Chem. 12, 1–131.
45 van der Drift, A.C.M., Poppema, A., Haverkate, F. and Nieuwenhuizen, W. (1983) in: Fibrinogen (Haverkate, F., Henschen, A., Nieuwenhuizen, W. and Straub, P.W., Eds.) Vol. 2, pp. 3–18, de Gruyter, Berlin.
46 Marguerie, G. and Stuhrmann, H.B. (1976) J. Mol. Biol. 102, 143–156.
47 Marx, J., Hudry-Clergeon, G., Capet-Antonini, F. and Bernard, L. (1979) Biochim. Biophys. Acta 578, 107–115.
48 Hantgan, R.R. and Hermans, J. (1979) J. Biol. Chem. 254, 11272–11281.
49 Müller, M., Lasarcyk, H. and Burchard, W. (1981) Int. J. Biol. Macromol. 3, 19–24.
50 Shah, G.A., Ferguson, I.A., Dhall, T.Z. and Dhall, D.P. (1982) Biopolymers 21, 1037–1047.
51 Wiltzius, P., Dietler, G., Känzig, W., Häberli, A. and Straub, P.W. (1982) Biopolymers 21, 2205–2223.
52 Janmey, P.A., Bale, M.D. and Ferry, J.D. (1983) Biopolymers 22, 2017–2019.
53 Montague, C.E. and Newman, J. (1984) Macromolec. 17, 1391–1396.
54 Bale, M.D., Müller, M.F. and Ferry, J.D. (1985) Biopolymers 24, 461–482.
55 Hall, C.E. and Slayter, H.S. (1959) J. Biophys. Biochem. Cytol. 5, 11–17.
56 Williams, R.C. (1981) J. Mol. Biol. 150, 399–408.
57 Slayter, H.S. (1983) Ann. N.Y. Acad. Sci. 408, 131–145.
58 Cohen, C., Weisel, J.W., Phillips Jr., G.N., Stauffacher, C.V., Fillers, J.P. and Daub, E. (1983) Ann. N.Y. Acad. Sci. 408, 194–213.
59 Gollwitzer, R., Bode, W., Schramm, H.-J., Typke, D. and Guckenberger, R. (1983) Ann. N.Y. Acad. Sci. 408, 214–225.
60 Telford, J.N., Nagy, J.A., Hatcher, P.A. and Scheraga, H.A. (1980) Proc. Natl. Acad. Sci. (U.S.A.) 77, 2372–2376.
61 Price, T.M., Strong, D.D., Rudee, M.L. and Doolittle, R.F. (1981) Proc. Natl. Acad. Sci. (U.S.A.) 78, 200–204.
62 Norton, P.A. and Slayter, H.S. (1981) Proc. Natl. Acad. Sci. (U.S.A.) 78, 1661–1665.
63 Erickson, H.P. and Fowler, W.E. (1983) Ann. N.Y. Acad. Sci. 408, 146–163.
64 Mosesson, M.W., Hainfeld, J., Wall, J. and Haschemeyer, R.H. (1981) J. Mol. Biol. 153, 695–718.
65 Hewat, E.A., Tranqui, L. and Wade, R.H. (1983) J. Mol. Biol. 170, 203–222.
66 Fowler, W.E., Fretto, L.J., Erickson, H.P. and McKee, P.A. (1980) J. Clin. Invest. 66, 50–56.
67 Weisel, J.W., Stauffacher, C.V., Bullitt, E. and Cohen, C. (1985) Science 230, 1388–1391.
68 Müller, M.F., Ris, H. and Ferry, J.D. (1984) J. Mol. Biol. 174, 369–384.
69 Stewart, G.J. and Niewiarowski, S. (1969) Biochim. Biophys. Acta 194, 462–469.
70 Cohen, C., Slayter, H., Goldstein, L., Kucera, J. and Hall, C. (1966) J. Mol. Biol. 22, 385–388.
71 Fowler, W.E., Erickson, H.P., Hantgan, R.R., McDonagh, J. and Hermans, J. (1981) Science 211, 287–289.
72 Freyssinet, J.-M., Torbet, J. and Hudry-Clergeon, G. (1984) Biochimie 66, 81–85.
73 Privalov, P.L. and Medved, L.V. (1982) J. Mol. Biol. 159, 665–683.
74 Medved, L.V., Privalov, P.L. and Ugarova, T.P. (1982) FEBS Lett. 146, 339–342.
75 Medved, L.V., Gorkun, O.V. and Privalov, P.L. (1983) FEBS Lett. 160, 291–295.
76 Bettelheim, F.R. and Bailey, K. (1952) Biochim. Biophys. Acta 9, 578–579.

77 Lorand, L. and Middlebrook, W.R. (1952) Biochim. Biophys. Acta 9, 581–582.
78 Blombäck, B. and Yamashina, I. (1958) Ark. Kem. 12, 299–319.
79 Henschen, A. (1962) Acta Chem. Scand. 16, 1037–1038.
80 Clegg, J.B. and Bailey, K. (1962) Biochim. Biophys. Acta 63, 525–527.
81 Henschen, A. and Edman, P. (1972) Biochim. Biophys. Acta 263, 351–367.
82 Kehl, M., Lottspeich, F. and Henschen, A. (1982) Hoppe-Seyler's Z. Physiol. Chem. 363, 1501–1505.
83 Lottspeich, F. and Henschen, A. (1977) Hoppe-Seyler's Z. Physiol. Chem. 358, 935–938.
84 Blombäck, B., Gröndahl, N.J., Hessel, B., Iwanaga, S. and Wallén, P. (1973) J. Biol. Chem. 248, 5806–5820.
85 Sharp, J.J., Cassman, K.G. and Doolittle, R.F. (1972) FEBS Lett. 25, 334–336.
86 Chung, D.W., Chan, W.-Y. and Davie, E.W. (1983) Biochemistry 22, 3250–3256.
87 Kant, J.A., Lord, S.T. and Crabtree, G.R. (1983) Proc. Natl. Acad. Sci. (U.S.A.) 80, 3953–3957.
88 Mosesson, M.W., Finlayson, J.S. and Umfleet, R.A. (1972) J. Biol. Chem. 247, 5223–5227.
89 Chung, D.W. and Davie, E.W. (1984) Biochemistry 23, 4232–4236.
90 Henschen, A. and Lottspeich, F. (1977) Hoppe-Seyler's Z. Physiol. Chem. 358, 1643–1646.
91 Hessel, B., Makino, M., Iwanaga, S. and Blombäck, B. (1979) Eur. J. Biochem. 98, 521–534.
92 Watt, K.W.K., Takagi, T. and Doolittle, R.F. (1979) Biochemistry 18, 68–76.
93 Chung, D.W., Que, B.G., Rixon, M.W., Mace Jr., M. and Davie, E.W. (1983) Biochemistry 22, 3244–3250.
94 Blombäck, B., Hessel, B., Iwanaga, S., Reuterby, J. and Blombäck, M. (1972) J. Biol. Chem. 247, 1496–1512.
95 Takagi, T. and Doolittle, R.F. (1975) Biochemistry 14, 5149–5156.
96 Cottrell, B.A. and Doolittle, R.F. (1976) Biochem. Biophys. Res. Commun. 71, 754–761.
97 Doolittle, R.F., Watt, K.W.K., Cottrell, B.A., Strong, D.D. and Riley, M. (1979) Nature (London) 280, 464–468.
98 Henschen, A., Lottspeich, F. and Hessel, B. (1979) Hoppe-Seyler's Z. Physiol. Chem. 360, 1951–1956.
99 Kaiser, C., Seydewitz, H.H. and Witt, I. (1984) Thromb. Res. 33, 543–548.
100 Rixon, M.W., Chan, W.-Y., Davie, E.W. and Chung, D.W. (1983) Biochemistry 22, 3237–3244.
101 Semeraro, N., Collen, D. and Verstraete, M. (1977) Biochim. Biophys. Acta 492, 204–214.
102 Henschen, A. and Lottspeich, F. (1980) Haematologica 65, 535–541.
103 Timpl, R., Fietzek, P.P., van Delden, V. and Landrath, G. (1978) Hoppe-Seyler's Z. Physiol. Chem. 359, 1553–1560.
104 Martinelli, R.A., Inglis, A.S., Rubira, M.R., Hageman, T.C., Hurrell, J.G.R., Leach, S.J. and Scheraga, H.A. (1979) Arch. Biochem. Biophys. 192, 27–32.
105 Henschen, A., Lottspeich, F., Töpfer-Petersen, E., Kehl, M. and Timpl, R. (1980) in: Protides of the Biological Fluids (Peeters, H., Ed.) Vol. 28, pp. 47–50, Pergamon, Oxford.
106 Chung, D.W., Rixon, M.W., McGillivray, R.T.A. and Davie, E.W. (1981) Proc. Natl. Acad. Sci. (U.S.A.) 78, 1466–1470.
107 Chung, D.W., Rixon, M.W. and Davie, E.W. (1982) in: Proteins in Biology and Medicine (Bradshaw, R.A., Hill, R.L., Tang, J., Chi-chuan, L., Tien-chin, T. and Chen-lu, T., Eds.) pp. 309–328, Academic Press, New York.
108 Kehl, M. and Henschen, A. (1982) in: Fibrinogen (Henschen, A., Graeff, H. and Lottspeich, F., Eds.) Vol. 1, pp. 109–114, de Gruyter, Berlin.
109 Crabtree, G.R., Comeau, C.M., Fowlkes, D.M., Fornace Jr., A.J., Malley, J.D. and Kant, J.A. (1985) J. Mol. Biol. 185, 1–19.
110 Crabtree, G.R. and Kant, J.A. (1982) Cell 31, 159–166.
111 Strong, D.D., Moore, M., Cottrell, B.A., Bohonus, V.L., Pontes, M., Evans, B., Riley, M. and Doolittle, R.F. (1985) Biochemistry 24, 92–101.
112 Henschen, A. (1964) Ark. Kem. 22, 355–373.
113 Blombäck, B., Blombäck, M., Henschen, A., Hessel, B., Iwanaga, S. and Woods, K.R. (1968) Nature (London) 218, 130–134.

114 Blombäck, B., Hessel, B. and Hogg, D. (1976) Thromb. Res. 8, 639–658.
115 Gårdlund, B., Hessel, B., Marguerie, G., Murano, G. and Blombäck, B. (1977) Eur. J. Biochem. 77, 595–610.
116 Henschen, A. (1978) Hoppe-Seyler's Z. Physiol. Chem. 359, 1757–1770.
117 Hoeprich Jr., P.D. and Doolittle, R.F. (1983) Biochemistry 22, 2049–2055.
118 Henschen, A., Lottspeich, F. and Hessel, B. (1978) Hoppe-Seyler's Z Physiol. Chem. 359, 1607–1610.
119 Blombäck, B., Blombäck, M., Finkbeiner, W., Holmgren, A., Kowalska-Loth, B. and Olovson, G. (1974) Thromb. Res. 4, 55–75.
120 Töpfer-Petersen, E., Lottspeich, F. and Henschen, A. (1976) Hoppe-Seyler's Z. Physiol. Chem. 357, 1509–1513.
121 Töpfer-Petersen, E. (1980) in: Fibrinogen, Fibrin and Fibrin Glue (Schimpf, K., Ed.) pp. 43–45, Schattauer, Stuttgart.
122 Mizuochi, T., Taniguchi, T., Asami, Y., Takamatsu, J., Okude, M., Iwanaga, S. and Kobata, A. (1982) J. Biochem. 92, 283–293.
123 Townsend, R.R., Hilliker, E., Li, Y.-T., Laine, R.A., Bell, W.R. and Lee, Y.C. (1982) J. Biol. Chem. 257, 9704–9710.
124 Kuyas, C., Haeberli, A. and Straub, P.W. (1982) Thromb. Haemostas. 47, 19–21.
125 Townsend, R.R., Heller, D.N., Fenselau, C.C. and Lee, Y.C. (1984) Biochemistry 23, 6389–6392.
126 Blombäck, B., Blombäck, M., Edman, P. and Hessel, B. (1966) Biochim. Biophys. Acta 115, 371–396.
127 Seydewitz, H.H., Kaiser, C., Rothweiler, H. and Witt, I. (1984) Thromb. Res. 33, 487–498.
128 Kudryk, B., Okada, M., Redman, C.M. and Blombäck, B. (1982) Eur. J. Biochem. 125, 673–682.
129 Seydewitz, H.H. and Witt, I. (1985) Thromb. Res. 40, 29–39.
130 Krust, B., Galabru, J. and Hovanessian, A.G. (1983) Biochem. Biophys. Res. Commun. 117, 350–357.
131 Humble, E., Heldin, P., Forsberg, P.-O. and Engström, L. (1984) J. Biochem. 95, 1435–1443.
132 Jevons, F.R. (1963) Biochem. J. 89, 621–624.
133 Jollès, P., Loucheux-Lefebvre, M.-H. and Henschen, A. (1978) J. Mol. Evol. 11, 271–277.
134 Doolittle, R.F., Goldbaum, D.M. and Doolittle, L.R. (1978) J. Mol. Biol. 120, 311–325.
135 Parry, D.A.D. (1978) J. Mol. Biol. 120, 545–551.
136 Yu, S., Redman, C.M., Goldstein, J. and Blombäck, B. (1980) Biochem. Biophys. Res. Commun. 96, 1032–1038.
137 Nickerson, J.M. and Fuller, G.M. (1981) Proc. Natl. Acad. Sci. (U.S.A.) 78, 303–307.
138 Crabtree, G.R. and Kant, J.A. (1981) J. Biol. Chem. 256, 9718–9723.
139 Uzan, G., Besmond, C., Kahn, A. and Marguerie, G. (1982) Biochem. Int. 4, 271–278.
140 Olaisen, B., Teisberg, P. and Gedde-Dahl Jr., T. (1982) Hum. Genet. 61, 24–26.
141 Henry, I., Uzan, G., Weil, D., Nicolas, H., Kaplan, J.C., Marguerie, C., Kahn, A. and Junien, C. (1984) Am. J. Hum. Genet. 36, 760–768.
142 Humphries, S.E., Imam, A.M.A., Robbins, T.P., Cook, M., Carritt, B., Ingle, C. and Williamson, R. (1984) Hum. Genet. 68, 148–153.
143 Kant, J.A., Fornace Jr., A.J., Saxe, D., Simon, M.I., McBride, O.W. and Crabtree, G.R. (1985) Proc. Natl. Acad. Sci. (U.S.A.) 82, 2344–2348.
144 Rixon, M.W., Chung, D.W. and Davie, E.W. (1985) Biochemistry 24, 2077–2086.
145 Fornace Jr., A.J., Cummings, D.E., Comeau, C.M., Kant, J.A. and Crabtree, G.R. (1984) J. Biol. Chem. 259, 12826–12830.
146 Leven, R.M., Schick, P.K. and Budzynski, A.Z. (1985) Blood 65, 501–504.
147 Belloc, F., Hourdille, P., Fialon, P., Boisseau, M.R. and Soria, J. (1985) Thromb. Res. 38, 341–351.
148 Teige, B., Gogstad, G., Brosstad, F. and Olaisen, B. (1985) Blood 65, 120–126.
149 Mosesson, M.W., Homandberg, G.A. and Amrani, D.L. (1984) Blood 63, 990–995.
150 Francis, C.W., Nachman, R.L. and Marder, V.J. (1984) Thromb. Haemostas. 51, 84–88.
151 Yu, S., Sher, B., Kudryk, B. and Redman, C.M. (1984) J. Biol. Chem. 259, 10574–10581.
152 Alving, B.M., Chung, S.I., Murano, G., Tang, D.B. and Finlayson, J.S. (1982) Arch. Biochem. Biophys. 217, 1–9.

234

153 Galanakis, D.K., Henschen, A., Keeling, M., Kehl, M., Dismore, R. and Peerschke, E. (1983) Ann. N.Y. Acad. Sci. 408, 644–648.

154 Nickerson, J.M. and Fuller, G.M. (1981) Biochemistry 20, 2818–2821.

155 Kirsch, R.E. and Franks, J.J. (1982) Hepatology 2, 205–208.

156 Fuller, G.M. and Ritchie, D.G. (1982) Ann. N.Y. Acad. Sci. 389, 308–322.

157 Fuller, G.M., Otto, J.M., Woloski, B.M., McGary, C.T. and Adams, M.A. (1985) J. Cell Biol. 101, 1481–1486.

158 Sanders, K.D. and Fuller, G.M. (1983) Thromb. Res. 32, 133–145.

159 Bell, W.R., Kessler, C.M. and Townsend, R.R. (1983) Br. J. Haematol. 53, 599–610.

160 Qureshi, G.D., Guzelian, P.S., Vennart, R.M. and Evans, H.J. (1985) Biochim. Biophys. Acta 844, 288–295.

161 Princen, H.M.G., Moshage, H.J., Emeis, J.J., de Haard, H.J.W., Nieuwenhuizen, W. and Yap, S.H. (1985) Thromb. Haemostas. 53, 212–215.

162 Princen, H.M.G., Moshage, H.J., de Haard, H.J.W., van Gemert, P.J.L. and Yap, S.H. (1984) Biochem. J. 220, 631–637.

163 Kampschmidt, R.F. and Mesecher, M. (1985) Proc. Soc. Exp. Biol. Med. 179, 197–200.

164 Collen, D., Tytgat, G.N., Claeys, H. and Piessens, R. (1972) Br. J. Haematol. 22, 681–700.

165 Nieuwenhuizen, W., Emeis, J.J. and Vermond, A. (1982) Thromb. Haemostas. 48, 59–61.

166 Martinez, J., Palascak, J. and Peters, C. (1977) J. Lab. Clin. Med. 89, 367–377.

167 Kehl, M., Lottspeich, F. and Henschen, A. (1981) Hoppe-Seyler's Z. Physiol. Chem. 362, 1661–1664.

168 Henschen, A., Kehl, M. and Southan, C. (1984) in: Variants of Human Fibrinogen (Beck. E.A. and Furlan, M., Eds.) pp. 273–320, Huber, Bern.

169 Canfield, R.E., Dean, J., Nossel, H.L., Butler Jr., V.P. and Wilner, G.D. (1976) Biochemistry 15, 1203–1209.

170 Kockum, C. and Frebelius, S. (1980) Thromb. Res. 19, 589–598.

171 Gaffney, P.J., Joe, F., Mahmoud, M., Fossati, C.A. and Spitz, M. (1980) Thromb. Res. 19, 815–822.

172 Stehle, G., Harenberg, J., Schmidt-Gayk, H. and Zimmermann, R. (1983) J. Clin. Chem. Clin. Biochem. 21, 91–95.

173 Walenga, J.M., Hoppensteadt, D., Emanuele, R.M. and Fareed, J. (1984) Sem. Thromb. Hemostas. 10, 219–227.

174 Butt, R.W., deBoer, A.C. and Turpie, A.G.G. (1984) J. Immunoass. 5, 245–266.

175 Bilezikian, S.B., Nossel, H.L., Butler Jr., V.P. and Canfield, R.E. (1975) J. Clin. Invest. 56, 438–445.

176 LaGamma, K.S. and Nossel, H.L. (1978) Thromb. Res. 12, 447–454.

177 Butler Jr., V.P., Weber, D.A., Nossel, H.L., Tse-Eng, D., LaGamma, K.S. and Canfield, R.E. (1982) Blood 59, 1006–1012.

178 Soria, J., Soria, C. and Ryckewaert, J.J. (1980) Thromb. Res. 20, 425–435.

179 Amiral, J., Walenga, J.M. and Fareed, J. (1984) Sem. Thromb. Hemostas. 10, 228–242.

180 Martinelli, R.A. and Scheraga, H.A. (1979) Anal. Biochem. 96, 246–249.

181 Koehn, J.A. and Canfield, R.E. (1981) Anal. Biochem. 116, 349–356.

182 Lewis, S.D. and Shafer, J.A. (1984) Thromb. Res. 35, 111–120.

183 Ebert, R.F. and Bell, W.R. (1985) Anal. Biochem. 148, 70–78.

184 Fenton, J.W. (1981) Ann. N.Y. Acad. Sci. 370, 468–495.

185 Chang, J.-Y. (1985) Eur. J. Biochem. 151, 217–224.

186 Iwanaga, S., Henschen, A. and Blombäck, B. (1966) Acta Chem. Scand. 20, 1183–1185.

187 Blombäck, B. (1958) Ark. Kem. 12, 321–335.

188 Blombäck, B., Hogg, D.H., Gårdlund, B., Hessel, B. and Kudryk, B. (1976) Thromb. Res. 8, Suppl. II, 329–346.

189 Blombäck, B., Hessel, B., Hogg, D. and Therkildsen, L. (1978) Nature (London) 275, 501–505.

190 Hurlet-Jensen, A., Cummins, H.Z., Nossel, H.L. and Liu, C.Y. (1982) Thromb. Res. 27, 419–427.

191 Martinelli, R.A. and Scheraga, H.A. (1980) Biochemistry 19, 2343–2350.

192 Kehl, M., Lottspeich, F. and Henschen, A. (1982) in:Fibrinogen (Henschen, A., Graeff, H. and Lottspeich, F., Eds.) Vol. 1, pp. 217–226, de Gruyter, Berlin.

193 Higgins, D.L, Lewis, S.D. and Shafer, J.A. (1983) J. Biol. Chem. 258, 9276–9282.

194 Hanna, L.S., Scheraga, H.A., Francis, C.W. and Marder, V.J. (1984) Biochemistry 23, 4681–4687.

195 Southan, C. and Henschen, A. (1985) in: Fibrinogen (Henschen, A., Hessel, B., McDonagh, J. and Saldeen, T., Eds.) Vol. 3, pp. 73–82, de Gruyter, Berlin.

196 Lewis, S.D., Shields, P.P. and Shafer, J.A. (1985) J. Biol. Chem. 260, 10192–10199.

197 Kehl, M., Lottspeich, F. and Henschen, A. (1983) in: Fibrinogen (Haverkate, F., Henschen, A., Nieuwenhuizen, W. and Straub, P.W., Eds.) Vol. 2, pp. 183–193, de Gruyter, Berlin.

198 Nagy, J.A., Meinwald, Y.C. and Scheraga, H.A. (1982) Biochemistry 21, 1794–1806.

199 Nagy, J.A., Meinwald, Y.C. and Scheraga, H.A. (1985) Biochemistry 24, 882–887.

200 Liu, C.Y., Nossel, H.L. and Kaplan, K.L. (1979) J. Biol. Chem. 254, 10421–10425.

201 Wilner, G.D., Danitz, M.P., Mudd, M.S., Hsieh, K.-H. and Fenton, J.W. (1981) J. Lab. Clin. Med. 97, 403–411.

202 Kaminski, M. and McDonagh, J. (1983) J. Biol. Chem. 258, 10530–10535.

203 Francis, C.W., Markham Jr., R.E., Barlow, G.H., Florack, T.M., Dobrzynski, D.M. and Marder, V.J. (1983) J. Lab. Clin. Med. 102, 220–230.

204 Liu, C.Y., Handley, D.A. and Chien, S. (1985) Anal. Biochem. 147, 49–56.

205 Kaminski, M. and McDonagh, J. (1985) in: Fibrinogen (Henschen, A., Hessel, B., McDonagh, J. and Saldeen, T., Eds.) Vol. 3, pp. 51–63, de Gruyter, Berlin.

206 Stocker, K., Fischer, H. and Meier, J. (1982) Toxicon 20, 265–273.

207 Shainoff, J.R. and Dardik, B.N. (1979) Science 204, 200–202.

208 Dyr, J.E., Blombäck, B. and Kornalik, F. (1983) Thromb. Res. 30, 185–194.

209 Hermans, J. and McDonagh, J. (1982) Sem. Thromb. Hemostas. 8, 11–24.

210 Fowler, W.E., Hantgan, R.R., Hermans, J. and Erickson, H.P. (1981) Proc. Natl. Acad. Sci. (U.S.A.) 78, 4872–4876.

211 Preissner, K.T., Rötker, J., Selmayr, E., Fasold, H. and Müller-Berghaus, G. (1985) Biochim. Biophys. Acta 829, 358–364.

212 Shainoff, J.R. (1985) in: Fibrinogen (Henschen, A., Hessel, B., McDonagh, J. and Saldeen, T., Eds.) Vol. 3, pp. 91–100, de Gruyter, Berlin.

213 Graeff, H., Hafter, R. and von Hugo, R. (1979) Thromb. Res. 16, 575–576.

214 Smith, G.F. (1980) Biochem. J. 185, 1–11.

215 Müller-Berghaus, G., Mahn, I., Krell, W. and Bernhard, J.C. (1982) in: Fibrinogen (Henschen, A., Graeff, H. and Lottspeich, F., Eds.) Vol. 1, pp. 237–248, de Gruyter, Berlin.

216 Alkjaersig, N. and Fletcher, A.P. (1983) Biochem. J. 213, 75–83.

217 Knoll, D., Hantgan, R., Williams, J., McDonagh, J. and Hermans, J. (1984) Biochemistry 23, 3708–3715.

218 Holm, B., Brosstad, F., Kierulf, P. and Godal, H.C. (1985) Thromb. Res. 39, 595–606.

219 Olexa, S.A., Budzynski, A.Z., Doolittle, R.F., Cottrell, B.A. and Greene, T.C. (1981) Biochemistry 20, 6139–6145.

220 Gogstad, G.O. and Brosstad, F. (1983) Thromb. Res. 30, 441–448.

221 Belitser, V.A., Lugovskoy, E.V., Musjalkovskaja, A.A. and Gogolinskaja, G.K. (1982) Thromb. Res. 27, 261–269.

222 Nieuwenhuizen, W., Voskuilen, M., Vermond, A., Haverkate, F. and Hermans, J. (1982) Biochim. Biophys. Acta 707, 190–192.

223 Olexa, S.A. and Budzynski, A.Z. (1981) J. Biol. Chem. 256, 3544–3549.

224 Horwitz, B.H., Váradi, A. and Scheraga, H.A. (1984) Proc. Natl. Acad. Sci. (U.S.A.) 81, 5980–5984.

225 Southan, C., Thompson, E., Panico, M., Etienne, T., Morris, H.R. and Lane, D.A. (1985) J. Biol. Chem. 260, 13095–13101.

226 Pandya, B.V., Cierniewski, C.S. and Budzynski, A.Z. (1985) J. Biol. Chem. 260, 2994–3000.

227 Laudano, A.P. and Doolittle, R.F. (1981) Science 212, 457–459.

228 Furlan, M., Rupp, C. and Beck, E.A. (1983) Biochim. Biophys. Acta 742, 25–32.

229 Hsieh, K.-H., Mudd, M.S. and Wilner, G.D. (1981) J. Med. Chem. 24, 322–327.
230 Matthias, F.R., Reinicke, R. and Heene, D.L. (1977) Thromb. Res. 10, 365–384.
231 Heene, D.L., Matthias, F.R., Wegrzynowicz, Z. and Hocke, G. (1979) Thromb. Haemostas. 41, 677–686.
232 York, L.L. and Blombäck, B. (1976) Thromb. Res. 8, 607–618.
233 von Hugo, R., Hafter, R., Stemberger, A. and Graeff, H. (1977) Hoppe-Seyler's Z. Physiol. Chem. 358, 1359–1363.
234 Hörmann, H. and Henschen, A. (1979) Thromb. Haemostas. 41, 691–694.
235 Olexa, S.A. and Budzynski, A.Z. (1980) Proc. Natl. Acad. Sci. (U.S.A.) 77, 1374–1378.
236 Belitser, V.A., Pozdnjakova, T.M. and Ugarova, T.P. (1980) Thromb. Res. 19, 807–814.
237 Thiel, W., Delvos, U. and Müller-Berghaus, G. (1985) Thromb. Haemostas. 54, 533–538.
238 Plow, E.F. (1977) Eur. J. Biochem. 80, 55–64.
239 Matsushima, A., Takiuchi, H., Saito, Y. and Inada, Y. (1980) Biochim. Biophys. Acta 625, 230–236.
240 Kaye, N.M.C. and Jollès, P. (1978) Mol. Cell. Biochem. 20, 173–182.
241 Shimizu, A., Saito, Y., Matsushima, A. and Inada, Y. (1983) J. Biol. Chem. 258, 7915–7917.
242 Gilman, P.B., Keane, P. and Martinez, J. (1984) J. Biol. Chem. 259, 3248–3253.
243 Diaz-Mauriño, T., Castro, C. and Albert, A. (1982) Thromb. Res. 27, 397–403.
244 Blombäck, B., Okada, M., Forslind, B. and Larsson, U. (1984) Biorheology 21, 93–104.
245 Bale, M.D., Müller, M.F. and Ferry, J.D. (1985) Proc. Natl. Acad. Sci. (U.S.A.) 82, 1410–1413.
246 Mihalyi, E. and Donovan, J.W. (1985) Biochemistry 24, 3443–3448.
247 Lee, F.H., Fujimoto, S. and Sehon, A.H. (1978) Cancer Immunol. Immunother. 5, 187–193.
248 Hui, K.Y., Haber, E. and Matsueda, G.R. (1985) Thromb. Haemostas. 54, 524–527.
249 Kudryk, B., Rohoza, A., Ahadi, M., Chin, J. and Wiebe, M.E. (1984) Mol. Immunol. 21, 89–94.
250 Scheefers-Borchel, U., Müller-Berghaus, G., Fuhge, P., Eberle, R. and Heimburger, N. (1985) Proc. Natl. Acad. Sci. (U.S.A.) 82, 7091–7095.
251 Koppert, P.W., Huijsmans, C.M.G. and Nieuwenhuizen, W. (1985) Blood 66, 503–507.
252 Ehrlich, P.H., Sobel, J.H., Moustafa, Z.A. and Canfield, R.E. (1983) Biochemistry 22, 4184–4192.
253 Sobel, J.H., Koehn, J.A., Friedman, R. and Canfield, R.E. (1982) Thromb. Res. 26, 411–424.
254 Whitaker, A.N., Elms, M.J., Masci, P.P., Bundesen, P.G., Rylatt, D.B., Webber, A.J. and Bunce, I.H. (1984) J. Clin. Pathol. 37, 882–887.
255 Doolittle, R.F., Cassman, K.G., Chen, R., Sharp, J.J. and Wooding, G.L. (1972) Ann. N.Y. Acad. Sci. 202, 114–126.
256 Cottrell, B.A., Strong, D.D., Watt, K.W.K. and Doolittle, R.F. (1979) Biochemistry 18, 5405–5409.
257 Fretto, L.J., Ferguson, E.W., Steinman, H.M. and McKee, P.A. (1978) J. Biol. Chem. 253, 2184–2195.
258 Corcoran, D.H., Ferguson, E.W., Fretto, L.J. and McKee, P.A. (1980) Thromb. Res. 19, 883–888.
259 Nussenzweig, V., Seligmann, M., Pelmont, J. and Grabar, P. (1961) Ann. Inst. Pasteur, 100, 377–389.
260 Marder, V.J., Budzynski, A.Z., and James, H.L. (1972) J. Biol. Chem. 247, 4775–4781.
261 Gårdlund, B., Kowalska-Loth, B., Gröndahl, N.J. and Blombäck, B. (1972) Thromb. Res. 1, 371–388.
262 Mosesson, M.W., Finlayson, J.S. and Galanakis, D.K. (1973) J. Biol. Chem. 248, 7913–7929.
263 Hessel, B. (1975) Thromb. Res. 7, 75–87.
264 Collen, D., Kudryk, B., Hessel, B. and Blombäck, B. (1975) J. Biol. Chem. 250, 5808–5817.
265 Takagi, T. and Doolittle, R.F. (1975) Biochemistry 14, 940–946.
266 Harfenist, E.J. and Canfield, R.E. (1975) Biochemistry 14, 4110–4117.
267 Furlan, M., Kemp, G. and Beck, E.A. (1975) Biochim. Biophys. Acta 400, 95–111.
268 Henschen, A. and Lottspeich, F. (1976) Hoppe-Seyler's Z. Physiol. Chem. 357, 1801–1803.
269 Birken, S., Agosto, G., Lahiri, B. and Canfield, R. (1984) Thromb. Haemostas. 51, 16–21.
270 Müller, E. and Henschen, A. (1986) in: Fibrinogen (Lane, D.A., Henschen, A. and Jasani, M.K., Eds.) Vol. 4, pp. 137–144, de Gruyter, Berlin.
271 Nossel, H.L. (1981) Nature (London) 291, 165–167.
272 Haverkate, F. and Timan, G. (1977) Thromb. Res. 10, 803–812.

273 Henschen, A., Lottspeich, F., Kehl, M., Southan, C. and Lucas, J., (1982) in: Fibrinogen (Henschen, A., Graeff, H. and Lottspeich, F., Eds.) Vol. 1, pp. 67–82, de Gruyter, Berlin.

274 Purves, L.R., Lindsey, G.G. and Franks, J.J. (1978) S. Afr. J. Sci. 74, 202–209.

275 Britton, D.W., Lawrie, J.S. and Kemp, G.D. (1982) Thromb. Res. 27, 167–173.

276 Dang, C.V., Bell, W.R., Ebert, R.F. and Starksen, N.F. (1985) Arch. Biochem. Biophys. 238, 452–457.

277 Gaffney, P.J. and Whitaker, A.N. (1979) Thromb. Res. 14, 85–94.

278 Olexa, S.A., Budzynski, A.Z. and Marder, V.J. (1979) Biochim. Biophys. Acta 576, 39–50.

279 Gaffney, P.J. and Joe, F. (1979) Thromb. Res. 15, 673–687.

280 Francis, C.W., Marder, V.J. and Barlow, G.H. (1980) J. Clin. Invest. 66, 1033–1043.

281 Francis, C.W. and Marder, V.J. (1982) Sem. Thromb. Hemostas. 8, 25–35.

282 Graeff, H. and Hafter, R. (1982) Sem. Thromb. Hemostas. 8, 57–68.

283 Hurlet-Jensen, A., Koehn, J.A. and Nossel, H.L. (1983) Thromb. Res. 29, 609–617.

284 Carroll, R.C., Lockhart, M.S. and Taylor Jr., F.B., (1984) J. Lab. Clin. Med. 103, 695–703.

285 Wilner, G.D., Mudd, M.S., Hsieh, K.-H. and Thomas, D.W. (1982) Biochemistry 21, 2687–2692.

286 Matsushima, A., Takahama, Y., Inada, Y. (1982) Thromb. Res. 27, 111–115.

287 Cierniewski, C.S., Janiak, A., Nowak, P. and Augustyniak, W. (1982) Thromb. Haemostas. 48, 33–37.

288 Matsumoto, T., Nishijima, Y., Teramura, Y., Fujino, K., Hibino, M. and Hirata, M., (1985) Thromb. Res. 38, 297–302.

289 Hunt, F.A., Rylatt, D.B., Hart, R.A. and Bundesen, P.G. (1985) Br. J. Haematol. 60, 715–722.

290 Gaffney, P.J. and Perry, M.J. (1985) Thromb. Haemostas. 53, 301–302.

291 Connaghan, D.G., Francis, C.W., Lane, D.A. and Marder, V.J. (1985) Blood 65, 589–597.

292 Kudryk, B., Robinson, D., Netré, C., Hessel, B., Blombäck, M. and Blombäck, B. (1982) Thromb. Res. 25, 277–291.

293 Walenga, J.M., Fareed, J., Mariani, G., Messmore Jr., H.L., Bick, R.L. and Emanuele, R.M. (1984) Sem. Thromb. Hemostas. 10, 252–263.

294 Gollwitzer, R., Kulbe, G.E., Gabrijelčič and Linke, R.P. (1986) in: Fibrinogen (Lane, D.A., Henschen, A. and Jasani, M.K., Eds.) Vol. 4, pp. 297–302, de Gruyter, Berlin.

295 Kennel, S.J. and Lankford, P.K. (1983) Clin. Chem. 29, 778–781.

296 Mirshahi, M., Soria, J., Soria, C., Perrot, J.Y., Bernadou, A. and Boucheix, C. (1986) in: Fibrinogen (Lane, D.A., Henschen, A., and Jasani, M.K., Eds.) Vol. 4, pp. 271–277, de Gruyter, Berlin.

297 Plow, E.F. and Edgington, T.S. (1982) Sem. Thromb. Hemostas. 8, 36–56.

298 Stegnar, M. and Chen, J.P. (1984) Thromb. Haemostas. 52, 315–320.

299 Garman, A.J. and Smith, R.A.G. (1982) Thromb. Res. 27, 311–320.

300 Lucas, M.A., Fretto, L.J. and McKee, P.A. (1983) J. Biol. Chem. 258, 4249–4256.

301 Suenson, E., Lützen, O. and Thorsen, S. (1984) Eur. J. Biochem. 140, 513–522.

302 Sakata, Y., Mimuro, J. and Aoki, N. (1984) Blood 63, 1393–1401.

303 Váradi, A. and Patthy, L. (1984) Biochemistry 23, 2108–2112.

304 Bok, R.A. and Mangel, W.F. (1985) Biochemistry 24, 3279–3286.

305 Soria, J., Soria, C., Dunn, F., Deguchi, K., Mirshahi, M., Lijnen, R., Nieuwenhuizen, W., Haverkate, F., Samama, M. and Caen, J. (1985) in: Fibrinogen (Henschen, A., Hessel, B., McDonagh, J. and Saldeen, T., Eds.) Vol. 3, pp. 313–322, de Gruyter, Berlin.

306 Bingenheimer, C., Gramse, M., Egbring, R. and Havemann, K. (1981) Hoppe-Seyler's Z. Physiol. Chem. 362, 853–863.

307 Plow, E.F., Gramse, M. and Havemann, K. (1983) J. Lab. Clin. Med. 102, 858–869.

308 Sterrenberg, L., van Liempt, G.J., Nieuwenhuizen, W. and Hermans, J. (1984) Thromb. Haemostas. 51, 398–402.

309 Sterrenberg, L., Haak, H.L., Brommer, E.J.P. and Nieuwenhuizen, W. (1985) Haemostasis. 15, 126–133.

310 Bang, N.U., Chang, M.L., Mattler, L.E., Burck, P.J., Van Frank, R.M., Zimmerman, R.E., Marks, C.A. and Boxer, L.J. (1981) Ann. N.Y. Acad. Sci. 370, 568–587.

311 Moran, J.B. and Geren, C.R. (1981) Biochim. Biophys. Acta 659, 161–168.
312 Ouyang, C., Hwang, L.-J. and Huang, T.-F. (1983) Toxicon 21, 25–33.
313 Sapru, Z.Z., Tu, A.T. and Bailey, G.S. (1983) Biochim. Biophys. Acta 747, 225–231.
314 Evans, H.J. (1984) Biochim. Biophys. Acta 802, 49–54.
315 Malinconico, S.M., Katz, J.B. and Buzynski, A.Z. (1984) J. Lab. Clin. Med. 104, 842–854.
316 Arocha-Piñango, C.L., Perales, J. and Carvajal, Z. (1981) Thromb. Haemostas. 45, 233–236.
317 Scherer, R., Simon, J., Abd-el-fattah, M. and Ruhenstroth-Bauer, G. (1980) Clin. Exp. Immunol. 40, 49–59.
318 Abiko, T., Onodera, I. and Sekino, H. (1979) Biochem. Biophys. Res. Commun. 89, 813–821.
319 Mehta, J., Wargovich, T., Nichols, W.W., Saldeen, K., Wallin, R. and Saldeen, T. (1985) Am. J. Physiol. 249, 457–462.
320 Eriksson, M., Saldeen, K., Saldeen, T., Strandberg, K. and Wallin, R. (1983) Int. J. Microcirc. Clin. Exp. 2, 337–345.
321 Nichols, W.W., Mehta, J., Wargovich, T., Saldeen, K., Wallin, R. and Saldeen, T. (1985) Thromb. Res. 38, 223–229.
322 Gartner, T.K. and Bennett, J.S. (1985) J. Biol. Chem. 260, 11891–11894.
323 Wallén, P., Bergsdorf, N. and Rånby, M. (1982) Biochim. Biophys. Acta 719, 318–328.
324 Bányai, L., Váradi, A. and Patthy, L. (1983) FEBS Letts. 163, 37–41.
325 Kagitani, H., Tagawa, M., Hatanaka, K., Ikari, T., Saito, A., Bando, H., Okada, K. and Matsuo, O. (1985) FEBS Lett. 189, 145–149.
326 Harpel, P.C., Chang, T.-S. and Verderber, E. (1985) J. Biol. Chem. 260, 4432–4440.
327 Nieuwenhuizen, W. and Keyser, J. (1985) Thromb. Res. 38, 663–670.
328 Gurewich, V., Pannell, R., Louie, S., Kelley, P., Suddith, R.L. and Greenlee, R. (1984) J. Clin. Invest. 73, 1731–1739.
329 Kasai, S., Arimura, H., Nishida, M. and Suyama, T. (1985) J. Biol. Chem. 260, 12377–12381.
330 Takada, Y., Makino, Y. and Takada A. (1985) Thromb. Res. 39, 289–296.
331 Lijnen, H.R., van Hoef, B. and Collen, D. (1984) Eur. J. Biochem. 144, 541–544.
332 Chibber, B.A.K., Morris, J.P. and Castellino, F.J. (1985) Biochemistry 24, 3429–3434.
333 Takada, A., Takada, Y. and Sugawara, Y. (1985) Thromb. Res. 37, 465–475.
334 Ichinose, A., Mimuro, J., Koide, T. and Aoki, N. (1984) Thromb. Res. 33, 401–407.
335 Kluft, C., Los, P. and Jie, A.F.H. (1984) Thromb. Res. 33, 419–425.
336 Petersen, T.E., Thøgersen, H.C., Skorstengaard, K., Vibe-Pedersen, K., Sahl, P., Sottrup-Jensen, L. and Magnusson, S. (1983) Proc. Natl. Acad. Sci. (U.S.A.) 80, 137–141.
337 Niewiarowska, J. and Cierniewski, C.S. (1982) Thromb. Res. 27, 611–618.
338 Holm, B. and Brosstad, F. (1983) in: Fibrinogen (Haverkate, F., Henschen, A., Nieuwenhuizen, W. and Straub, P.W., Eds.) Vol. 2, pp. 323–335, de Gruyter, Berlin.
339 Okada, M., Blombäck, B., Chang, M.-D. and Horowitz, B. (1985) J. Biol. Chem. 260, 1811–1820.
340 Hörmann, H. (1985) in: Plasma Fibronectin (McDonagh, J., Ed.) pp. 99–120, Dekker, New York.
341 Jilek, F. and Hörmann, H. (1981) Thromb. Res. 21, 265–272.
342 Ku, C.S.L. and Fiedel, B.A. (1983) J. Exp. Med. 158, 767–780.
343 Wisløff, F., Michaelsen, T.E. and Godal, H.C. (1984) Thromb. Res. 35, 81–90.
344 Wilf, J., Gladner, J.A. and Minton, A.P. (1985) Thromb. Res. 37, 681–688.
345 Whitaker, A.N., McFarlane, J.R., Rowe, E.A., Lee, K. and Masci, P.P. (1985) Thromb. Haemostas. 53, 80–85.
346 Vanstapel, M.J., de Wolf-Peeters, C., de Vos, R. and Desmet, V.J. (1984) Liver 4, 148–155.
347 Diaz-Mauriño, T., Blanco, R. and Albert, A. (1984) Biochim. Biophys. Acta 799, 45–50.
348 Marguerie, G., Benabid, Y. and Suscillon, M. (1979) Biochim. Biophys. Acta 579, 134–141.
349 Nieuwenhuizen, W., Vermond, A. and Hermans, J. (1983) Thromb. Res. 31, 81–86.
350 Tufty, R.M. and Kretsinger, R.H. (1975) Science 187, 167–169.
351 Dang, C.V., Ebert, R.F. and Bell, W.R. (1985) J. Biol. Chem. 260, 9713–9719.
352 Scully, M.F. and Kakkar, V.V. (1983) Thromb. Res. 30, 297–300.
353 Marx, G. and Eldor, A. (1985) Am. J. Hematol. 19, 151–159.
354 Kanaide, H., Uranishi, T. and Nakamura, M. (1982) Am. J. Hematol. 13, 229–237.

355 Kornecki, E., Lee, H., Merlin, F., Hershock, D., Tuszynski, G.P. and Niewiarowski, S. (1984) Thromb. Res. 34, 35–49.

356 Marguerie, G.A., Thomas-Maison, N., Ginsberg, M.H. and Plow, E.F. (1984) Eur. J. Biochem. 139, 5–11.

357 Nachman, R.L., Leung, L.L.K., Kloczewiak, M. and Hawiger, J. (1984) J. Biol. Chem. 259, 8584–8588.

358 Hawiger, J., Kloczewiak, M., Timmons, S. and Lukas, T.J. (1985) in: Fibrinogen (Henschen, A., Hessel, B., McDonagh, J. and Saldeen, T., Eds.) Vol. 3, pp. 345–368, de Gruyter, Berlin.

359 Peerschke, E.I.B. (1985) Sem. Hematol. 22, 241–259.

360 Tuszynski, G.P., Srivastava, S., Switalska, H.I., Holt, J.C., Cierniewski, C.S. and Niewiarowski, S. (1985) J. Biol. Chem. 260, 12240–12245.

361 Bale, M.D., Westrick, L.G. and Mosher, D.F. (1985) J. Biol. Chem. 260, 7502–7508.

362 Rampling, M.W., Whittingstall, P. and Linderkamp, O. (1984) Clin. Hemorrh. 4, 533–543.

363 Maeda, N., Imaizumi, K., Sekiya, M. and Shiga, T. (1984) Biochim. Biophys. Acta 776, 151–158.

364 Wautier, J.L., Pintigny, D., Wautier, M.P., Paton, R.C., Galacteros, F., Passa, P. and Caen, J.P. (1983) J. Lab. Clin. Med. 101, 911–920.

365 Dejana, E., Languino, L.R., Polentarutti, N., Balconi, G., Ryckewaert, J.J., Larrieu, M.J., Donati, M.B., Mantovani, A. and Marguerie, G. (1985) J. Clin. Invest. 75, 11–18.

366 Delvos, U., Preissner, K.T. and Müller-Berghaus, G. (1985) Thromb. Haemostas. 53, 26–31.

367 Olander, J.V., Bremer, M.E., Marasa, J.C. and Feder, J. (1985) J. Cell. Physiol. 125, 1–9.

368 Watanabe, K. and Tanaka, K. ((1983) Atherosclerosis 48, 57–70.

369 Copley, A.L. (1984) Biorheology 21, 135–153.

370 Hogg, N. (1983) J. Exp. Med. 157, 473–485.

371 Gonda, S.R. and Shainoff, J.R. (1982) Proc. Natl. Acad. Sci. (U.S.A.) 79, 4565–4569.

372 Colvin, R.B. (1983) Ann. N.Y. Acad. Sci. 408, 621–633.

373 Dejana, E., Vergara-Dauden, M., Balconi, G., Pietra, A., Cherel, G., Donati, M.B., Larrieu, M.-J. and Marguerie, G. (1984) Eur. J. Biochem. 139, 657–662.

374 Jeleńska, M., Kopeć, M., Rochowska, M. and Skurzak, H. (1985) in: Fibrinogen (Henschen, A., Hessel, B., McDonagh, J. and Saldeen, T., Eds.) Vol. 3, pp. 405–411, de Gruyter, Berlin.

375 Strong, D.D., Laudano, A.P., Hawiger, J. and Doolittle, R.F. (1982) Biochemistry 21, 1414–1420.

376 Chhatwal, G.S., Lämmler, C. and Blobel, H. (1983) IRCS Med. Sci. 11, 1015–1016.

377 Lämmler, C., Chhatwal, G.S. and Blobel, H. (1983) Med. Microbiol. 172, 149–153.

378 Reuterswärd, A., Miörner, H., Wagner, M. and Kronvall, G. (1985) Act. Pat. M.B. 93, 77–82.

379 Kühnemund, O., Havliček, J., Knöll, H., Sjöquist, J. and Köhler, W. (1985) Act. Pat. M. B. 93, 201–209.

380 Whitnack, E. and Beachey, E.H. (1985) J. Bacteriol. 164, 350–358.

381 Gati, W.P. and Straub, P.W. (1978) J. Biol. Chem. 253, 1315–1321.

382 Carrell, N.A., Holahan, J.R., White, G.C. and McDonagh, J. (1983) Thromb. Haemostas. 49, 47–50.

383 Brosstad, F., Teige, B., Olaisen, B., Gravem, K., Godal, H.C. and Stormorken, H. (1983) in: Fibrinogen (Haverkate, F., Henschen, A., Nieuwenhuizen, W. and Straub, P.W., Eds.) Vol. 2, pp. 145–153, de Gruyter, Berlin.

384 Tesch, R., Trolp, R. and Witt, I. (1979) Thromb. Res. 16, 239–243.

385 Galanakis, D.K. (1984) Clin. Lab. Med. 4, 395–418.

386 Galanakis, D.K. (1985) in: Fibrinogen (Henschen, A., Hessel, B., McDonagh, J. and Saldeen, T., Eds.) Vol. 3, pp. 147–152, de Gruyter, Berlin.

387 Francis, J.L. and Armstrong, D.J. (1982) Haemostasis 11, 223–228.

388 Francis, J.L. and Armstrong, D.J. (1983) Med. Lab. Sci. 40, 165–175.

389 Hamulyák, K., Nieuwenhuizen, W., Devilée, P.P. and Hemker, H.C. (1983) Thromb. Res. 32, 301–310.

390 Martinez, J., MacDonald, K.A. and Palascak, J.E. (1983) Blood 61, 1196–1202.

391 Francis, J.L., Watson, N.J. and Simmonds, V.J. (1984) Thromb. Res. 34, 187–197.

392 Lütjens, A., te Velde, A.A., v.d.Veen, E.A. and v.d.Meer, J. (1985) Diabetologia 28, 87–89.

393 Ney, K.A., Pasqua, J.J., Colley, K.J., Guthrow, C.E. and Pizzo, S.V. (1985) Diabetes 34, 462–470.
394 Beck, E.A. (1982) in: Hemostasis and Thrombosis, Basic Principles and Clinical Practice (Colman, R.W., Hirsch, J., Marder, V.J. and Salzman, E.W., Eds.) pp. 185–209, Lippincott, New York.
395 Mammen, E.F. (1983) Sem. Thromb. Hemostas. 9, 1–9 and 57–72.
396 Henschen, A. (1985) in: Protides of the Biological Fluids (Peeters, H., Ed.) Vol. 33, pp. 107–110, Pergamon, Oxford.
397 Henschen, A., Lottspeich, F., Kehl, M. and Southan, C. (1983) Ann. N.Y. Acad. Sci. 408, 28–43.
398 Soria, J., Soria, C., Samama, M., Henschen, A. and Southan, C. (1982) in: Fibrinogen (Henschen, A., Graeff, H. and Lottspeich, F., Eds.) Vol. 1, pp. 129–143, de Gruyter, Berlin.
399 Southan, C., Henschen, A. and Lottspeich, F. (1982) in: Fibrinogen (Henschen, A., Graeff, H. and Lottspeich, F., Eds.) Vol. 1, pp. 153–166, de Gruyter, Berlin.
400 Henschen, A., Kehl, M. and Deutsch, E. (1983) Hoppe-Seyler's Z. Physiol. Chem. 364, 1747–1751.
401 Liu, C.Y., Koehn, J.A. and Morgan, F.J. (1985) J. Biol. Chem. 260, 4390–4396.
402 Southan, C., Lane, D.A., Bode, W. and Henschen, A. (1985) Eur. J. Biochem. 147, 593–600.
403 Southan, C., Lane, D.A., Knight, I., Ireland, H. and Bottomley, J. (1985) Biochem. J. 229, 723–730.
404 Blombäck, M., Blombäck, B., Mammen, E.F. and Prasad, A.S. (1968) Nature (London) 218, 134–137.
405 Kaudewitz, H., Henschen, A., Soria, J. and Soria, C. (1986) in: Fibrinogen (Lane, D.A., Henschen, A. and Jasani, M.K., Eds.) Vol. 4, pp. 91–96, de Gruyter, Berlin.
406 Reber, P., Furlan, M., Rupp, C., Kehl, M., Henschen, A., Mannucci, P.M. and Beck, E.A. (1986) in: Fibrinogen (Lane, D.A., Henschen, A. and Jasani, M.K., Eds.) Vol. 4, pp. 97–102, de Gruyter, Berlin.
407 Flute, P.T. (1977) Br. Med. Bull. 33, 253–259.
408 Wehinger, H., Klinge, O., Alexandrakis, E., Schürmann, J., Witt, J. and Seydewitz, H.H. (1983) Eur. J. Pediat. 141, 109–112.
409 Uzan, G., Courtois, G., Besmond, C., Frain, M., Sala-Trepat, J., Kahn, A. and Marguerie, G. (1984) Biochem. Biophys. Res. Commun. 120, 376–383.
410 Hemmendorff, B., Brandt, J. and Andersson, L.-O. (1981) Biochim. Biophys. Acta 667, 15–22.
411 York, J.L. (1983) Thromb. Res. 31, 203–209.
412 Söderqvist, T. and Blombäck, B. (1971) Naturwissenschaften 58, 16–23.
413 Dayhoff, M.O. (1972) in: Atlas of Protein Sequence and Structure, Vol. 5, pp. 1–D 418, National Biomedical Research Foundation, Washington, DC.
414 Henschen, A. and Lottspeich, F. (1977) Thromb. Res. 11, 869–880.
415 Doolittle, R.F. (1984) in: The Plasma Proteins (Putnam, F.W., Ed.) Vol. 4, pp. 317–360, Academic Press, New York.
416 Doolittle, R.F. (1981) Science 214, 149–159.
417 Skrzynia, C., Reisner, H.M. and McDonagh, J. (1982) Blood 60, 1089–1095.
418 Curtis, C.G. and Lorand, L. (1976) Methods Enzymol. 45, 177–191.
419 Lorand, L., Credo, R.B. and Janus, T.J. (1981) Methods Enzymol. 80, 333–341.
420 Kazama, M., McDonagh, J., Wagner, R.H., Langdell, R.D. and McDonagh, R.P. (1976) Hemostasis 5, 329–340.
421 Cooke, R.D. and Holbrook, J.J. (1974) Biochem. J. 141, 79–84.
422 McDonagh, J., Waggoner, W.G., Hamilton, E.G., Hindenach, B. and McDonagh, R.P. (1976) Biochim. Biophys. Acta 446, 345–357.
423 Schwartz, M.L., Pizzo, S.V., Hill, R.L. and McKee, P.A. (1973) J. Biol. Chem. 248, 1395–1407.
424 Miraglia, C.C. and Greenberg, C.S. (1985) Anal. Biochem. 144, 165–171.
425 Godal, H.C., Gravem, K., Brosstad, F. and Nyvold, N. (1984) Thromb. Res. 35, 577–582.
426 Ikematsu, S., McDonagh, R.P., Reisner, H.M., Skrzynia, C. and McDonagh, J. (1981) J. Lab. Clin. Med. 97, 662–671.
427 Kiesselbach, T.H. and Wagner, R.H. (1972) Ann. N.Y. Acad. Sci. 202, 318–328.
428 McDonagh, J., McDonagh, R.P., Delage, J.M. and Wagner, R.H. (1969) J. Clin. Invest. 48, 940–946.

429 Lopaciuk, S., Lovette, K.M., McDonagh, J., Chuang, H.Y.K. and McDonagh, R.P. (1976) Thromb. Res. 8, 453–465.

430 Henriksson, P., Becker, S., Lynch, G. and McDonagh, J. (1985) J. Clin. Invest. 76, 528–534.

431 Losowsky, M.S. and Walls, W.D. (1971) Br. J. Haematol. 20, 377–383.

432 Hedner, U., Henriksson, P. and Nilsson, I.M. (1975) Scand. J. Haematol. 14, 114–119.

433 Nagy, J.A., Henriksson, P. and McDonagh, J. (1985) Thromb. Haemostas., 54, 274.

434 Chung, S.I., Lewis, M.C. and Folk, J.E. (1974) J. Biol. Chem. 249, 940–950.

435 Carrell, N., Erickson, H. and McDonagh, J. (1982) Circulation 66, 174.

436 Bohn, H. (1978) Mol. Cell. Biochem. 20, 67–75.

437 Takagi, T. and Doolittle, R.F. (1974) Biochemistry 13, 750–756.

438 Seelig, G.F. and Folk, J.E. (1980) J. Biol. Chem. 255, 8881–8886.

439 Curtiss, C.G., Brown, K.L., Credo, R.B., Domanik, R.A., Gray, A., Stenberg, P. and Lorand, L. (1974) Biochemistry 13, 3774–3780.

440 Lewis, B.A., Freyssinet, J.M. and Holbrook, J.J. (1978) Biochem. J. 169, 397–402.

441 Nakamura, S., Iwanaga, S. and Suzuki, T. (1975) J. Biochem. 78, 1247–1266.

442 Holbrook, J.J., Cooke, R.D. and Kingston, I.B. (1973) Biochem. J. 135, 901–903.

443 Folk, J.E. and Cole, P.W. (1966) J. Biol. Chem. 241, 3238–3240.

444 Drenth, J., Jansonius, J.N., Koekoek, R., Swen, H.M. and Wolthers, B.G. (1968) Nature (London) 218, 929–932.

445 Sarasua, M., Koehler, K.A., Skrzynia, C. and McDonagh, J. (1982) J. Biol. Chem. 257, 14102–14109.

446 Credo, R.B., Curtis, C.G. and Lorand, L. (1978) Proc. Natl. Acad. Sci. (U.S.A.) 75, 4234–4237.

447 Credo, R.B., Curtis, C.G. and Lorand, L. (1981) Biochemistry 20, 3770–3778.

448 Janus, T.J., Lewis, S.D., Lorand, L. and Shafer, J.A. (1983) Biochemistry 22, 6269–6272.

449 Folk, J.E. (1983) Adv. Enzymol. 54, 1–56.

450 Gorman, J.J. and Folk, J.E. (1984) J. Biol. Chem. 259, 9007–9010.

451 Laki, K. and Lorand, L. (1948) Science 108, 280.

452 Schwartz, M.L., Pizzo, S.V., Hill, R.L. and McKee, P.A. (1971) J. Clin. Invest. 50, 1506–1513.

453 Kopéc, M., Teisseyre, E., Dudek-Wojciechowska, G., Kloczewiak, M., Pankiewicz, A. and Latallo, Z. (1973) Thromb. Res. 2, 283–291.

454 Shen, L.L., McDonagh, R.P., McDonagh, J. and Hermans, J. (1977) J. Biol. Chem. 252, 6184–6189.

455 Kanaide, H. and Shainoff, J.R. (1975) J. Lab. Clin. Med. 85, 574–597.

456 Tamaki, T. and Aoki, N. (1982) J. Biol. Chem. 257, 14767–14772.

457 Sakata, Y. and Aoki, N. (1982) J. Clin. Invest. 69, 536–542.

458 Mosher, D.F. and Johnson, R.B. (1983) Ann. N.Y. Acad. Sci. 408, 583–593.

459 Iwanaga, S., Suzuki, K. and Hashimoto, S. (1978) Ann. N.Y. Acad. Sci. 312, 56–73.

460 McDonagh, R.P., McDonagh, J., Petersen, T.E., Thøgersen, H.C., Skorstengaard, K., Sottrup-Jensen, L. and Magnusson, S. (1981) FEBS Lett. 127, 174–178.

461 Bale, M.D., Westrick, L.G. and Mosher, D.F. (1985) J. Biol. Chem. 260, 7502–7508.

462 Hada, M., Kato, M., Ikematsu, S., Fujimaki, M. and Fukutake, K. (1982) Thromb. Res. 25, 163–168.

463 Mosher, D.F. (1984) Mol. Cell. Biochem. 58, 63–68.

464 Greenberg, C.S. and Shuman, M.A. (1984) J. Biol. Chem. 259, 14721–14727.

465 Cohen, I., Glaser, T., Veis, A. and Bruner-Lorand, J. (1981) Biochim. Biophys. Acta 676, 137–147.

466 Grinnell, F. (1984) J. Cell Biochem. 26, 107–116.

467 Duckert, F. (1972) Ann. N.Y. Acad. Sci. 202, 190–199.

468 Board, P.G., Reid, M. and Serjeantson, S. (1984) Hum. Genet. 67, 406–408.

469 Duckert, F., Jung, E. and Shmerling, D.H. (1960) Thromb. Diath. Haemorrh. 5, 179–186.

470 Lorand, L., Losowsky, M.S. and Miloszewski, K.J.M. (1980) Progr. Hemostas. Thromb. 5, 245–290.

R.F.A. Zwaal and H.C. Hemker (Eds.), *Blood Coagulation*
© 1986 Elsevier Science Publishers B.V. (Biomedical Division)

CHAPTER 8

Fibrinolysis and thrombolysis

D. COLLEN and H.R. LIJNEN

*Center for Thrombosis and Vascular Research, University of Leuven, Campus
Gasthuisberg, Herestraat 49, B-3000 Leuven (Belgium)*

1. Introduction

Mammalian blood contains an enzymatic system capable of dissolving blood clots, which is called the fibrinolytic enzyme system. Most of the components of the fibrinolytic enzyme system have been identified between 1930 and 1950. The highlights of this evolution have been reviewed by Astrup [1], Fearnley [2] and Collen [3].

The fibrinolytic system which is schematically represented below comprises a proenzyme, plasminogen, which can be activated to the active enzyme plasmin, that will degrade fibrin, by several different types of plasminogen activators. Inhibition of the fibrinolytic system may occur at the level of the activators or at the level of plasmin.

$$\text{Activator(s)} \leftarrow \text{Antiactivator(s)}$$
$$\downarrow$$
$$\text{Plasminogen} \rightarrow \text{Plasmin} \leftarrow \text{Antiplasmin(s)}$$
$$\downarrow$$
$$\text{Fibrin} \rightarrow \text{Fibrin degradation products}$$

2. Main components of the fibrinolytic system

(a) Plasminogen

(i) Physicochemical properties

Human plasminogen is a single-chain glycoprotein with a molecular weight of about 92 000, containing about 2% carbohydrate. The plasminogen molecule consists of 790 amino acids, it contains 24 disulfide bridges and 5 homologous triple loop structures or 'kringles' [4]. Native plasminogen has NH_2-terminal glutamic acid ('Glu-plasminogen') but is easily converted by limited plasmic digestion to modified forms with NH_2-terminal lysine, valine or methionine [5], commonly designated 'Lys-plasminogen'. This conversion occurs by hydrolysis of the Arg 67-Met 68, Lys 76-Lys 77 or Lys 77-Val 78 peptide bonds.

Affinity chromatography on lysine-Sepharose using gradient elution with 6-aminohexanoic acid separates plasminogen in 2 fractions, called type I and type II in the order of their elution from lysine-Sepharose [6]. Type I plasminogen contains a glucosamine-based carbohydrate chain on Asn 288 and a galactosamine-based carbohydrate chain on Thr 345, while type II plasminogen has only the latter [7]. These differences in carbohydrate composition play a role in their interaction with α_2-antiplasmin and fibrin, type II showing the strongest interaction with both [8]. Each of these two fractions can be separated in about 6 forms with different isoelectric points [5,9] due to differences in sialic acid content.

The concentration of plasminogen in plasma is about 2 μM [10].

(ii) Activation to plasmin

Lys-plasminogen forms are converted to plasmin by cleavage of a single Arg-Val bond [10] corresponding to the Arg 560-Val 561 bond. The two-chain plasmin molecule is composed of a heavy chain or A-chain, originating from the NH_2-terminal part of plasminogen and a light chain or B-chain constituting the COOH-terminal part [9]. The B-chain was found to contain an active site similar to that of trypsin, composed of His 602, Asp 645 and Ser 740 [4].

Rickli and Otavsky [11] demonstrated the release of an amino-terminal peptide from human plasminogen by urokinase. In view of the great sensitivity of the Arg 67-Met 68 bond to plasmin it was suggested that the major pathway for activation of plasminogen is via Lys-plasminogen generated by plasmic cleavage of Glu-plasminogen [12,13]. Activation of Glu-plasminogen in the presence of the physiological plasmin inhibitor α_2-antiplasmin however generates inhibited Glu-plasmin [14]. The exact mechanism of activation of plasminogen in vivo thus remains unsettled.

Several groups have studied the kinetics of the activation of plasminogen by tissue-type plasminogen activator (t-PA) in the presence or the absence of fibrin. The activation obeys Michaelis–Menten kinetics with more favourable kinetic constants in the presence of fibrin than in its absence [15–18]. The plasminogen-activating properties of one- and two-chain forms of t-PA were found to be very similar [19]. Hoylaerts et al. [17] found a marked decrease of K_m (from 65 to 0.16 μM) while the catalytic rate constant did not change significantly (k_{cat} from 0.06 to 0.1/sec) in the presence of fibrin. Except for the study of Nieuwenhuizen et al. [20] all authors report a K_m value in the absence of fibrin which is far above the plasminogen concentration in plasma (1.5–2 μM), which precludes systemic activation of plasminogen by t-PA.

Recently it was shown that the kinetic properties of recombinant t-PA for the activation of plasminogen are very similar to those of the natural t-PA [21].

(iii) Lysine-binding sites

The plasminogen molecule contains structures, called lysine-binding sites which interact specifically with certain amino acids such as lysine, 6-aminohexanoic acid and *trans*-4-aminomethylcyclohexane-1-carboxylic acid (tranexamic acid) [6,22,23]. Plasminogen contains one binding site with high affinity for 6-aminohexanoic acid ($K_d = 9\ \mu M$), and about four with low affinity ($K_d = 5$ mM) [24]. These lysine-binding sites are located in the plasmin A-chain [22]. The high-affinity lysine-binding site has been shown to be comprised within the first kringle structure of plasminogen [25].

Plasminogen can specifically bind to fibrin through its lysine-binding sites. Both in purified systems [26] and in plasma [27] Lys-plasminogen has a higher affinity for fibrin than Glu-plasminogen. The presence of 6-aminohexanoic acid abolishes the adsorption of plasminogen to fibrin. The lysine-binding sites in plasminogen mediate its interaction with fibrin and with α_2-antiplasmin [28] and histidine-rich glycoprotein [29]. On the basis of these interactions it was suggested that the lysine-binding sites play a crucial role in the regulation of fibrinolysis [3,30].

(b) Plasminogen activators and inhibitors of plasminogen activators

Plasminogen activation may occur via different pathways but all mechanisms of plasminogen activation studied so far occur by hydrolysis of the Arg 560-Val 561 peptide bond in plasminogen yielding the two-chain plasmin molecule. Some of these activators are counterbalanced by inhibitors.

(i) 'Intrinsic' activation

In the so-called intrinsic or humoral pathway of plasminogen activation all the components involved (factor XII, prekallikrein, high molecular weight kininogen...) are present in precursor form in the blood (see Ch. 5A). Kluft distinguishes between a factor XII-dependent and a factor XII-independent activator activity [31]. Inhibitors of 'intrinsic' plasminogen activation occur in human plasma: C_1-inactivator [32], and an inhibitor of factor XII_a-induced fibrinolysis [33]. Its biological role, however, is not well established.

(ii) Urokinase and pro-urokinase

Urokinase is a trypsin-like serine protease composed of 2 polypeptide chains (M_r 20000 and 34000) connected by a single disulfide bridge. It is isolated from human urine or cultured human embryonic kidney cells. Urokinase activates plasminogen directly to plasmin. It may occur in 2 molecular forms designated S_1 (M_r 31600, low molecular weight urokinase) and S_2 (M_r 54000, high molecular weight urokinase), the former being a proteolytic degradation product of the latter [34]. The complete primary structure of high molecular weight urokinase has been elucidated [35]; the light chain contains 157 amino acids and the heavy chain 253.

Evidence that urokinase is secreted in an inactive form (pro-urokinase) which can be activated by plasmin, was already provided in 1973 [36], but the mechanism of activation remained unknown. Recently several groups have apparently simultaneously and independently isolated a single-chain form of urokinase [37–40]. Most groups found that single-chain urokinase is a proenzyme which, following limited digestion with plasmin, is converted to fully active two-chain urokinase [37–41].

Urokinase differs from the tissue-type plasminogen activator both in its antigenic characteristics [42] and in its enzyme specificity, particularly with respect to the activation of fibrin-associated plasminogen [15,17]. From turnover studies of urokinase in rabbits [43,44] and in squirrel monkeys [44] it has been concluded that urokinase is rapidly removed from the blood by clearance and degradation in the liver. Recognition by the liver does not require a functional active site and is not mediated via carbohydrate side chains.

Inactivation by plasma protease inhibitors does not seem to play a significant role in the inhibition of urokinase in vivo [44], although recently a new fast-acting inhibitor of urokinase (and of t-PA) has been detected in very low concentrations in the blood [45].

Urokinase has successfully been used for thrombolytic therapy but its exact place in the management of the several clinical forms of thrombosis remains to be further established [46–48].

(iii) Streptokinase

Streptokinase is a non-enzyme protein with M_r 47 000, produced by Lancefield group C strains of β-hemolytic streptococci, which activates the fibrinolytic system indirectly [49]. Streptokinase initially forms a 1:1 stoichiometric complex with plasminogen which then undergoes a transition, allowing formation of a complex, which exposes an active site in the modified plasminogen moiety. This complex then enzymatically converts plasminogen to plasmin [49].

Human plasma contains antibodies directed against streptokinase, which most probably result from previous infections with β-hemolytic streptococci. The amount of streptokinase antibodies varies over a wide range [50]. Because streptokinase reacts with antibodies and is thereby rendered biochemically inert, sufficient amounts of streptokinase must be infused to neutralize the antibodies before fibrinolytic activation is obtained [51].

Streptokinase is at present the most widely used thrombolytic agent but its optimal dose regimen and exact place in the treatment of thromboembolic disease are still debated [48].

(iv) Tissue-type plasminogen activator

The first satisfactory purification of human tissue-type plasminogen activator (t-PA) has been obtained from uterine tissues [42]. t-PA has been purified from the culture fluid of a stable human melanoma cell line [52]. Sufficient amounts were obtained to study its biochemical and biological properties.

Recently, the gene of human t-PA has been cloned and expressed [53]. Human t-PA, obtained by expression of recombinant DNA coding for its entire sequence in eukaryotic cells, was shown to be indistinguishable from the natural activator isolated from human melanoma cell cultures, with respect to biochemical properties, turnover in vivo and specific thrombolytic effect [54].

(a) Physicochemical properties. Native t-PA is a serine protease with a molecular weight of about 70 000, composed of one polypeptide chain containing 527 amino acids, 35 cysteine residues and 4 potential N-glycosylation sites (Asn 118, 186, 218 and 448) [53]. Upon limited plasmic action the molecule is converted to a two-chain activator linked by one disulfide bond [52,55]. This occurs by cleavage of the Arg 275-Ile 276 peptide bond yielding a heavy chain (M_r 31 000) derived from the NH_2-terminal part of the molecule and a light chain (M_r 28 000) comprising the COOH-terminal region. The heavy chain contains 2 regions of 82 amino acids each (residues 92-173 and 180-261) which share a high degree of homology with the 5 kringles of plasminogen and with similar kringles in prothrombin and urokinase.

The catalytic site located in the light chain of t-PA is composed of His 322, Asp 371 and Ser 478. The amino acid sequences surrounding these residues are highly homologous to corresponding parts of other serine proteases [53]. Comparison of the primary structures of high molecular weight urokinase and t-PA has revealed a high degree of homology between the two proteins, except that t-PA contains a 43-residue-long amino-terminal region, which has no counterpart in urokinase; this segment was shown to be homologous with the finger domains responsible for the fibrin affinity of fibronectin. Limited proteolysis of this region leads to a loss of the fibrin affinity of the enzyme [56].

The one-chain and two-chain forms of t-PA have virtually the same fibrinolytic and plasminogen-activating properties [19,55]. The one-chain activator is quickly converted to a two-chain form on the fibrin surface and therefore it was suggested that physiological fibrinolysis induced by native one-chain plasminogen activator nevertheless occurs mainly via a two-chain derivative [19].

(b) Release and inhibition. The mean antigen level of t-PA in human plasma at rest was found to be 6.6 ± 2.9 ng/ml of which one third represents free t-PA [57]. This level increases about 3-fold by exhaustive physical exercise, venous occlusion or infusion of 1-deamino-8-D-arginine vasopressin [57]. t-PA occurs in plasma as a free active form and as complexes with α_2-antiplasmin and α_1-antitrypsin [58]. In another study the baseline activity of t-PA in plasma was determined to be 0.05 ± 0.03 IU/ml or 0.2 ± 0.1 ng/ml [59].

The mechanism of the release of t-PA remains unknown. Cash [60] had speculated that t-PA release may be under neurohumoral control and that a plasminogen activator-releasing hormone (PARH) would constitute the major pathway for its release from the endothelial cells. This hormone could, however, not be identified in bovine pituitary or hypothalamic extracts [61]. From infusion experiments of bovine protein C in dogs, Comp and Esmon have concluded that activated protein C might be involved in the release of t-PA in vivo [62]. This could, however, not be confirmed in squirrel monkeys using human protein C [63].

The mechanisms involved in the removal of t-PA from the blood are multiple and poorly understood. One main mechanism is through clearance by the liver, which results in a $t_{1/2}$ of a few minutes [64]. ^{125}I-Labeled t-PA was found to disappear from the plasma of human volunteers with a half-life of 3–4 min [65].

In several pathological conditions (liver disease, pancreatitis, ... but not in myocardial infarction or venous thrombosis) up to 50% of the patients develop a (transient) fast inhibitory activity for t-PA [43]. Inhibition of t-PA is associated with the formation of a complex with M_r 110000–130000, which could not be identified as a complex of t-PA with any of the known plasma protease inhibitors. From the molecular weight of t-PA (70000) and of this complex (120000) a molecular weight estimate of about 50000 for the inhibitor may be assumed. Assuming formation of a 1:1 stoichiometric complex of t-PA with this inhibitor, the second-order rate constant has been estimated at 10^7/M/sec [66]. A positive correlation was found between inhibition of t-PA and of urokinase [43]. Several other laboratories have recently obtained evidence for the existence of a rapidly acting inhibitor of t-PA at low concentrations in plasma of healthy individuals [67–69], or at higher levels in pathological plasma samples [45,70]. Its exact pathophysiological role is not known.

(c) Mechanism of action. t-PA is a poor enzyme in the absence of fibrin, but fibrin strikingly enhances the activation rate of plasminogen [15]. This has been explained by an increased affinity of fibrin-bound t-PA for plasminogen without significantly influencing the catalytic efficiency of the enzyme [17]. The kinetic data of Hoylaerts et al. [17] support a mechanism in which t-PA and plasminogen adsorb to a fibrin clot in a sequential and ordered way yielding a ternary complex. Fibrin essentially increases the local plasminogen concentration by creating an additional interaction between t-PA and its substrate. The high affinity of t-PA for plasminogen in the presence of fibrin thus allows efficient activation on the fibrin clot, while no efficient plasminogen activation by t-PA occurs in plasma.

(c) α_2-Antiplasmin

For a long time it was accepted that there were essentially two functionally important plasmin inhibitors in plasma: an immediately reacting one and a slowly reacting one identical with α_2-macroglobulin and α_1-antitrypsin respectively [71]. Later, however, a new plasmin inhibitor occurring in human plasma has been described and called α_2-antiplasmin [72–75]. Upon activation of plasminogen in plasma, the formed plasmin is first preferentially bound to this inhibitor; only upon complete activation of plasminogen (concentration about 1.5 μM), resulting in saturation of this plasmin inhibitor (concentration about 1 μM), is the excess plasmin neutralized by α_2-macroglobulin.

(i) Physicochemical properties

α_2-Antiplasmin is a single-chain glycoprotein with an M_r of 70000 containing about 14% carbohydrate. The molecule consists of about 500 amino acids and contains 3 disulfide bridges. The NH$_2$-terminal amino acid sequence is Asn-Gln-Glu-Gln-Val- and the COOH-terminal sequence -Pro-Lys [76,77]. α_2-Antiplasmin belongs to the same protein family as anti-thrombin III, α_1-antitrypsin and ovalbumin [77].

The concentration of the inhibitor in normal plasma determined by electroimmunoassay is about 7 mg/100 ml (about 1μM) [73,76]. The half-life of purified biologically intact iodine-labeled α_2-antiplasmin was found to be about 2.6 days, while the plasmin–α_2-antiplasmin complex disappeared from plasma with a half-life of approximately 0.5 days [78].

The inhibitor in normal plasma is heterogeneous, consisting of functionally active and inactive material. Complete activation of the plasminogen present in normal plasma converted only about 0.7 of the antigen material into a complex with plasmin, while 0.3 of the inhibitor-related antigen appeared to be functionally inactive [74]. Human plasma contains a form of the inhibitor which binds to plasminogen and one which does not bind (about 0.4 of the total) but still remains an active plasmin inhibitor [79–81]. Both forms are immunochemically indistinguishable. It has been shown that the non-plasminogen-binding form lacks a 26-residue peptide from the COOH-terminal end of α_2-antiplasmin [82]. This peptide was found to inhibit the interaction of α_2-antiplasmin with plasmin suggesting that it contains the plasminogen-binding site(s) [82].

From studies of the ratio of both forms in the plasma of pregnant women subjected to extensive plasmapheresis, Wiman et al. [83] concluded that the plasminogen-binding form of α_2-antiplasmin is primarily synthesized, and that it becomes partly converted to the non-plasminogen-binding form in the circulating blood.

(ii) Mechanism of the interaction with plasmin

In purified systems [73,76] and in plasma [72,74] α_2-antiplasmin forms a 1:1 stoichiometric complex with plasmin which is devoid of protease or esterase activity. α_2-Antiplasmin, like many other plasma proteinase inhibitors, has a broad in vitro inhibitory spectrum, but its physiological role as an inhibitor of proteinases other than plasmin seems negligible.

(a) Kinetics of the reaction. The kinetics of the inhibition of human plasmin by α_2-antiplasmin have been extensively studied [84,85]. The disappearance of plasmin activity after addition of excess α_2-antiplasmin does not follow first-order kinetics. Most of the plasmin is very rapidly inactivated, but the process only slowly proceeds towards completion. This time course of the reaction is compatible with a kinetic model composed of two successive reactions: a very fast reversible second-order reaction, followed by a slower irreversible first-order reaction:

$$P + A \underset{k_{-1}}{\overset{k_1}{\rightleftharpoons}} PA \xrightarrow{k_2} PA'$$

in which P represents plasmin, A α_2-antiplasmin, PA the reversible but inactive complex formed in the first step, PA' the irreversible inactive complex formed by an intramolecular transition in the second step and k_1, k_{-1} and k_2 the rate constants.

The second-order rate constant k_1 is 2–4 × 10^7/M/sec [83]. This is among the fastest protein–protein reactions so far described. Such rate constants approach the theoretical values for a diffusion-controlled process. The dissociation constant of the reversible complex is 2 × 10^{-10} M. The half-time of the first-order transition PA → PA' was determined to be 166 sec corresponding to a k_2 value of 4.2 × 10^{-3}/sec [83].

Plasmin molecules which have a synthetic substrate bound to their active site or 6-aminohexanoic acid bound to their lysine-binding site(s) [79,83] do not react or react only very slowly with α_2-antiplasmin. The first step of the process is thus clearly dependent on the presence of a free lysine-binding site and active site in the plasmin molecule. Later work [84] in which plasminogen fragments containing lysine-binding site(s) were allowed to compete with plasmin for the binding of α_2-antiplasmin indicated that mainly the high-affinity lysine-binding site(s) situated in triple loops 1–3 of the plasmin A-chain is responsible for the interaction with α_2-antiplasmin [28].

(b) Mechanism of complex formation. Plasmin and α_2-antiplasmin form a stoichiometric 1:1 complex with a molecular weight of about 140 000 by strong interaction between the light (B) chain of plasmin and the inhibitor. Upon reduction this complex is dissociated in two parts: an intact plasmin A-chain (M_r 60 000) and a very stable complex between the plasmin B-chain and α_2-antiplasmin (M_r 80 000), provided that the complex formation is performed in excess α_2-antiplasmin [76,85]. Wiman and Collen [85] demonstrated the release of a non-disulfide-bonded peptide (M_r 8000) concomitantly with complex formation. In this study the peptide moieties of the plasmin–α_2-antiplasmin complex were separated and characterized. NH_2- and COOH-terminal amino acid sequence analysis suggested that complex formation occurs by plasmic attack at a specific leucyl-methionyl peptide bond in the COOH-terminal portion of the inhibitor. Recent evidence (unpublished) suggests however that the reactive site peptide bond might consist of Arg-Met. A strong bond is formed between the active site seryl residue in plasmin and the specific arginyl residue in the inhibitor. Indirect evidence that an ester bond may play a role in stabilizing the plasmin–α_2-antiplasmin complex has been reported [87].

3. Mechanism of physiological fibrinolysis

The specific molecular interactions between the components of the fibrinolytic system described above enabled us to formulate a molecular model for the regulation of fibrinolysis [3,30]. When fibrin is formed, plasminogen activator and plasminogen adsorb to the clot in a sequential and ordered way. Fibrin essentially increases the local plasminogen concentration by creating an additional interaction between t-PA and its substrate. In the presence of fibrin the affinity of t-PA for plasminogen is high, indicating that efficient activation can occur. Plasmin formed on the fibrin surface has both its lysine-binding sites and active site occupied and is thus only slowly inactivated by α_2-antiplasmin. Efficient fibrinolysis in vivo however seems to require a continuous replacement at the fibrin surface of inactivated plasmin molecules by plasminogen molecules. In this respect, the finding that binding of plasminogen to fibrin is enhanced by the presence of t-PA [88] might be relevant. In plasma no efficient plasminogen activation by t-PA occurs and α_2-antiplasmin rapidly binds free plasmin thereby protecting fibrinogen. These interactions thus indicate that the fibrinolytic process is triggered by and confined to fibrin.

Although these molecular interactions between the components of the fibrinolytic system are rather well established, less is known about the dynamics of clot dissolution in vivo. It has been shown that the rate of fibrinolysis depends on the amount of t-PA incorporated in a clot [89,90]. Not only the concentration of t-PA and of the fast reacting t-PA inhibitor but also their distribution between the clot and the surrounding plasma are important determinants for fibrinolysis [90].

As a consequence of this molecular model for fibrinolysis, thrombolysis is expected to be more fibrin-specific with the use of plasminogen activators with an affinity for fibrin (t-PA and possibly pro-urokinase) as compared to the presently used streptokinase or urokinase (without specific affinity for fibrin).

4. Thrombolytic properties of tissue-type plasminogen activator

(a) In vivo animal studies

The thrombolytic effect of t-PA and urokinase was compared in rabbits with an experimental pulmonary embolus [91]. t-PA caused thrombolysis at lower doses than urokinase (on a molar basis); thrombolysis with t-PA was achieved without extensive plasminogen activation in the circulating blood and without hemostatic breakdown.

In dogs with an experimental thrombosis of the femoral vein, urokinase infusion at a rate of 2500 IU/kg/h for 4 h did not induce significant lysis [92]. With 25 000 IU of urokinase/kg/h for 4 h about 30% lysis was obtained but this was associated with defibrinogenation. Infusion of 2500 urokinase equivalent units of t-PA/kg/h for 4 h caused 20–45% lysis without causing any fibrinogen breakdown.

In a preliminary report, Sampol et al. [93] reported successful recanalization with porcine t-PA in dogs with femoral vein thrombosis. Carlin et al. [94] induced lysis of intravascular fibrin deposits in the lungs of rats following infusion of human t-PA.

In rabbits with experimental jugular vein thrombosis the extent of thrombolysis by t-PA is mainly determined by the dose of t-PA and its delivery in the vicinity of the thrombus and much less by the age of the thrombus or the molecular form of the activator [95].

Agnelli et al. [96] used a quantitative bleeding model in rabbits to demonstrate that t-PA, in contrast to streptokinase, did not provoke hemorrhage at thrombolytic doses.

At present, 4 studies with t-PA in animal models for myocardial infarction have been completed [97–100]. Bergmann et al. [97] produced a thrombus in the left anterior descending (LAD) coronary artery with a copper coil. Intravenous or intracoronary infusion of t-PA, obtained from cell culture fluid, at a rate of 10 000 IU/min produced coronary reperfusion of 1–2-h-old occlusions within 10 min. In addition intermediary metabolism and nutritional myocardial blood flow were restored and thrombolysis was obtained without inducing a systemic fibrinolytic state.

Van de Werf et al. [98] compared the thrombolytic effect of recombinant t-PA with that of urokinase in dogs with a 1-h-old LAD occlusion introduced with a copper coil. Intravenous infusion in 9 dogs of 1000 IU (10 μg)/kg/min of t-PA obtained by recombinant DNA technology (rt-PA) elicited reperfusion within 14 min without producing systemic fibrinolysis or distal coronary embolization. Infusion of urokinase at the same rate elicited thrombolysis in 7 of 10 dogs within an average of 19 min. However, distal coronary embolization occurred in 2 dogs and systemic fibrinolysis was observed in all. In 3 dogs treated with urokinase thrombolysis was obtained only with subsequent intracoronary infusion. Restoration of myocardial perfusion and metabolism assessed with positron-emission tomography was consistently noted in dogs treated with rt-PA.

Gold et al. [99] studied the thrombolytic potency and infarct-sparing potential of rt-PA in open chested, anesthetized dogs. Localized coronary thrombosis was produced in the LAD by endothelial injury and instillation of thrombin and fresh blood. After 2 h of stable thrombotic occlusion, rt-PA was infused intravenously. At 5 μg/kg/min, time to reperfusion was greater than 40 min. However, at higher infusion rates a linear, dose-dependent time to coronary reperfusion was obtained ($r=0.88$): at 10 μg/kg/min reperfusion occurred after 31 min; at 15 μg/kg/min it was 26 min; and at 25 μg/kg/min, lysis was obtained within 13 min. Thrombolysis was not associated with alterations either in plasma hemostatic factors (fibrinogen, plasminogen and α_2-antiplasmin) or in systemic blood pressures. Epicardial electrographic measurements revealed a significant reduction in ST elevation in all reperfused hearts.

Gold et al. [99] also performed a randomized-blinded study using 15 μg/kg/min of rt-PA versus saline in 18 dogs with 30 min of coronary thrombosis. Reperfusion in the treated group occurred after 28 min. No evidence of thrombolysis occurred in the saline-treated group within 240 min. Myocardial infarct size was determined by triphenyl tetrazolium chloride staining and planimetry. Infarction involved 2.5% of the left ventricular wall in the rt-PA group, but 16% of the left ventricle in the saline group.

Flameng et al. [100] produced occlusive thrombi in the LAD of 16 open chest baboons. In 6 control animals, occlusive thrombosis persisting over a period of 4 h as evidenced by coronary arteriography, resulted in large transmural infarction (63% of the perfusion area). In 10 animals rt-PA was infused systemically at a rate of 1000 IU (10 μg)/kg/min for 30 min after 30–80 min of coronary thrombosis. Reperfusion occurred within 30 min in 9 animals. In the rt-PA group mean duration of occlusion before reperfusion was 77 min. Recanalization resulted in an overall reduction of infarct size to 38%. Residual infarction was related to the duration of occlusion ($r=0.80$). Reperfusion was associated with reduced reflow: myocardial blood flow in the reperfusion area of the LAD was only 70% of normal after 4 h in spite of perfect angiographic refilling. The infusion of rt-PA was not associated with systemic activation of the fibrinolytic system, fibrinogen breakdown or clinically evident bleeding.

From all these studies it is concluded that intravenous injection of t-PA may recanalize thrombosed coronary vessels without inducing a systemic fibrinolytic state. Timely reperfusion results in infarct sparing and restoration of nutritional blood flow.

(b) In vivo human studies

The first patients were treated with t-PA in 1981. Intravenous administration of human t-PA (7.5 mg over 24 h) induced complete lysis of a 6-week-old renal and iliofemoral thrombosis in a renal allograft recipient [101]. Thrombolysis was achieved without systemic fibrinolytic activation or hemostatic breakdown, and was not associated with bleeding. The second case was a 73-year-old man with the nephrotic syndrome, who developed an ascending thrombosis of the iliofemoral vein after removal of an infarcted femoral-popliteal graft and mid-thigh amputation of the right leg. Venography showed thrombotic masses in the vena cava, and selective venography revealed a thrombus of the right renal vein. t-PA, 5 mg, given intravenously over 24 h, resulted in resolution of the thrombosis in the iliac vein, vena cava, and renal vein. No side effects were noted, and again this thrombolytic therapy was not associated with consumption of fibrinogen, plasminogen, α_2-antiplasmin or factor V [101].

In 4 patients with deep vein thrombosis over extended segments of the iliac and femoral veins, intravenous infusion of 5–15 mg of t-PA over 24–36 h did however not result in thrombolysis (unpublished).

Van de Werf et al. [102] performed a pilot study with t-PA obtained from cell culture fluid in 7 patients with acute myocardial infarction. Coronary thrombolysis, confirmed angiographically, was induced within 19–50 min with intravenous or intracoronary t-PA in 6 of the 7 patients. Circulating fibrinogen, plasminogen and α_2-antiplasmin were not depleted by t-PA, in contrast to the case in the 2 patients subsequently given streptokinase. In the one patient in whom lysis was not inducible with t-PA, it was also not inducible with streptokinase. These observations indicate that clot-selective coronary thrombolysis can be induced in patients with evolving myocardial infarction by means of t-PA, without concomitant induction of a systemic lytic state. In two of these patients positron-emission tomography revealed an improved regional palmitate accumulation following coronary reperfusion with t-PA [103].

From all these studies it thus appears that specific thrombolysis without systemic activation of the fibrinolytic system can be achieved with t-PA. Limited experience in treatment of patients with myocardial infarction suggests that the potentially widely available recombinant t-PA offers a promising practical approach for coronary thrombolysis. Coronary thrombolysis is however not a goal in itself but is employed to prevent necrosis and dysfunction of jeopardized myocardial cells. There is ample evidence in animals that the infarct size is smaller and the myocardial function better when an occluded coronary artery is reopened within at most a couple of hours [104]. The proof that coronary reperfusion is of real benefit to patients with acute myocardial infarction in terms of morbidity or mortality is however still lacking [105–107]. To this end several large-scale trials are required.

5. *Thrombolytic effect of pro-urokinase*

In vitro, pro-urokinase (pro-UK) is a true proenzyme, inactive in plasma but slowly activated in the presence of a fibrin clot. The single-chain proenzyme has a higher specific thrombolytic activity and/or a better fibrin selectivity than two-chain urokinase [40,41,108].

In a standardized radiolabeled clot lysis assay, pro-UK purified from a transformed human kidney cell line, was found to lyse clots in a similar way as t-PA, with equivalent efficacy and fibrin specificity [108]. Using pro-UK obtained by recombinant DNA technology in a system composed of a radioactive human plasma clot immersed in human plasma, Zamarron et al. [41] observed a similar fibrinolytic effect of pro-UK and two-chain urokinase, while t-PA caused equivalent degrees of clot lysis at 10-fold lower concentrations. With pro-UK significant clot lysis could be obtained without systemic activation of the fibrinolytic system. With two-chain urokinase, all concentrations which caused significant clot lysis also caused extensive fibrinolytic activation in the plasma. Whereas t-PA is progressively inactivated upon prolonged incubation in plasma, pro-UK retains its potential fibrinolytic activity for at least 24 h [41,108]. Two-chain urokinase is inactivated in plasma within a few hours.

In rabbits and squirrel monkeys, pro-UK was found to have an equally short half-life as active urokinase (3–6 min), due to clearance and degradation by the liver [43,44]. Its proenzyme nature as such does therefore not result in a prolonged thrombolytic effect in vivo.

Clot lysis induced by pro-UK, as well as by two-chain urokinase and t-PA, is very variable from one species to another when assayed in an in vitro system consisting of ^{125}I-labeled autologous plasma clots immersed in plasma [109]. In general good reactivity towards t-PA is paralleled by good reactivity towards pro-UK and active urokinase.

Several groups have compared the thrombolytic effect of single-chain pro-UK and two-chain active urokinase in animal models [108,110,111]. By intravenous administration of 3000 IU of urokinase/kg body weight in dogs with an experimental thrombosis, Sumi et al. [110] obtained complete thrombolysis within 1.5 h with pro-UK, whereas the lysis time was more than 3 h in the group treated with two-chain urokinase. Gurewich et al. [108] studied the thrombolytic effect of pro-

UK of human kidney cell origin in rabbits and dogs with pulmonary embolus. In rabbits the mean extent of thrombolysis after 5 h was 6%, 17% and 53% following infusion of saline, two-chain urokinase and pro-UK respectively. Infusion of two-chain urokinase was accompanied by systemic fibrinogenolysis whereas pro-UK did not cause significant fibrinogen degradation. Dogs were found to be about 10 times more sensitive to human urokinase than rabbits, but otherwise similar results were obtained as in rabbits.

The thrombolytic properties of recombinant pro-UK (rec-pro-UK), recombinant active urokinase (rec-UK) and natural urinary urokinase (nat-UK) were compared in rabbits with a radiolabeled thrombus in the jugular vein [111]. The thrombolytic agents were infused intravenously over a period of 4 h and the extent of thrombolysis was measured 2 h later as the difference between the radioactivity introduced in the clot and that recovered in the vein segment at the end of the experiment. Significant thrombolysis with nat-UK and rec-UK was only obtained with 240 000 IU/kg or more, and this was associated with a marked systemic activation of the fibrinolytic system, as evidenced by consumption of plasminogen and α_2-antiplasmin and fibrinogen breakdown. Infusion of rec-pro-UK induced thrombolysis at a dose of 60 000 IU/kg or more and without associated activation of the fibrinolytic system. The specific thrombolytic activity of t-PA was however 2–4-fold higher than that of rec-pro-UK.

From these studies it is concluded that pro-UK has a better fibrin selectivity than active urokinase. However, in order to establish its potential value as a thrombolytic agent, more studies are required.

References

1 Astrup, T. (1956) Blood 11, 781–806.
2 Fearnley, G.R. (1973) Adv. Drug. Res. 7, 107–163.
3 Collen, D. (1980) Thromb. Haemostas. 43, 77–89.
4 Sottrup-Jensen, L., Petersen, T.E. and Magnusson, S. (1978) in: Atlas of Protein Sequence and Structure, Vol. 5, Suppl. 3, p. 91.
5 Wallén, P. and Wiman, B. (1970) Biochim. Biophys. Acta 221, 20–30.
6 Brockway, W.J. and Castellino, F.J. (1972) Arch. Biochem. Biophys. 151, 194–199.
7 Hayes, M.L. and Castellino, F.J. (1979) J. Biol. Chem. 254, 8768–8771.
8 Lijnen, H.R., Van Hoef, B. and Collen, D. (1981) Eur. J. Biochem. 120, 149–154.
9 Summaria, L., Arzadon, L., Bernabe, P. and Robbins, K.C. (1972) J. Biol. Chem. 247, 4691–4702.
10 Robbins, K.C., Summaria, L., Hsieh, B. and Shah, R.J. (1967) J. Biol. Chem. 242, 2333–2342.
11 Rickli, E.E. and Otavsky, W.I. (1973) Biochim. Biophys. Acta 295, 381–384.
12 Wallén, P. and Wiman, B. (1975) in: Proteases and Biological Control (Reich, E., Rifkin, D.B. and Shaw, E., Eds.) pp. 291–303, Cold Spring Harbor Laboratory, Cold Spring Harbor, NY.
13 Violand, B.N. and Castellino, F.J. (1976) J. Biol. Chem. 251, 3906–3912.
14 Wiman, B. and Collen, D. (1979) J. Biol. Chem. 254, 9291–9297.
15 Camiolo, S.M., Thorsen, S. and Astrup, T. (1971) Proc. Soc. Exp. Biol. Med. 138, 277–280.
16 Lucas, M.A., Straight, D.L., Fretto, L.J. and McKee, P.A. (1983) J. Biol. Chem. 258, 12171–12177.
17 Hoylaerts, M., Rijken, D.C., Lijnen, H.R. and Collen, D. (1982) J. Biol. Chem. 257, 2912–2919.
18 Rånby, M. (1982) Biochim. Biophys. Acta 704, 461–469.

19 Rijken, D.C., Hoylaerts, M. and Collen, D. (1982) J. Biol. Chem. 257, 2920–2925.
20 Nieuwenhuizen, W., Voskuylen, M., Traas, D.W., Hoegee-de Nobel, B. and Verheijen, J.H. (1985) in: Fibrinogen, Structure and Function (Henschen, A., Hessel, B., McDonagh, J. and Saldeen, T., Eds.), Vol. 3, de Gruyter, Berlin, pp. 331–342.
21 Zamarron, C., Lijnen, H.R. and Collen, D. (1984) J. Biol. Chem. 259, 2080–2083.
22 Rickli, E.E. and Otavsky, W.I. (1975) Eur. J. Biochem. 9, 441–447.
23 Hoylaerts, M., Lijnen, H.R. and Collen, D. (1981) Biochim. Biophys. Acta 673, 75–85.
24 Markus, G., De Pasquale, J.L. and Wissler, F.C. (1978) J. Biol. Chem. 253, 727–732.
25 Vali, Z. and Patthy, L. (1982) J. Biol. Chem. 257, 2104–2110.
26 Thorsen, S. (1975) Biochim. Biophys. Acta 393, 55–65.
27 Rákóczi, I., Wiman, B. and Collen, D. (1978) Biochim. Biophys. Acta 540, 295–300.
28 Wiman, B., Lijnen, H.R. and Collen, D. (1979) Biochim. Biophys. Acta 579, 142–154.
29 Lijnen, H.R., Hoylaerts, M. and Collen, D. (1980) J. Biol. Chem. 255, 10214–10222.
30 Wiman, B. and Collen, D. (1978) Nature (London) 272, 549–550.
31 Kluft, C. (1980) in: Synthetic Substrates in Clinical Blood Coagulation Assays (Lijnen, H.R., Collen, D. and Verstraete, M., Eds.) pp. 113–122, Nijhoff, The Hague.
32 Kluft, C. (1977) Haemostasis 6, 351–369.
33 Hedner, U. and Martinsson, G. (1978) Thromb. Res. 12, 1015–1023.
34 White, W.F., Barlow, G.H. and Mozen, M.N. (1966) Biochemistry 5, 2160–2169.
35 Gunzler, W.A., Steffens, G.J., Otting, F., Kim, S.M.A., Frankus, E. and Flohé, L. (1982) Hoppe-Seyler's Z. Physiol. Chem. 363, 1155–1165.
36 Bernik, M.B. (1973) J. Clin. Invest. 52, 823–834.
37 Wun, T.C., Ossowski, L. and Reich, E. (1982) J. Biol. Chem. 257, 7262–7268.
38 Nielsen, L.S., Hansen, J.G., Skriver, L., Wilson, E.L., Kaltoft, K., Zeuthen, J. and Danø, K. (1982) Biochemistry 21, 6410–6415.
39 Sumi, H., Kosugi, T., Matsuo, O. and Mihara, H. (1982) Acta Haematol. Jpn. 45, 119–128.
40 Husain, S., Gurewich, V. and Lipinski, B. (1983) Arch. Biochem. Biophys. 220, 31–38.
41 Zamarron, C., Lijnen, H.R., Van Hoef, B. and Collen, D. (1984) Thromb. Haemostas. 52, 19–23.
42 Rijken, D.C., Wijngaards, G., Zaal-De Jong, M. and Welbergen, J. (1979) Biochim. Biophys. Acta 580, 140–153.
43 Matsuo, O., Kosugi, T. and Mihara, H. (1978) Haemostasis 7, 367–372.
44 Collen, D., De Cock, F. and Lijnen, H.R. (1984) Thromb. Haemostas. 52, 24–26.
45 Juhan-Vague, I., Moerman, B., De Cock, F., Aillaud, M.F. and Collen, D. (1984) Thromb. Res. 33, 523–530.
46 Kakkar, V.V. and Scully, M.F. (1978) Br. Med. Bull. 34, 191–199.
47 Paoletti, R. and Sherry, S. (1977) Thrombosis and Urokinase, Academic Press, London.
48 Verstraete, M. (1980) in: Fibrinolysis (Kline, D.L. and Reddy, N.N., Eds.) pp. 129–149, CRC Press, Cleveland, OH.
49 Kosow, D.P. (1975) Biochemistry, 14, 4459–4465.
50 Verstraete, M., Vermylen, J., Amery, A. and Vermylen, C. (1966) Br. Med. J. 5485, 454–456.
51 Johnson, A.J. and McCarty, W.R. (1959) J. Clin. Invest. 38, 1627–1643.
52 Rijken, D.C. and Collen, D. (1981) J. Biol. Chem. 256, 7035–7041.
53 Pennica, D., Holmes, W.E., Kohr, W.J., Harkins, R.N., Vehar, G.A., Ward, C.A., Bennett, W.F., Yelverton, E., Seeburg, P.H., Heyneker, H.L., Goeddel, D.V. and Collen, D. (1983) Nature (London) 301, 214–221.
54 Collen, D., Stassen, J.M., Marafino, B.J., Builder, S., De Cock, F., Ogez, J., Tajiri, D., Pennica, D., Bennett, W.F., Salwa, J. and Hoyng, C.F. (1984) J. Pharmacol. Exp. Ther., 231, 146–152.
55 Wallén, P., Bergsdorf, N. and Rånby, M. (1982) Biochim. Biophys. Acta 719, 318–328.
56 Banyai, L., Varadi, A. and Patthy, L. (1983) FEBS Lett. 163, 37–41.
57 Rijken, D.C., Juhan-Vague, I., De Cock, F. and Collen, D. (1983) J. Lab. Clin. Med. 101, 274–284.
58 Rijken, D.C., Juhan-Vague, I. and Collen, D. (1983) J. Lab. Clin. Med. 101, 285–294.
59 Wiman, B., Mellbring, G. and Rånby, M. (1983) Clin. Chim. Acta 127, 279–288.
60 Cash, J.D. (1978) in: Progress in Chemical Fibrinolysis and Thrombolysis (Davidson, J.F., Rowan, R.M., Samama, M.M. and Desnoyers, P.C., Eds.) Vol. 3, pp. 65–75, Raven, New York.

61 Colucci, M., Stassen, J.M., Salwa, J. and Collen, D. (1984) Br. J. Haematol., 58, 337–346.
62 Comp, P.C. and Esmon, C.T. (1981) J. Clin. Invest. 68, 1221–1228.
63 Colucci, M., Stassen, J.M. and Collen, D. (1984) J. Clin. Invest. 74, 200–204.
64 Korninger, C., Stassen, J.M. and Collen, D. (1981) Thromb. Haemostas. 46, 658–661.
65 Nilsson, T., Wallén, P. and Mellbring, G. (1984) Haemostasis 14, 90 (abstr.).
66 Wiman, B., Chmielewska, J. and Rånby, M. (1984) J. Biol. Chem. 259, 3644–3647.
67 Chmielewska, J., Rånby, M. and Wiman, B. (1983) Thromb. Res. 31, 427–436.
68 Kruithof, E.K.O., Ransijn, A. and Bachmann, F. (1983) in: Progress in Fibrinolysis (Davidson, J.F., Bachmann, F., Bouvier, C.A. and Kruithof, E.K.O., Eds.) Vol. VI, pp. 365–369, Churchill Livingstone, Edinburgh.
69 Verheijen, J.H., Chang, G.T.G. and Kluft, C. (1984) Thromb. Haemostas. 51, 392–395.
70 Wijngaards, G. and Groeneveld, E. (1982) Haemostasis 12, 571.
71 Schwick, H.G., Heimburger, N. and Haupt, H. (1966) Z. Inn. Med. 21, 1–6.
72 Collen, D. (1976) Eur. J. Biochem. 69, 209–216.
73 Moroi, M. and Aoki, N. (1976) J. Biol. Chem. 251, 5956–5965.
74 Müllertz, S. and Clemmensen, I. (1976) Biochem. J. 159, 545–553.
75 Bagge, L., Bjork, I., Saldeen, T. and Wallin, R. (1976) Forens. Sci. 7, 83–86.
76 Wiman, B. and Collen, D. (1977) Eur. J. Biochem. 78, 19–26.
77 Lijnen, H.R., Wiman, B. and Collen, D. (1982) Thromb. Haemostas. 48, 311–314.
78 Collen, D. and Wiman, B. (1979) Blood 53, 313–324.
79 Christensen, U. and Clemmensen, I. (1978) Biochem. J. 175, 635–641.
80 Wiman, B. (1980) Biochem. J. 191, 229–232.
81 Kluft, C. and Los, N. (1981) Thromb. Res. 21, 65–71.
82 Sasaki, T., Morita, T. and Iwanaga, S. (1983) Thromb. Haemostas. 50, 170 (abstr.).
83 Wiman, B., Nilsson, T. and Cedergren, B. (1982) Thromb. Res. 28, 193–200.
84 Christensen, U. and Clemmensen, I. (1977) Biochem. J. 163, 389–391.
85 Wiman, B. and Collen, D. (1978) Eur. J. Biochem. 84, 573–578.
86 Wiman, B. and Collen, D. (1979) J. Biol. Chem. 254, 9291–9297.
87 Nilsson, T. and Wiman, B. (1982) FEBS Lett. 142, 111–114.
88 Tran-Chang, C., Wyss, P., Kruithof, E.K.O., Hauert, J. and Bachmann, F. (1984) Haemostasis 14, 17 (abstr.).
89 Brommer, E.J.P. (1984) Thromb. Res. 34, 109–115.
90 Zamarron, C., Lijnen, H.R. and Collen, D. (1984) Thromb. Res. 35, 335–345.
91 Matsuo, O., Rijken, D.C. and Collen, D. (1981) Nature (London) 291, 590–591.
92 Korninger, C., Matsuo, O., Suy, R., Stassen, J.M. and Collen, D. (1982) J. Clin. Invest. 69, 573–580.
93 Sampol, J., Mercier, C., Houel, F., David, G. and Daver, J. (1983) in: Progress in Fibrinolysis (Davidson, J.F., Bachmann, F., Bouvier, C.A. and Kruithof, E.K.O., Eds.) Vol. VI, pp. 463–466, Churchill Livingstone, Edinburgh.
94 Carlin, G., Einarsson, M. and Saldeen, T. (1983) in: Progress in Fibrinolysis (Davidson, J.F., Bachmann, F., Bouvier, C.A. and Kruithof, E.K.O., Eds.) Vol. VI, pp. 471–474, Churchill Livingstone, Edinburgh.
95 Collen, D., Stassen, J.M. and Verstraete, M. (1983) J. Clin. Invest. 71, 368–376.
96 Agnelli, G., Buchanan, M.R., Fernandez, F., Bonen, B., Van Rijn, J., Hirsch, J. and Collen, D. (1985) Circulation 72, 178–182.
97 Bergmann, S.R., Fox, K.A.A., Ter-Pogossian, M.M., Sobel, B.E. and Collen, D. (1983) Science 220, 1181–1183.
98 Van de Werf, F., Bergmann, S.R., Fox, K.A.A., De Geest, H., Hoyng, C.F., Sobel, B.E. and Collen, D. (1984) Circulation 69, 605–610.
99 Gold, H.K., Fallon, J.T., Yasuda, T., Khaw, B.A., Guerrero, J.L., Vislosky, J.M., Leinbach, R.C., Harper, C., Hoyng, C., Grossbard, E. and Collen, D. (1983) Circulation 68, Suppl. III, 150 (abstr.).
100 Flameng, W., Van de Werf, F., Vanhaecke,J., Verstraete, M. and Collen, D. (1985) J. Clin. Invest., 75, 84–90.

101 Weimar, W., Stibbe, J., Van Seyen, A.J., Billiau, A., De Somer, P. and Collen, D. (1981) Lancet 2, 1018–1020.

102 Van de Werf, F., Ludbrook, P.A., Bergmann, S.R., Tiefenbrunn, A.J., Fox, K.A.A., De Geest, H., Verstraete, M., Collen, D. and Sobel, B.E. (1984) New Engl. J. Med. 310, 609–613.

103 Sobel, B.E., Geltman, E.M., Tiefenbrunn, A.J., Jaffe, A.S., Spadaro, J.J., Collen, D. and Ludbrook, P.A. (1984) Circulation 69, 983–990.

104 Bergmann, S.R., Lerch, R.A., Fox, K.A.A. et al. (1982) Am. J. Med. 73, 573–581.

105 Anderson, J.L., Marshall, H.W., Bray, B.E. et al. (1983) New Engl. J. Med. 308, 1312–1318.

106 Khaja, F., Walton, J.A., Brymer, J.F. et al. (1983) New Engl. J. Med. 308, 1305–1311.

107 Kennedy, J.W., Ritchie, J.L., David, K.B. and Fritz, J.K. (1983) New Engl. J. Med. 309, 1477–1482.

108 Gurewich, V., Pannell, R., Louie, S., Kelley, P., Suddith, R.L. and Greenlee, R. (1984) J. Clin. Invest. 73, 1731–1739.

109 Lijnen, H.R., De Wreede, K., Demarsin, E. and Collen, D. (1984) Thromb. Haemostas. 52, 31–33.

110 Sumi, H., Toki, N., Sasaki, K. and Mihara, H. (1983) in: Progress in Fibrinolysis (Davidson, J.F., Bachmann, F., Bouvier, C.A. and Kruithof, E.K.O., Eds.) Vol. VI, pp. 165–167, Churchill Livingstone, Edinburgh.

111 Collen, D., Stassen, J.M., Blaber, M., Winkler, M. and Verstraete M. (1984) Thromb. Haemostas. 52, 27–30.

R.F.A. Zwaal and H.C. Hemker (Eds.), *Blood Coagulation*
© 1986 Elsevier Science Publishers B.V. (Biomedical Division)

Inhibitors: antithrombin III and heparin

MICHAEL J. GRIFFITH

Department of Pathology, University of North Carolina, Chapel Hill, NC (U.S.A.)

1. Introduction

Antithrombin III appears to be the primary plasma inhibitor of thrombin. The correlation between thrombotic disorders and a deficiency in functional plasma antithrombin III levels [1] suggests that antithrombin III is intimately involved in the regulation of hemostasis in vivo. Heparin is an effective plasma anticoagulant; an activity of heparin which can be attributed, at least in part, to a rate-enhancing effect on blood coagulation protease inhibition by antithrombin III [2,3].

In the present chapter, the biochemistry of antithrombin III and heparin is reviewed and discussed. The focus is on the structural and functional properties of both which appear to be important in terms of the rate of protease inhibition in purified component reaction systems. The objective is to define the current base of knowledge regarding the properties of antithrombin III and heparin in vitro which can then be applied to the more complex roles of these molecules in vivo. Antithrombin III is a single-chain α_2-glycoprotein ($M_r = 58\,000$) which has been isolated from mammalian, avian, reptilian and amphibian plasma [3–13]. The primary structure of human antithrombin III has been reported [14]. Three disulfide bonds have been found linking Cys8 to Cys128, Cys21 to Cys95, and Cys239 to Cys422 and 4 glucosamine-based oligosaccharide units are attached to Asn96, Asn135, Asn155 and Asn192 [14]. The carbohydrate content of human antithrombin III is ~9% by weight [9,10] and consists of *N*-acetylglucosamine, mannose, galactose and sialic acid in molar ratios of approximately 1:1:0.6:1 [15]. Microheterogeneity in human antithrombin III has been detected by isoelectric focusing [10,16–18] with p*I* values of 3 major forms of the protein in the range of 4.9–5.3 [10]. Absorbtion ($E_{280}^{1\%}$ coefficient values for human antithrombin III of 5.7–6.5 have been reported [6,9,10] while the value calculated from the amino acid composition [14] is 6.2. The hydrodynamic properties of human antithrombin III, i.e. frictional ratio and intrinsic viscosity, suggest that the protein is asymmetrical [6,10], with an estimated axial ratio of ~4.5 [10]. The secondary structure of human antithrombin III appears to consist of ~10% α-helix, 30–40% β-structure and the remainder random conformation [10,19].

The antithrombin III concentration in pooled normal human plasma has been estimated in several studies [20–28]. Conrad and coworkers [28] have estimated the plasma concentration of antithrombin III to be ~2.5 μM (0.15 mg/ml) while Murano and coworkers [27] have found the level to be somewhat lower, ~2.1 μM (0.125 mg/ml). It is not certain, however, to what extent the presence of heparin cofactor A in human plasma [29] has affected the estimated concentrations of antithrombin III reported to date.

The early procedures described for the isolation of antithrombin III from human plasma were associated with relatively low yields of the purified protein [3–5]. Both the yield of purified protein and the ease with which the purification procedure is performed have been greatly improved by the use of heparin–agarose affinity chromatography [6,8]. Several hereditary abnormal antithrombin III molecules have been identified [30–37], however only in the case of antithrombin III Toyama has the site of structural mutation been characterized [38]. In addition to thrombin [3], purified antithrombin III inhibits factor X_a [39,40], factor IX_a [41,42] factor XI_a [43], factor XII_a [44], kallikrein [45–48], plasmin [49,50], urokinase [51], C1 esterase [52] and trypsin [53,54]. The rates of inhibition of these serine proteases by antithrombin III are increased to varying degrees by heparin. Factor VII_a does not appear to be inhibited at an appreciable rate by antithrombin III in the absence of heparin [40,55,56] while in the presence of heparin a measurable rate of inhibition has been observed [56]. Protease inhibition by antithrombin III involves the formation of a stable 1:1 molar complex between the active site of the protease and a site referred to as the reactive site of antithrombin III [5]. The reactive site (peptide bond) of antithrombin III (Arg385–Ser386) appears to be the same for thrombin [57], factors IX_a and X_a [158] and trypsin [59].

In the following section the mechanism of protease inhibition by antithrombin III is discussed within the context of the standard mechanism of protease inhibition by protein inhibitors. Heparin structure–function relationships are then discussed as they pertain to antithrombin III binding and to the catalysis of antithrombin III–protease reactions. The interaction of heparin with antithrombin III is subsequently discussed in terms of the effects of heparin binding on antithrombin III structure and the structural properties of antithrombin III which appear to be important for heparin binding. A section has been devoted to the description/derivation of possible kinetic mechanisms of action of heparin in catalyzing antithrombin III–protease reactions and to the discussion of the currently available evidence which supports these mechanisms. Finally, the structural and functional properties of heparin cofactor II, which appears to be similar to antithrombin III in both regards, are discussed. It is sincerely hoped that the work cited in this chapter adequately and accurately credits the many contributions which have been made to attain our present level óf understanding of antithrombin III and heparin. The limited scope of the present chapter has, however, excluded many significant contributions which are discussed elsewhere [23,60–68].

2. Antithrombin III–protease interaction

Serine protease inhibition by protein inhibitors has been extensively studied [69,70]. The 'standard mechanism' of protease inhibition is closely related to the catalytic pathway of substrate hydrolysis (proteolysis) described for serine proteases [71]. The underlying interactions between the 'reactive site', i.e. scissile peptide bond, of the inhibitor molecule and the active site of the target protease have been established through in-depth analysis of both structural and functional properties of the reactants and of the stable inhibitor–protease complex. The data obtained from X-ray crystallographic examination of inhibitor–protease complexes have provided a detailed picture of the nature of the bonds formed. For the most part, the nature of the bonds formed in the stable antithrombin III–protease complex is not known, although a number of interesting observations have been reported. The reaction sequence describing substrate hydrolysis by serine proteases and the standard mechanism of protease inhibition by protein inhibitors are briefly discussed below to provide a framework for discussion of protease inhibition by antithrombin III.

The reaction sequence describing substrate hydrolysis by serine proteases of the chymotrypsin family is shown schematically in Fig. 1. The initial interaction between the protease and substrate involves the formation of a dissociable 'Michaelis' complex wherein the susceptible peptide bond of the substrate becomes associated with the active site residues of the protease (see also Ch. 3). A pair of hydrogen bonds formed between the oxyanion hole of the protease and the carbonyl oxygen of the P_1 residue of the substrate distorts the carbonyl carbon for nucleophilic attack by the active site serine O^γ-oxygen and formation of the covalent tetrahedral adduct. Proton transfer from the active site histidine to the amide NH of the substrate results in the breakdown of the tetrahedral intermediate and formation of the acyl–enzyme intermediate and release of the leaving group. Deacylation of the acyl–enzyme intermediate occurs by reversing the order of the steps leading to formation of the acyl–enzyme with the exception that water of another nucleophile replaces the peptide leaving group in the sequence.

Serine protease inhibition by protein inhibitors, as described by the standard mechanism, follows the reaction sequence for substrate hydrolysis shown in Fig. 1, differing only in the relative rates at which the steps take place. While inhibitor hydrolysis can occur, the primary feature of the stable inhibitor–protease complex is the interaction between the carbonyl oxygen of the P_1 residue of the inhibitor with the oxyanion hole of the protease. The reactive site peptide bond of the inhibitor is intact and covalent bonding between the active serine O^γ-oxygen and the carbonyl carbon, i.e. tetrahedral intermediate formation, does not occur. As a consequence, the active site serine of the protease is not required for stable complex formation and the cleaved inhibitor retains inhibitory activity. Conformational changes during the formation of the stable inhibitor–protease complex are minimal indicating that the conformation of the reactive site residue of the inhibitor easily attains the transition-state conformation upon binding to the active site of the protease.

$$E + S \underset{k_{-1}}{\overset{k_1}{\rightleftharpoons}} E{:}S \underset{k_{-2}}{\overset{k_2}{\rightleftharpoons}} E{-}S \underset{k_{-3}}{\overset{k_3}{\rightleftharpoons}} E{-}S' \underset{k_{-4}}{\overset{k_4}{\rightleftharpoons}} E{-}P \underset{k_{-5}}{\overset{k_5}{\rightleftharpoons}} E{:}P \underset{k_{-6}}{\overset{k_6}{\rightleftharpoons}} E + P$$

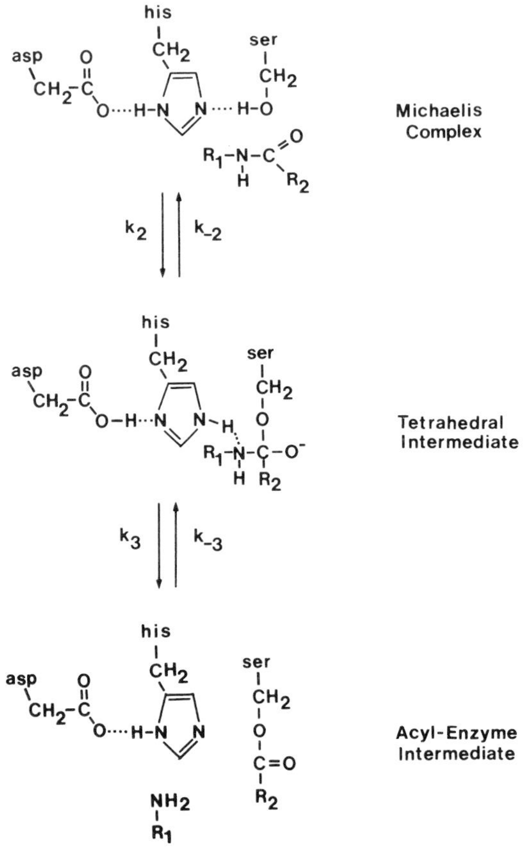

Fig. 1. Reaction sequence for substrate hydrolysis by serine proteases. The reaction sequence for substrate (S) hydrolysis by serine proteases (E) of the chymotrypsin family is shown at the top of the figure. E:S, dissociable Michaelis complex; E–S, covalent tetrahedral intermediate; E–S', covalent acyl–enzyme intermediate; E–P, enzyme–product tetrahedral intermediate; E:P, enzyme:product Michaelis complex; P, product of bond cleavage. The lower portion of the figure attempts to illustrate the bonds formed and broken in the reaction sequence leading to the formation of the acyl–enzyme intermediate. The active site aspartic acid (asp), histidine (his) and serine (ser) residues of the enzyme are shown. Noncovalent bonds are indicated by (···).

The reaction sequence describing protease inhibition by antithrombin III is not known. Several studies have been reported, however, which provide reasonable evidence that the reaction sequence shown in Fig. 1 is followed, but the standard mechanism of protease inhibition described above may not apply to protease inhibition by antithrombin III. The most extensively studied antithrombin III–protease reaction has been the antithrombin III–thrombin reaction. Therefore, the general observations related to thrombin inhibition by antithrombin III are the primary focus of the following discussion.

The antithrombin III–thrombin reaction was shown in early studies to follow apparent second-order kinetics at protein concentrations of ~10 μM [72]. Subsequently, Jesty demonstrated that the antithrombin III–thrombin reaction follows apparent pseudo-first-order kinetics in the presence of excess antithrombin III and that the reaction velocity is proportional to the antithrombin III concentration up to 20 μM [75]. From this it was concluded that the dissociation constant value for the antithrombin III–thrombin (Michaelis) complex, if formed, must exceed 10^{-4} M and that the apparent first-order rate constant value for the step leading to complex stabilization must be greater than 2/sec [73]. Recent work has shown that saturation kinetics for the antithrombin III–thrombin reaction are detectable only when the antithrombin III concentration exceeds 70 μM [74]. By using stopped-flow fluorimetry with thrombin-bound p-aminobenzamidine as a probe, Olson and Shore have demonstrated the formation of a weak antithrombin III–thrombin complex (K_d = 1.4 mM), followed by a first-order complex stabilization step (k = 10.4/sec) in the antithrombin III–thrombin reaction sequence [74]. Thus, it is reasonable to conclude that the mechanism of thrombin inhibition by antithrombin III involves at least two steps, one of which (Michaelis complex formation) is clearly an integral step found in the standard mechanism of protease inhibition.

The chemical nature of the bond(s) formed between antithrombin III and thrombin during the complex stabilization step in the antithrombin III–thrombin reaction sequence was initially addressed by Rosenberg and Damus [5]. The involvement of the active site serine of thrombin in the formation of a stable antithrombin III–thrombin complex was suggested from the observation that diisopropyl fluorophosphate-inactivated thrombin (DIP-thrombin) did not interact measurably with antithrombin III under a variety of experimental conditions [5]. However, the ability of the DIP-group to attain the transition state, tetrahedral intermediate structure and physically block antithrombin III binding, precluded this observation being taken as evidence for bond formation between the active site serine of thrombin and the reactive site carbonyl carbon of antithrombin III. The stability of the antithrombin III–thrombin complex to the denaturing conditions associated with SDS–polyacrylamide gel electrophoresis suggested, in the absence of direct evidence for covalent bond formation, that electrostatic/hydrophobic interactions between the proteins could aid in the resistance of the complex to denaturing agents [5]. Owen found in subsequent studies that the antithrombin III—thrombin complex is also stable in the presence of 6.0 M guanidine hydrochloride, but could be dissociated by incubation at pH 12.0 in the presence of 0.1% SDS or at pH 7.5 in the presence of 1.0 M hydroxylamine, 0.1% SDS [75]. These observations provide strong evidence for the formation of a covalent bond between antithrombin III and thrombin and suggest that the stable complex is analogous to the acyl–enzyme intermediate formed in the reaction scheme shown in Fig. 1.

Under nondenaturing conditions, at neutral pH, the antithrombin III–thrombin reaction appears to be at least partially reversible [73,76]. Based on the observation that the antithrombin III–thrombin reaction reaches an apparent equilibrium, Jesty found the apparent dissociation (equilibrium) constant value for the antithrombin III–thrombin complex to be 1.25×10^{-10} M [73]. This value was in good agreement with the dissociation constant value of 1.0×10^{-10} M calculated from the apparent second-order rate constant value measured for complex formation and the apparent first-order rate constant value for complex dissociation, thus suggesting that the antithrombin III–thrombin reaction is reversible [75]. Subsequent studies were reported which suggested that the reversibility of the antithrombin III–thrombin reaction is pH dependent [76]. Based on the apparent rates of active antithrombin III and thrombin dissociation from the antithrombin III–thrombin complex it was found that increasing amounts of inactive antithrombin III are released with thrombin as the pH of the solution is increased [76]. While the antithrombin III–thrombin reaction appeared to be reversible at pH 7.0, as indicated by equivalent rates of dissociation of thrombin and active antithrombin III, at pH 9.5, approximately 99% of the antithrombin III released from the complex was inactive. From these observations it has been suggested that thrombin inhibition by complex formation with antithrombin III does not require the formation of an acyl bond and concomitant cleavage of the antithrombin III molecule [76], but covalent bond formation, as in the tetrahedral intermediate, is not precluded. Similar studies reported more recently have not confirmed the dissociation of active antithrombin III from the antithrombin III–thrombin complex [77,78], thus suggesting that either the acyl–enzyme intermediate is the true form of the stable complex or that breakdown of the tetrahedral intermediate to the acyl–enzyme intermediate is very sensitive to the experimental conditions.

The inability of thrombin-cleaved antithrombin III to inactivate thrombin [79,80] suggests that the cleaved inhibitor does not readily attain the transition state conformation required for complex stabilization. Alternatively, if the acyl–enzyme intermediate is the stable form of the antithrombin III–thrombin complex, formation of an acyl bond between thrombin and the cleaved inhibitor might not be thermodynamically favorable. In related studies, Mahoney and coworkers found that anhydrotrypsin, i.e. trypsin in which the active site serine has been chemically modified to dehydroalanine, does not form a stable complex with either antithrombin III or α_1-antitrypsin [81]. This observation indicates that covalent bond formation between these inhibitors and the active site of trypsin is required for complex stabilization. It was also found, however, that dissociation of the α_1-antitrypsin–trypsin complex did not occur in the presence of hydroxylamine, nor was reactive site(s) peptide bond cleavage detected in the complex by amino terminal sequence analysis [81]. Interestingly, the α_1-antitrypsin–trypsin complex, like the antithrombin III–thrombin complex is stable under the conditions of SDS–polyacrylamide gel electrophoresis. While antithrombin III and α_1-antitrypsin appear to be structurally very similar [82], it is not clear to what extent the functional properties of the two inhibitors can be related to one another. At the least, the demonstration that the α_1-antitrypsin–trypsin complex is stable to denaturing conditions without evidence for acyl-bond formation provides indirect support for the possibility that acyl-bond formation may not be required for thrombin inhibition by antithrombin III.

It should be apparent from the discussion above that much of the antithrombin III–thrombin reaction sequence remains uncertain. Until X-ray crystallographic data on the antithrombin III–thrombin complex are obtained, the chemical nature of the bonds formed in the stable complex will not be known with certainty. If the data obtained from the study of the antithrombin III–trypsin complex are generally representative of antithrombin III–protease complexes, then the results obtained with anhydrotrypsin suggest that the antithrombin III–protease reaction sequence deviates from the standard mechanism of protease inhibition in that covalent bond formation is required for complex stabilization.

3. Heparin structure and function

Heparin is one of 6 structurally related glycosaminoglycans containing an alternating uronic acid (L-iduronic acid and/or D-glucuronic acid), hexosamine (D-glucosamine or D-galactosamine) carbohydrate backbone [83]. The general backbone of heparin [84] is composed of a repeating disaccharide of 1→4-linked uronic acid (α-L-iduronic acid or β-D-glucuronic acid) and α-D-glucosamine. The majority of the glucosamine residues have O-sulfate groups at C-6 and sulfated or acetylated amino groups. Most of the iduronic acid residues have O-sulfate groups at C-2, but glucuronic acid residues are nonsulfated. Commercial heparin preparations consist of molecules ranging in apparent molecular weight from ~5000 to ~30 000 [85] which also vary in degree of sulfation [86], N-acetylation [87] and in the ratio of iduronic acid to glucuronic acid [88]. Chondroitin-4-sulfate, chondroitin-6-sulfate and keratan sulfate, although structurally related to heparin, do not have measurable anticoagulant activity [89] and the anticoagulant activity of dermatan sulfate [89,90] appears to differ in mechanism from that of heparin [90]. Heparan sulfate differs from heparin in terms of iduronic acid:glucuronic acid ratio and degree of sulfation, but appears to have a mechanistically similar, albeit low, anticoagulant activity [90].

Commercial heparin preparations have been fractionated according to size, charge and affinity for antithrombin III in order to correlate heparin structure with function. The anticoagulant activity of heparin, measured in whole blood [91], plasma [92], or in related purified systems containing antithrombin III [93], has been shown to increase with increasing heparin size [94–114] and increasing degree of sulfation, i.e. increasing anionic charge density [100,103,115–121]. The affinity of heparin for antithrombin III has been shown to be a critical factor in the anticoagulant activity of heparin [102, 122,123]. Heparin with a high affinity for antithrombin III, representing approximately 1/3 of the heparin in commercial preparations, was found to have an anticoagulant activity ~10-fold higher than heparin with a low affinity for antithrombin III. The isolation of heparin fragments, prepared by chemical and/or enzymatic degradation, led to the preliminary characterization of the structural properties of heparin which are required for high-affinity binding to antithrombin III [124–127]. The results obtained in subsequent studies [110,128–139] have culminated in the identification of the monosaccharide sequence of an octasaccharide fragment of heparin which contains the antithrombin III-binding site [138]. While a recently reported study has indicated that the high-affinity antithrombin III (octasaccharide)-binding site is located at or near the nonreducing terminus of the heparin chain [140], there is also evidence that high molecular weight heparin may contain more than one antithrombin III-binding site per chain [108,112,141]. Further resolution of the critical functional groups within the antithrombin III-binding site can be anticipated, however, there appear to be additional structural properties of heparin beyond the antithrombin III-binding site which are related to the anticoagulant activity of molecules which remain to be quantitatively characterized.

4. Heparin–antithrombin III interaction

The results obtained in the initial investigation of antithrombin III structure and function suggested that there might be a functional link between the heparin-binding site and the reactive site, i.e. protease-binding site, of the antithrombin III molecule. Specifically, it was postulated that heparin binding via lysyl residues of antithrombin III causes a conformational change in the protein such that the reactive site arginine becomes more favorably exposed for rapid interaction with thrombin [5]. Thus, it was considered that the antithrombin III–protease reaction rate-enhancing effect of heparin was due to a direct effect of heparin on antithrombin III structure. A number of subsequent studies demonstrated changes in the spectral properties of antithrombin III in the presence of heparin. By UV double difference spectral analysis, Einarsson found that heparin binding to antithrombin III alters the environments of both tryptophan and tyrosine in the inhibitor and that ~1.8 moles of heparin are bound per mole of antithrombin III with an average dissociation constant value of 4.5×10^{-6} M [142]. It was also found that the fluorescence emission intensity of antithrombin III-bound 1-anilino-8-naphthalene-sulfonate (ANS), which binds noncompetitively with respect to heparin to antithrombin III, was decreased in the presence of heparin suggesting that heparin binding to antithrombin III alters the environment of the ANS-binding site [142]. Further evidence that heparin alters the environments of tryptophan and tyrosine was reported by Villanueva and Danishefsky who also showed by circular dichroism spectral analysis that heparin binding to antithrombin III results in a decrease in the β-structure of the molecule with an associated increase in random structure [19]. Both studies [19,142] were, however, complicated somewhat by the fact that unfractionated heparin was used. In particular, Einarsson and Andersson subsequently found that antithrombin III affinity-fractionated heparin binds to only one site on the protein with a dissociation constant value of 4.5×10^{-7} M, whereas unfractionated heparin appeared to be bound to two sites [143], as reported earlier [142]. This study also demonstrated that the intrinsic fluorescence emission of antithrombin III is increased by ~30% in the presence of heparin [143]. Additional studies were reported which indicated that the spectral changes in antithrombin III observed in the presence of high- (antithrombin III) affinity and low-affinity heparin fractions are different [144,145], even though both fractions appear to bind to the same site on antithrombin III [146]. While these studies and others [147–149] convincingly demonstrated that spectral changes in antithrombin III are associated with heparin binding, the evidence for a heparin-induced conformational change in the inhibitor was still somewhat circumstantial.

Evidence for a heparin-induced conformational change in antithrombin III was obtained after rigorous characterization of the protein fluorescence enhancement in the presence of heparin. Olson and Shore found that the fluorescence enhancement associated with heparin binding to antithrombin III is due to an alteration in the environment of buried tryptophan and concluded that this must result from a change in the conformation of antithrombin III [150]. Stopped flow fluorescence measurements indicated that heparin binding to antithrombin III is a two-step process in which rapid-equilibrium, low-affinity ($K_d = 4.3 \times 10^{-5}$ M) heparin binding induces a conformational change in the protein to increase the affinity for heparin by > 300-fold [151].

Several studies have been reported in which the structure–function relationships in antithrombin III related to heparin binding have been probed by chemical modification of the protein. Of particular interest is the observation that reduction of the Cys239–Cys422 disulfide bond in antithrombin III [152] results in a reduced affinity for heparin and a corresponding loss of heparin cofactor activity, i.e. antithrombin activity in the presence of heparin [153]. The antithrombin activity in the absence of heparin of reduced-antithrombin III is essentially unchanged, indicating that the reactive site region is not significantly affected by reduction of the Cys239–Cys422 bond [152,153]. While complete reduction and S-carbamidomethylation of antithrombin III results in a total loss of antithrombin activity, the general conformation of the molecule is not substantially changed [143,154]. Thus, in view of the two-step heparin-binding process [151], reduction of the Cys239–Cys422 disulfide bond may not affect the initial rapid equilibrium heparin–antithrombin III interaction, whereas the ability of antithrombin III to undergo the heparin-induced conformational change is lost.

The involvement of tryptophan in the binding of heparin by antithrombin III has been shown in several chemical modification studies [150,155–159]. Bjork and Nordling found that N-bromosuccinimide (NBS) modification of approximately 1 mole of tryptophan/mole of antithrombin III significantly decreases the rate of thrombin inhibition by the modified protein in the presence, but not in the absence of heparin [155]. It was also found that heparin partially protects antithrombin III from modification with NBS. Similar results were obtained when antithrombin III was modified by incubation with dimethyl(2-hydroxy-5-nitrobenzyl)sulfonium bromide (HNB) [156–158]. The fluorescence yield of solvent-exposed tryptophan, i.e. tryptophan susceptible to chemical modification, is not affected by heparin binding although a slight shift in the emission spectrum is observed [150]. These observations suggest that surface tryptophan, in close proximity to the heparin-binding site, is important for the high-affinity binding of heparin by antithrombin III.

Blackburn and coworkers recently reported that the Trp49 residue of antithrombin III is modified by HNB and suggested that the amino-terminal region of the protein may constitute a part of the heparin-binding domain [159]. A similar conclusion was reached by Koide and coworkers who found sequence homology in the amino-terminal regions of antithrombin III and histidine-rich glycoprotein [160], a protein which also binds heparin very tightly [161]. These investigators have also isolated a hereditary abnormal antithrombin III; antithrombin III Toyama, which inhibits thrombin at a normal rate in the absence, but not in the presence of heparin [37,162]. The amino acid substitution in antithrombin III Toyama is at residue 47 where cysteine has replaced the normal arginine residue [38], thus adding evidence that the amino-terminal region of antithrombin III is essential for heparin binding.

The involvement of lysine in the binding of heparin to antithrombin III was shown in the early work of Rosenberg and Damus [5]. Recent studies by Pecon and Blackburn have shown that incubation of antithrombin III with pyridoxal-5'-phosphate, followed by reduction with sodium borohydride, results in the modification of 3–4 moles of lysine/mole of protein [163]. Phosphopyridoxylated antithrombin III containing approximately 1 mole of modified lysine /mole of protein was obtained which had reduced activity in the presence, but not in the absence of heparin and did not show enhanced fluorescence in the presence of heparin. Fluorescence energy transfer from tryptophan to the bound phosphopyridoxyl group was also found [163] which suggests that the modified lysine is in close proximity to tryptophan, although the specific residues involved have not, as yet, been identified. While the specific lysyl residues involved in heparin binding to antithrombin III have not been identified directly, Villanueva has suggested that lysyl residues at positions 282, 286 and 289 may be involved [164]. These residues appear in an unstable helical segment (residues 281–292) of the molecule which has been identified as being important for heparin binding from the results of antithrombin III denaturation studies and secondary structure analysis [164–167]. Model building has shown that the lysyl residues in the helical segment can be aligned with sulfate groups in the antithrombin III-binding octasaccharide of heparin [164]. Identification of the phosphopyridoxylated-lysyl residue(s) of antithrombin III which appear to be essential for heparin binding could add support for the involvement of the helical segment in heparin binding.

5. *Kinetic mechanisms of action of heparin*

In 1959 Markwardt and Walsmann reported evidence for a catalytic role for heparin in the acceleration of thrombin inhibition by antithrombin III [168]. Subsequent work more rigorously demonstrated that non-stoichiometric amounts of heparin accelerate the reaction between antithrombin III and thrombin and thus a catalytic role for heparin was established [169]. The precise nature of the catalytic role, i.e. the mechanism of action, of heparin in accelerating thrombin inhibition by antithrombin III has not, as yet, been completely determined in spite of intense investigation. There is also reason to suspect that the mechanism of action of heparin is different for the various proteases inhibited by antithrombin III [107,109,113]. While it would seem reasonable that a rigorous analysis of the kinetics of the various heparin-catalyzed antithrombin III–protease reactions would resolve many of the questions related to the mechanism(s) of action of heparin, heparin is simply too heterogeneous to expect that the experimental results obtained in different laboratories, using different heparin preparations and fractions, would necessarily lead to similar interpretations of data and conclusions regarding the mechanism(s). In the discussion which follows, experimental results are considered within the context of two basic models for the mechanism of action of heparin. These models can be expressed mathematically and one or the other should provide a 'fit' for the kinetic data obtained with any highly fractionated heparin preparation.

The primary assumption which is made in deriving the models for the mechanism of action of heparin is that heparin is functionally similar to an enzyme which catalyzes a bireactant, i.e. two-substrate, reaction. This assumption appears to be valid for the general models wherein heparin catalyzes the antithrombin III–protease reaction by (1) simultaneously binding both antithrombin III and protease; a random-order bireactant reaction mechanism, or (2) by binding only antithrombin III; an ordered bireactant reaction mechanism. The purpose in making this assumption is to put the heparin-catalyzed antithrombin III–protease reaction system into the context of well-defined enzyme–substrate systems where the effects of varying substrate concentration on reaction rates are quantitatively related to one another [170].

(a) Random-order bireactant reaction mechanism

The random-order bireactant reaction mechanism is described by the equilibria shown below.

$$
\begin{array}{ccccc}
& K_P & & & \\
\text{H} & + & \text{P} & \rightleftharpoons & \text{H:P} \\
+ & & & & + \\
\text{I} & & & & \text{I} \\
K_I \updownarrow & & K_P \updownarrow \; K_I & k & K_C \\
\text{H:I} + \text{P} & \rightleftharpoons & \text{H:I:P} & \rightarrow \text{H:(I–P)} \rightleftharpoons \text{H} + \text{I–P}
\end{array}
$$

In this system, antithrombin III (I) and protease (P) bind randomly and independently to heparin (H). K_I and K_P are the heparin:antithrombin III and heparin:protease dissociation constants, respectively, and k is the apparent first-order rate constant for the rate-limiting step in product formation. K_C is the dissociation constant for heparin and the product of the reaction, the stable antithrombin III–protease complex (I–P). Assuming rapid equilibrium, the initial reaction velocity, v_i, is described by the following rate equation:

$$v_i = k \cdot [H]_t \cdot \frac{[P]}{K_P + [P]} \cdot \frac{[I]}{K_I + [I]} \tag{1}$$

Under any set of experimental conditions the reaction velocity is proportional to the total heparin concentration, $[H]_t$, and the fractional saturation of heparin with respect to both proteins. When the heparin concentration is much lower than the K_I and K_P values, the initial antithrombin III and protease concentrations are essentially equivalent to $[I]$ and $[P]$ respectively and saturation kinetics are observed when the protein concentrations are varied. When the heparin concentration is varied the initial protein concentrations are not always equivalent to $[I]$ and $[P]$ (in Eqn. 1). To provide a more general rate equation to be used when the initial reaction velocity is measured as a function of heparin concentration, Eqn. 1 is modified as shown in the following.

$$v_i = k \cdot [H]_t \cdot \frac{[H:P]}{[H]_t} \cdot \frac{[H:I]}{[H]_t} \tag{2}$$

The heparin:inhibitor concentration, $[H:I]$, at any initial inhibitor concentration, $[I]_t$, is calculated by solving the quadratic equation shown in the following.

$$[H:I] = (K_I + [I]_t + [H]_t - \sqrt{(K_I + [I]_t [H]_t)^2 - 4 \cdot [I]_t \cdot [H]_t})/2 \tag{3}$$

The heparin:protease concentration, $[H:P]$, is calculated in a similar manner. When the heparin concentration is sufficiently high, $[H:I] = [I]_t$ and $[H:P] = [P]_t$ and Eqn. 2 can be modified accordingly as shown in the following.

$$v_i = k \cdot [P]_t \cdot [I]_t / [H]_t \tag{4}$$

(b) Ordered bireactant reaction mechanism

The ordered bireactant reaction mechanism is described by the equilibria shown below.

$$K_I$$
$$H + I \rightleftharpoons H{:}I$$
$$+$$
$$P$$

$$\uparrow\downarrow K_P \ K_C \qquad\qquad K_C$$
$$\qquad\quad k$$
$$H{:}I{:}P \ \rightarrow \ H{:}(I\text{--}P) \rightleftharpoons H + I\text{--}P$$

In this system the protease binds only to the heparin:antithrombin III complex. While the dissociation constant, K_p value reflects the affinity of the protease for the complex, the binding of protease to the complex could involve only protease–antithrombin III interactions. In other words, heparin could be considered to be a positive allosteric effector which alters the conformation of antithrombin III to enhance protease binding. However, since protease–complex binding could also involve limited interactions with heparin, as well as with antithrombin III, K_p is defined simply as the dissociation constant for the protease from the protease:heparin:antithrombin III complex. Assuming rapid equilibrium, the initial reaction velocity for an ordered reaction mechanism is described by the following rate equation.

$$v_i = \frac{k \cdot [\mathrm{H}]_t \cdot [\mathrm{P}] \cdot [\mathrm{I}]}{K_I \cdot K_P + K_P \cdot [\mathrm{I}] + [\mathrm{P}] \cdot [\mathrm{I}]} \tag{5}$$

When the heparin concentration is much lower than the K_P and K_I values, the initial antithrombin III and protease concentrations are essentially equivalent to [I] and [P] respectively and saturation kinetics are observed when the protein concentrations are varied. When the protease concentration is much lower than the K_P value, the rate equation can be modified as shown in the following.

$$v_i = k \cdot [\mathrm{I}]_t \cdot \frac{[\mathrm{P}]_t}{K_P + [\mathrm{P}]_t} \cdot \frac{[\mathrm{H}{:}\mathrm{I}]}{[\mathrm{I}]_t} \tag{6}$$

Eqn. 6 relates the reaction velocity to the fractional saturation of antithrombin III with respect to heparin, where [H:I] is calculated according to Eqn. 3. When the antithrombin III concentration is, in addition, much lower than the K_I value, the rate equation is modified further as shown in the following.

$$v_i = k \cdot [\mathrm{I}]_t \cdot \frac{[\mathrm{P}]_t}{K_P + [\mathrm{P}]_t} \cdot \frac{[\mathrm{H}]_t}{K_I + [\mathrm{H}]_t} \tag{7}$$

To establish a reaction mechanism for an enzyme-catalyzed reaction system based solely on the results of kinetic studies is inherently difficult. The heparin-catalyzed antithrombin III–protease reaction systems are associated with several problems which make the interpretation of kinetic data more complicated. First, the heparin preparation must be relatively homogeneous with respect to size, affinity for antithrombin III and, probably, affinity for the protease. Kinetic analysis of a reaction system containing multiple forms of an enzyme catalyzing the reaction is difficult and a heterogeneous heparin preparation could result in similar difficulties in the analysis of the antithrombin III–protease reaction kinetics. Second, accurate measurement of the initial reaction velocity can also be difficult. At very low heparin concentration, the observed initial reaction velocity can be due to both the heparin-catalyzed and uncatalyzed antithrombin III–protease reactions. The observed initial velocity, therefore, must be correlated to correspond to the heparin-catalyzed reaction velocity only. At relatively high heparin concentration, the initial reaction velocity can be extremely fast and steps must be taken to obtain measurable reaction rates. In this regard, reversible active site reagents (e.g. synthetic substrates [171], p-aminobenzamidine [172], DAPA [173]) can be added to the reaction solution or the reaction temperature and/or protein concentrations can be lowered. Third, when the residual protease concentration is measured at timed intervals by removing samples from the reaction solution, the sampling procedure must immediately quench the antithrombin III–protease reaction. Polybrene binds very tightly to heparin and is often used to quench heparin-catalyzed antithrombin III–protease reactions. However, at very high heparin concentration the transient presence of even a trace amount of free heparin during the mixing/equilibration time could result in significant protease inhibition and an overestimation of the reaction velocity.

(c) Heparin-catalyzed antithrombin III–thrombin reaction

Early work suggested that the rate of thrombin inhibition by antithrombin III is accelerated by heparin when (1) heparin binds to thrombin [168,174–177], (2) when heparin binds to antithrombin III [5,20,72], or (3) when heparin simultaneously binds to both antithrombin III and thrombin [104,116,178–183]. The observation that heparin with a high affinity for antithrombin III is considerably more active than heparin with a low affinity for antithrombin III [102,122,123] provided compelling evidence that heparin binding to antithrombin III is an essential feature of the catalytic mechanism of action of heparin. Chemical modification of thrombin, however, was shown to decrease the rate of thrombin inhibition by antithrombin III in the presence, but not in the absence of heparin [175,185,186] and relatively low concentrations of active site blocked thrombin were found to competitively inhibit the heparin-catalyzed antithrombin III–thrombin reaction [186,187]. These results, in addition to the observation that thrombin binds with relatively high affinity to heparin in solution [188], provided good reason to believe that heparin binding to thrombin is an essential feature of the catalytic mechanism of action of heparin. Studies reported by Pomerantz and Owen strongly suggested that the catalytic mechanism of action of heparin involves the formation of a ternary complex of antithrombin III, thrombin and heparin [181]. Laurent and coworkers reached a similar conclusion based on the empirical relationship between heparin activity and heparin size [104]. While the results of relatively rigorous kinetic studies have argued for either a heparin–thrombin- [187] or a heparin–antithrombin III-binding model [189] for the kinetic mechanism of action of heparin, the weight of evidence from the above studies appears to favor the ternary complex (random order) model [104,116,178–183].

Heparin does not appear to have a significant effect on the apparent first-order rate constant value for the rate-limiting step in the antithrombin III–thrombin reaction sequence [74]. Results reported by Olson and Shore indicate that the primary effect of heparin on the antithrombin III–thrombin reaction is related to an increase in the apparent affinity of the proteins for one another [74]. While these results do not exclude the possibility that the heparin-induced conformational change in antithrombin III increases the affinity of antithrombin III for the active site of thrombin, the results of several recent kinetic studies suggest that the apparent increase in affinity is due to the simultaneous binding and effective concentration of both proteins by heparin [190–194].

The heparin-catalyzed antithrombin III–thrombin reaction is saturable with respect to both antithrombin III and thrombin [192]. In the presence of very low heparin concentration the apparent heparin:antithrombin III and heparin:thrombin dissociation constant values were found to be 100 nM and 36 nM, respectively, and the apparent first-order rate constant value was 800/min. Nearly identical kinetic parameter values were empirically derived in earlier work when the initial antithrombin III–thrombin reaction velocity was determined as a function of heparin concentration [191]. Over a 1000-fold heparin concentration range (5 nM–5μM), and in the presence of several different protein concentrations, the observed initial reaction velocity could be fit to the random-order bireactant reaction mechanism when K_I, K_P and k values of 100 nM, 35 nM and 800/min were used to calculate the initial reaction velocity according to Eqn. 2 [191]. The kinetically determined K_I value was also identical to the heparin:antithrombin III dissociation constant value measured by titration of the fluorescence enhancement in antithrombin III by heparin. The k value of 800/min (13/sec) is also in reasonable agreement with the k values of 5/sec and 10/sec determined by Olson and Shore for the antithrombin III–thrombin reaction in the presence and absence of heparin, respectively [74]. The kinetically determined K_P value, however, is approximately 20-fold lower than the heparin:thrombin dissociation constant value determined by equilibrium dialysis by Jordan and coworkers [190]. This difference can be explained by the difference between the apparent molecular weights of the heparin fractions used in the two studies [104,194].

Nesheim has shown that the kinetics of the heparin-catalyzed antithrombin III–thrombin reaction, determined over a range of heparin and protein concentrations, are described by a rate law [173] which is identical to that described by the rate equation for the random-order bireactant reaction mechanism (Eqn. 2). The reaction was shown to be second order overall and first order with respect to both antithrombin III and thrombin in the presence of excess heparin and zero order overall when the proteins were in excess, indicating that the reaction is saturable with respect to both proteins [173]. The first-order rate constant value was also estimated to be 2–2.5/sec. Pletcher and Nelsestuen, however, have suggested that the heparin-catalyzed antithrombin III–thrombin reaction is described by an ordered bireactant reaction mechanism [195]. The model proposed by these investigators requires that the direct binding of heparin to thrombin decreases the affinity of thrombin for the heparin:antithrombin III complex and thereby accounts for the decrease in the initial reaction velocity at high heparin concentration [195]. This model is essentially identical to that proposed by Jordan and coworkers [190] who found, using heparin:thrombin and heparin:antithrombin III dissociation constant values of 800 nM and 100 nM (determined by equilibrium dialysis), an apparent correlation between the binding of heparin to thrombin and the decrease in reaction velocity at high heparin concentration. It is worth noting, however, that the first-order rate constant values calculated (according to Eqn. 2) from the initial velocity data reported by Jordan and coworkers are on the order of 20 ± 4/sec over a heparin concentration range from 10 nM to $\sim$1000 nM. Given that these experiments were performed at 37°C, the first-order rate constant values would be expected to be approximately 2-fold lower at 25°C and thus consistent with values reported by other investigators [74]. The data in general are therefore also consistent with a random-order reaction mechanism.

Hoylaerts and coworkers have greatly simplified the kinetic analysis of the heparin-catalyzed antithrombin III–thrombin reaction by preparing covalent heparin–antithrombin III and heparin–thrombin complexes [194]. Apparent dissociation constant values for the interaction between thrombin and the covalent heparin–antithrombin III complex were found to be 7 nM, 100 nM and 6 μM when the molecular weights of the covalently bound heparins were 15 000, 4300 and 3200 respectively. The apparent first-order rate constant values obtained at saturation were, however, independent of the heparin size; $k = 2$/sec. Since active site-blocked thrombin inhibited the interaction between thrombin and the covalent heparin–antithrombin III complex (heparin mol. wt. = 15 000) with an apparent dissociation constant value of 4 nM, it was concluded that the rate-enhancing effect of heparin depends on noncovalent bonds between heparin and thrombin, i.e. the binding of thrombin to the covalent heparin–antithrombin III complex involves electrostatic interactions between thrombin and a site on the heparin chain adjacent to antithrombin III [194]. While these results are consistent with the random-order bireactant reaction mechanism model, the model was extended by evidence that thrombin diffuses along the heparin chain to interact with antithrombin III [194]. Thus, increasing the chain length of heparin results in reaction rate enhancement due to a higher probability of interaction between thrombin and heparin in solution.

(d) Heparin-catalyzed antithrombin III–factor X_a reaction

While much less data are available on the kinetics of the heparin-catalyzed antithrombin III–factor X_a reaction at least two lines of evidence suggest that an ordered bireactant reaction mechanism is followed. First, very low molecular weight heparin fragments, which bind tightly to antithrombin III, enhance the antithrombin III–factor X_a reaction rate, but have little effect on the rate of thrombin inhibition [107,109,113,134,190]. Second, while the heparin-catalyzed antithrombin III–factor X_a reaction is saturable with respect to both antithrombin III and factor X_a [193,196], the reaction velocity increases with increasing heparin concentration as described by the ordered bireactant rate equation (Eqn. 7) [190,196]. Jordan and coworkers reported an apparent second-order rate constant, k''_{app}, value for the antithrombin III–factor X_a reaction of 3×10^8/M/min in the presence of saturating (with respect to antithrombin III) heparin concentrations [190]. Under the experimental conditions used, i.e. very low protein concentration, $k''_{app}=k/K_P$. While the K_P value was not measured in this study, values of 160 nM [193] and 1.5 μM (Griffith, unpublished) have been observed with heparin preparations with apparent molecular weights of 11 000 and 7000 respectively. Thus, k values from 0.8 to 7.5/sec can be estimated for the heparin-catalyzed antithrombin III–factor X_a reaction from the data reported by Jordan and coworkers [190]. Pletcher and Nelsestuen have reported an apparent K_P value of 100 nM and an apparent first-order rate constant value of 0.7/sec for the heparin-catalyzed antithrombin III–factor X_a reaction [195]. The apparent differences in K_P values observed with different molecular weight heparin preparations suggest that the binding of factor X_a to the heparin–antithrombin III complex involves interactions with both heparin and antithrombin III in the complex. This possibility is supported by the observation that arginine-modified factor X_a is inhibited by antithrombin III at a much slower rate than native factor X_a in the presence, but not in the absence of heparin [197]. Active site-blocked factor X_a, at relatively high concentration, has very little effect on the heparin-catalyzed antithrombin III–factor X_a reaction [195] which strongly suggests that the K_P value for the interaction between factor X_a and the heparin–antithrombin III complex reflects interactions with both antithrombin III and heparin.

Further analysis of the kinetics of the various heparin-catalyzed antithrombin III–protease reactions can be expected to extend the proposed models for the mechanism of action of heparin. Existing evidence suggests that thrombin, factor IX_a and factor XI_a are inhibited by a random-order reaction mechanism in the presence of heparin, whereas factor X_a, factor XII_a, kallikrein and plasmin are inhibited by heparin–antithrombin III by an ordered reaction mechanism [107,109,113,134,190]. Resolution of these models is very much dependent on the use of highly characterized, homogeneous heparin preparations. Given this, rigorous analysis of the antithrombin III–protease reaction kinetics, to include K_I, K_P and k determinations, coupled with independently measured heparin:antithrombin III and heparin:protease dissociation constant values should provide further insight into the mechanism(s) of action of heparin.

6. Heparin cofactor II

In 1974 Briginshaw and Shanberge demonstrated that there are at least two distinct thrombin inhibitors in human plasma which react with thrombin at an accelerated rate in the presence of heparin [29,198]. These inhibitors, termed heparin cofactor A and heparin cofactor B, differed in terms of apparent molecular weight and affinity for DEAE–cellulose [29]. In the absence of heparin, heparin cofactor A was shown to inhibit thrombin 30–40-fold more slowly than did heparin cofactor B [198]. While the rate of factor X_a inhibition by heparin cofactor B was accelerated by heparin, there was no inhibition of factor X_a by heparin cofactor A in the presence or absence of heparin [198]. The evidence strongly suggested that heparin cofactor B was identical to antithrombin III while heparin cofactor A was a previously unrecognized antithrombin–heparin cofactor in human plasma.

Several studies reported in the past few years [199–202] have confirmed the original observations made by Briginshaw and Shanberge [29,198]. Tollefsen and Blank found that radiolabeled thrombin is incorporated into complexes with apparent molecular weights of 96 000 and 85 000 when incubated with human plasma in the presence of heparin [199]. The 85 000 mol. wt. complex, immunologically identified as the complex between antithrombin III and thrombin, was the predominate complex formed at low heparin concentration while the 96 000 mol. wt. complex predominated at high heparin concentration. The 96 000 mol. wt. complex was also found to form in normal quantities when radiolabeled thrombin was incubated with plasma which was immunodepleted with respect to all of the known protease inhibitors [199]. Other studies indicated that the plasma levels of apparent antithrombin III activity exceed the levels of antithrombin III antigen in antithrombin III-deficient patients [201,202]. The discrepancy between activity and antigen levels was shown to be due to the presence of a second heparin cofactor in human plasma [201] which appeared to correspond to heparin cofactor A [202]. The second heparin cofactor appears to account for 20–35% of the total antithrombin III–heparin cofactor activity in human plasma [199,201,202].

The second heparin cofactor has been purified to homogeneity from human plasma [203] and from Cohn fraction IV [200]. Heparin cofactor II [203] and antithrombin BM [200,204] are essentially identical in amino acid composition and functional properties and are very likely one and the same protein. The term heparin cofactor II is used herein. Unlike antithrombin III, purified heparin cofactor II does not appear to inhibit factor X_a [200,203], plasmin or trypsin [200] at appreciable rates in the presence or in the absence of heparin. The apparent molecular weight of heparin cofactor II is ~65 600 and consists of approximately 10% (w/w) carbohydrate [203]. The amino-terminal amino acid sequence of heparin cofactor II does not appear to be similar to that of antithrombin III [204,205] and there is little evidence for long stretches of structural identity between the two proteins as determined by tryptic peptide mapping [205]. A significant degree of structural similarity has been found between the carboxy-terminal regions of heparin cofactor II and antithrombin III [205]. Specifically, of the 36 residues identified in the reactive site peptide of heparin cofactor II, i.e. the peptide formed by thrombin cleavage, 19 residues could be aligned with residues in the primary structure of the reactive site peptide from antithrombin III [205]. Thus it appears that heparin cofactor II, like antithrombin III is a member of the superfamily of proteins consisting of α_1-antitrypsin, α_1-chymotrypsin and ovalbumin which share a common genetic ancestry [82].

The rate of thrombin inhibition by heparin cofactor II is accelerated by dermatan sulfate as well as by heparin [206,207]. Earlier studies indicated that the anticoagulant activity of dermatan sulfate [89,90] is not dependent on the presence of antithrombin III, thus suggesting a different anticoagulant mechanism of action for dermatan sulfate than that for heparin [90]. It now appears that the anticoagulant activity of dermatan sulfate is related to the accelerated rate of thrombin inhibition by heparin cofactor II [208]. Both heparin and dermatan sulfate can be fractionated by affinity for heparin cofactor II to obtain high-activity material [206]. At the present time there are very little data regarding the mucopolysaccharide structure required for high-affinity binding to heparin cofactor II. There appears to be some degree of segregation of heparin with high heparin cofactor II activity from heparin with high antithrombin III activity when commercial grade heparin is fractionated by affinity for heparin cofactor II [206]. Hurst and coworkers have found essentially no difference between the heparin cofactor II–thrombin reaction rate-enhancing effects of heparins with high and very low affinity for antithrombin III [209]. These results suggest that there are differences between the heparin structure required for binding to the two inhibitors. The ability of dermatan sulfate to accelerate the heparin cofactor II–thrombin reaction while having little, if any, effect on the antithrombin III–thrombin reaction, further suggests that there are differences in the mucopolysaccharide structure required for binding to heparin cofactor II and antithrombin III. However, since the dermatan sulfate- and heparin-binding sites on heparin cofactor II may be different further investigation is required to determine the correlation between mucopolysaccharide structure and function with respect to heparin cofactor II.

The heparin-catalyzed heparin cofactor–thrombin reaction appears to follow a random-order bireactant reaction mechanism similar to that described for the heparin-catalyzed antithrombin III–thrombin reaction [210]. In the presence of catalytic amounts of heparin, the heparin cofactor II–thrombin reaction is saturable with respect to both heparin cofactor II and thrombin. The apparent heparin:heparin cofactor II dissociation constant value was, however, -4-fold higher than that determined for heparin antithrombin III [210] which is consistent with earlier studies where the affinity of heparin cofactor II for heparin was shown to be lower than that for antithrombin III [200,202,203,207]. There is essentially no difference between the apparent heparin:thrombin dissociation constant values determined from the kinetics of the heparin-catalyzed heparin cofactor II–thrombin and antithrombin III–thrombin reactions [207]. This observation is consistent with the random-order bireactant reaction mechanism which requires that inhibitor and protease bind independently to heparin and, therefore, the apparent affinity of thrombin for heparin should not be different when determined from the kinetics of the two inhibitor–thrombin reactions if a random-order mechanism applies to both reactions. There is also qualitative evidence that the heparin cofactor II–thrombin reaction rate increases with increasing heparin size [206] which is again consistent with a random-order reaction mechanism. In the absence of heparin, the heparin cofactor II–thrombin reaction rate appears to be approximately 20-fold slower than the antithrombin III–thrombin reaction rate [205] as originally observed by Briginshaw and Shanberge [198], although Tollefsen and coworkers have observed similar rates of thrombin inhibition by heparin cofactor II and antithrombin III [203]. At saturation with respect to both proteins, the heparin-catalyzed heparin cofactor II–thrombin reaction velocity was found to be ~4-fold slower than that observed for the antithrombin III–thrombin reaction under similar conditions [210]. This result must be qualified since the heparin preparation used in the study was fractionated by affinity for antithrombin III and could contain heparin molecules unable to bind to heparin cofactor II.

At the present time the physiological role of heparin cofactor II is not known. Assay procedures for the specific measurement of heparin cofactor II activity levels in plasma have been recently described [211,212]. The normal range for heparin cofactor II appears to be much larger than that for antithrombin III. Normal levels of heparin cofactor II have been found in patients with hereditary antithrombin III deficiency [202,211] and in patients with deep vein thrombosis [211]. Patients with liver disease or with disseminated intravascular coagulation have reduced levels of heparin cofactor II which parallel the reduction in antithrombin III levels [211]. Heparin cofactor II, therefore, appears to be involved in protease inhibition in patients with DIC, but the specific protease(s) inhibited by heparin cofactor II in vivo remains to be determined. Identification of the heparin cofactor II–protease complexes presumably formed during DIC could provide valuable insight into the physiological role of heparin cofactor II.

References

1 Egeberg, O. (1965) Thromb. Diath. Haemorr. 13, 516–530.
2 Brinkhous, K.M., Smith, H.P., Warner, E.D. and Seegers, W.H. (1939) Am. J. Physiol. 125, 683–687.
3 Abildgaard, U. (1968) Scand. J. Clin. Lab. Invest. 21, 89–91.
4 Heimburger, N., Haupt, H. and Schwick, H.G. (1971) in: Proceedings of the International Research Conference on Proteinase Inhibitors (Fritz, H. and Tschesche, H., Eds.) pp. 1–22, de Gruyter, Berlin.
5 Rosenberg, R.D. and Damus, P.S. (1973) J. Biol. Chem. 248, 6490–6505.
6 Miller-Andersson, M., Borg, H. and Andersson, L. (1974) Thromb. Res. 5, 439–452.
7 Damus, P.S. and Wallace, G.A. (1974) Biochem. Biophys. Res. Commun. 61, 1147–1153.
8 Thaler, E. and Schmer, G. (1975) Br. J. Haematol. 31, 233–243.
9 Kurachi, K., Schmer, G., Hermodson, M.A., Teller, D.C. and Davie, E.W. (1976) Biochemistry 15, 368–373.
10 Nordenman, B., Nystrom, C. and Bjork, I. (1977) J. Biochem. 78, 195–203.
11 Koide, T. (1979) J. Biochem. 86, 1841–1850.

protein to aggregate even under these conditions. SDS–polyacrylamide gel electrophoresis after reduction showed that bovine protein C is composed of two polypeptide chains, a light chain and a heavy chain, with apparent molecular weights
of 21 000 and 41 000, respectively (Fig. 1). The carbohydrate content of bovine
protein C is about 18%. Recently, Miletich et al. [20] showed the presence of
5–15% of single-chain protein C in human plasma, indicating that the protein is
synthesized as a single chain. In the newly synthesized molecule, the COOH-terminal of the light chain is linked to the NH$_2$-terminal of the heavy chain by the
dipeptide Lys-Arg, according to the recently determined nucleotide sequences for
human and bovine protein C [21,22].

The complete amino acid sequence has been determined both for the light chain
[23] and the heavy chain [24] of bovine protein C (Fig. 2). The light chain is composed of 155 amino acid residues. It contains one carbohydrate chain, attached to
an asparagine residue in position 97 [23]. The heavy chain is composed of 260 amino
acid residues and its 3 carbohydrate chains are attached to asparagine residues in

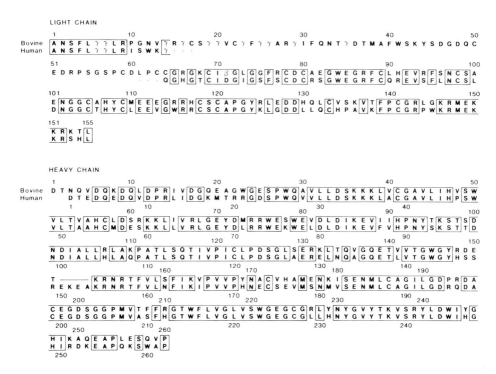

Fig. 2. Amino acid sequence of the light and heavy chains of bovine and human protein C. The sequence for bovine protein C is from protein [23,24] and cDNA [22] sequence data. The sequence for
the NH$_2$-terminal part of the light chain of human protein C is from protein sequence data [12] and
the remaining sequence from cDNA sequence data [21]. The standard IUPAC one-letter code for amino
acid residues was used. γ, γ-carboxyglutamic acid residues; β, β-hydroxyaspartic acid residue. The boxes
enclose residues identical in the two proteins.

positions 93, 154 and 170 [24]. These carbohydrate assignments are in agreement with the distribution of carbohydrate obtained by radioactivity-labelling experiments which showed that 75% of the carbohydrate is present in the heavy chain, and 25% in the light chain [19]. It should be pointed out that residue 172 in the heavy chain is a cysteine – which is probably in disulphide linkage with cysteine 186 (see below). The attachment of carbohydrate to the asparagine residue 170 is thus an exception to the rule that carbohydrate-carrying asparagine residues invariably have a serine or a threonine residue in the position two steps away in the COOH–terminal direction, a rule followed by the 3 other carbohydrate attachments in bovine protein C.

The light chain of bovine protein C contains two different post-translationally modified amino acids: γ-carboxyglutamic acid and β-hydroxyaspartic acid. γ-Carboxyglutamic acid is formed in a vitamin K-dependent carboxylation reaction (cf. Ch. 4) and is found in all vitamin K-dependent plasma proteins [25], as well as in a small protein present in bone tissue [26,27]. There are 11 γ-carboxyglutamic acid residues (in positions 6, 7, 14, 16, 19, 20, 23, 25, 26, 29 and 35) in the light chain of bovine protein C. Since there is no unmodified glutamic acid residue within this segment, all the glutamic acid residues present in the polypeptide chain, up to a position corresponding to the last γ-carboxyglutamic acid residue have been carboxylated during the biosynthesis of the bovine protein C light chain. This pattern is characteristic for all proteins studied so far that contain γ-carboxyglutamic acid.

The second post-translationally modified amino acid present in the light chain of bovine protein C is β-hydroxyaspartic acid. Before its discovery in protein C [28], this amino acid was an unknown constituent of proteins. It was not identified with the conventional method for amino acid sequencing, and in the report of the sequence of the light chain of bovine protein C [23], there was no certain assignment for the amino acid in position 71, although it was suggested that the unusual amino acid might be a derivative of cysteine. Isolation of a heptapeptide corresponding to the relevant part of the light chain – including position 71 – and analysis by ^{1}H-NMR spectroscopy, mass spectrometry and comparisons with the synthetic compound, revealed that the unusual amino acid is *erythro*-β-hydroxyaspartic acid [28].

In contrast to γ-carboxyglutamic acid, which is totally destroyed by acid hydrolysis, β-hydroxyaspartic acid can be measured by amino acid analysis after acid hydrolysis of the protein [29]. Such analysis has shown that bovine protein C contains approximately 1 mole of β-hydroxyaspartic acid/mole of protein [29], which is consistent with the finding of β-hydroxyaspartic acid in position 71 in the light chain, and in no other position in either the light or heavy chains of protein C. β-Hydroxyaspartic acid has also been demonstrated in several other vitamin K-dependent plasma proteins including human protein C (unpublished). Bovine coagulation factor VII [30], bovine and human factor IX, and factor X [29–32], contain about 1 mole of β-hydroxyaspartic acid/mole of protein, whereas bovine protein S contains 2–3 residues [29]. In contrast to this, prothrombin, which is the quantitatively predominant vitamin K-dependent protein in plasma, does not contain any β-hydroxyaspartic acid [29,30]. A number of non-vitamin K-dependent proteins have also been analysed, but so far none has been found to contain β-hydroxyaspartic acid [29].

According to sequence similarity, β-hydroxyaspartic acid occupies a position in human and bovine factors IX and X [31,32] that corresponds to position 71 of the light chain of bovine protein C. The mRNA nucleotide sequences coding for human protein C [21], bovine protein C [22], human factor IX [33], bovine factor IX [34], and human factor X [35], all have a triplet coding for aspartic acid at the position for the β-hydroxyaspartic acid residue, proving that β-hydroxyaspartic acid is formed by a post-translational hydroxylation of aspartic acid. In the analyses of β-hydroxyaspartic acid-containing proteins [29], it was frequently found that the amount of β-hydroxyaspartic acid recovered was less than an integer value when expressed as moles/mole of protein, and also that the amount varied between different preparations of the same protein [29]. The explanation for these findings is not entirely clear, but might be that unhydroxylated forms of the proteins exist. It is possible that they represent different functional forms of the protein, although that remains to be shown.

The amino acid sequence of the first 44 residues of the light chain of bovine protein C, which is the Gla domain of the protein, is very similar to the corresponding parts of other vitamin K-dependent plasma proteins. The percentage of identical residues varies between 59% and 67% in comparison with bovine factor IX, factor X and prothrombin [23]. The remaining part of the light chain (residues 45–155) shows only a low degree of similarity to the corresponding part of prothrombin (8% identical residues). On the other hand, the similarity to factor IX and factor X is much stronger with 38% and 47% identical residues, respectively [23].

The heavy chain of bovine protein C is clearly homologous to other serine proteases. Sequence comparison with bovine factor IX, factor X, thrombin, and chymotrypsin shows sequence identities amounting to between 35% and 40%, and the critical parts of a serine protease, such as the active site serine and the charge relay system are all present in bovine protein C [24].

The light chain of bovine protein C contains 17 half-cysteine residues and the heavy chain 7. The pairing of cysteines has not been determined for protein C, but at least one disulphide bridge links the light and the heavy chains, as reduction is required for separation of the chains. If the disulphide bridging in the heavy chain is homologous to that in bovine chymotrypsin A [36], then the following cysteine residues form intra-heavy-chain bridges: 41–57, 172–186 and 197–225. Cysteine 122 is thus left unpaired, and is presumably the link between the light and heavy chains. The large number of cysteine residues present in the light chain, most of which must be in intra-chain disulphides, suggests that the light chain has a very compact structure. There is no disulphide connection, however, between the Gla domain and the rest of the light chain, as the Gla domain can be released from bovine protein C by limited digestion with chymotrypsin [37].

Human protein C has a molecular weight of 62 000, when estimated by SDS–polyacrylamide gel electrophoresis [12]. It contains about 23% carbohydrate, including mannose, galactose, glucosamine and sialic acid. Reduction and SDS–polyacrylamide gel electrophoresis reveal a light and a heavy chain with estimated molecular weights of 41 000 and 21 000, respectively. As discussed, protein C is synthesized as a single-chain molecule and converted to its circulating two-chain state post-translationally [20–22]. An extensive sequence similarity exists between human protein C and its bovine counterpart, as shown by Foster and Davie [21] who determined the sequence of a cloned cDNA coding for human protein C (Fig. 2).

4. Activation of protein C

Interest in protein C has intensified over the last couple of years owing to the elucidation of its mode of activation. Within the framework of such studies, pioneered by Esmon and Owen [38] with the identification of a cofactor for protein C activation, new concepts were introduced relating to the regulation of blood coagulation and the role of protein C in this process (Fig. 3). It also provided an explanation for the puzzling fact that thrombin, the main procoagulant in plasma, when infused in low doses into an experimental animal, induces a state characterized by anticoagulation and even bleeding rather than thrombosis [39,40].

Protein C was first shown to be activated to a serine protease by incubation with trypsin, after which [^{3}H]DFP was incorporated in its heavy chain [41]. Subsequently, Kisiel et al. demonstrated that thrombin activated bovine protein C by cleavage at the arginine residue in position 14 of the heavy chain [19], and the human protein by cleavage at arginine 12 in its heavy chain [12]. The activation peptides from human and bovine protein C show little sequence similarity except that both have several negatively charged amino acids.

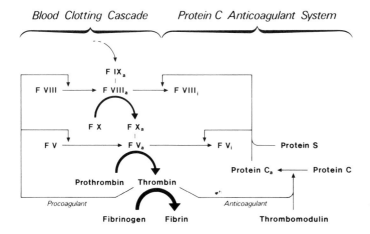

Fig. 3. Blood clotting cascade and the protein C anticoagulant system.

The in vitro activation of protein C by thrombin is very slow, and is slower in the presence of Ca^{2+} ions than in their absence [42]. Consistent with this was the finding that only the zymogen form of protein C was obtained when the protein was purified from serum [19]. Thus it was considered doubtful whether thrombin was the physiological activator of protein C. It was suspected either that an unidentified protease was the activator of protein C in vivo, or that some cofactor not present in plasma had to be implicated. Studies on the rate of activation of protein C in the presence of platelets indicated that they had at most a minor effect [43].

Soon after bovine protein C was first purified, it was demonstrated that a monospecific antiserum against bovine protein C reacted with autoprothrombin IIA – i.e., the anticoagulant formed from 'prothrombin complex' upon incubation with thrombin [14], which was first described by Mammen et al. in 1960 [45]. Several reports dealing with the properties of the inhibitor, published by Seegers and co-workers demonstrated the potential role of activated protein C as an anticoagulant [46–48]. In 1970, Marciniak [49] demonstrated that the precursor of the anticoagulant activity was not identical to prothrombin, and that the anticoagulant activity elicited in vivo by small amounts of thrombin had properties in common with autoprothrombin IIA [49,50]. Thus, in retrospect thrombin apparently activates protein C rapidly in vivo, contrasting to the very slow activation of protein C in vitro, suggesting that thrombin requires a cofactor for the activation of protein C – a cofactor which is present in vivo, but absent when thrombin is formed by the coagulation of plasma in vitro.

(a) Thrombomodulin, a cofactor for protein C activation

The mode of activation of protein C was resolved when Esmon and Owen demonstrated rapid activation of protein C by thrombin in the microcirculation [38,51]. They perfused the capillary bed in the myocardium, using the Langendorf heart preparation, and showed that protein C was activated at least 20 000 times more rapidly by thrombin during perfusion than when an identical mixture of protein C and thrombin was incubated in vitro under otherwise identical conditions. In an elegant series of experiments, it was shown that the effect was due to a reversible high-affinity binding of thrombin to a receptor on the surface of endothelial cells. The receptor, now called thrombomodulin, is an integral membrane protein that binds thrombin reversibly with high affinity. The isolated thrombomodulin was half-saturated at a thrombin concentration of 0.48 nM, and the K_m for the protein C activation by the thrombin–thrombomodulin complex was 0.72 μM [51] which is higher than the physiological protein C concentration in plasma (approximately 100 nM). However, no corresponding measurements have yet been made, either with intact endothelial cells or in vivo. The half-life of the thrombin–thrombomodulin complex in the microcirculation is approximately 15 min. DIP-thrombin (diisopropylfluorophosphate (DFP)-inactivated thrombin) bound equally well ($K_i = 0.56$ nM) as active thrombin to the receptor, indicating that the active site was not involved in binding [50]. Attempts to activate protein C by thrombin employing endothelial cells in tissue culture only led to an approximately 30-fold increase in the rate of activation attributable to the endothelial cells [51]. In this context, the enormous endothelial cell surface to blood volume ratio in the microcirculation compared to that obtaining in larger blood vessels should be emphasized — i.e., the surface to volume ratio is at least 1000 times larger in the capillaries than in the larger blood vessels [52]. So far thrombomodulin has only been identified on endothelial cells [51].

Thrombomodulin has been purified from rabbit lungs by Esmon et al. [53]. After initial solubilization with detergent, affinity chromatography on DIP-thrombin insolubilized on agarose gave a homogenous preparation of thrombomodulin. Approximately 1 mg of thrombomodulin was obtained from one rabbit lung. The purified thrombomodulin, which requires the addition of a detergent to remain soluble, proved remarkably resistant to denaturing agents, provided that the disulphide bonds were not reduced. For instance, it remained active after heating in 6 M guanidine hydrochloride.

The purified thrombomodulin retained its cofactor activity after purification and thus did not have an obligatory phospholipid requirement, which is noteworthy since the substrate for the thrombin–thrombomodulin complex is a vitamin K-dependent Gla-containing protein. The rate of protein C activation was saturable both with respect to cofactor and thrombin concentration also in vitro, utilizing purified thrombomodulin. The rate of activation also depended on the Ca^{2+} ion concentration. To investigate the effect of Ca^{2+} ions on the activation of protein C in more detail, Esmon et al. [37] selectively removed the region containing γ-carboxyglutamic acid (Gla), by limited proteolysis using chymotrypsin, which cleaves the light chain of protein C at tryptophan 41. Contrary to what was expected, it was found that there was also a Ca^{2+} ion dependence for activation of the Gla-domainless protein C. Furthermore, whereas the half-maximum rate of activation was obtained at 250 μM Ca^{2+} for intact protein C, the half-maximum rate for the Gla-domainless protein was obtained already at 50 μM Ca^{2+} [37]. As already mentioned Ca^{2+} inhibits the rate of activation of protein C in the absence of thrombomodulin. This inhibitory effect was also obtained with the Gla-domainless protein. Half-maximum inhibitions were found at 50 μM and 250 μM Ca^{2+} for Gla-domainless and intact protein C, respectively. It has subsequently been demonstrated by equilibrium dialysis that not only the Gla-domainless protein C [13,54] has a single high-affinity Ca^{2+}-binding site, but also Gla-domainless factor IX [55] and factor X [13]. Saturation of the Ca^{2+} ion-binding site induces a conformational change in all 3 proteins. Indirect evidence suggests that the Gla-independent Ca^{2+}-binding site is located in the vicinity of the β-hydroxyaspartic acid residue in the light chain of protein C and factor X [13,55].

In contrast to experiments using purified thrombomodulin, activation studies performed with endothelial cells and intact or Gla-domainless protein C showed that activation of the intact protein proceeded much more rapidly than activation of the Gla-domainless protein [37]. Whether this is due to the Ca^{2+}-dependent interaction of the Gla region with phospholipid, or to direct recognition of the Gla residues by a receptor adjacent to the thrombomodulin, is discussed below.

(b) Inhibition of the procoagulant activity of thrombomodulin

When thrombin becomes bound to rabbit thrombomodulin, its specificity is altered in two ways, as outlined by Esmon et al. [56]. Free thrombin is a very slow protein C activator, whereas thrombin in complex with thrombomodulin activates protein C very rapidly. Secondly, and equally important, thrombin in complex with thrombomodulin has no or virtually no procoagulant activity. This 'modulation' of the thrombin specificity is fully expressed when an equimolar complex has been formed, and is completely reversible [56]. Accordingly, thrombin dissociated from the complex by an excess of DIP-thrombin regains full procoagulant activity. The activity of thrombin against low molecular weight substrates such as *p*-tosyl-L-arginine methyl ester is only marginally affected by complex formation with thrombomodulin [56]. Likewise, thrombin bound to thrombomodulin is inhibited by antithrombin III as readily as is free thrombin [5].

The thrombin procoagulant functions inhibited by thrombomodulin are fibrin formation, factor V activation, and platelet activation [56,57]. Due to the large endothelial cell surface exposed to the blood in the microcirculation, and thereby to the potentially high concentration of thrombin in complex with thrombomodulin, the inhibition of the thrombin procoagulant activity appears to be necessary to prevent thrombotization in the microvasculature. Superimposed on this effect is the anticoagulant effect of the thrombin–thrombomodulin complex manifested by the generation of activated protein C. The role of protein C in preventing thrombotization in the microcirculation is dramatically illustrated by the skin necroses which often afflict patients with protein C deficiency when they are put on Warfarin anticoagulant therapy (see below).

(c) Factor V_a and protein C activation

When human plasma is brought to coagulate in vitro by the addition of Ca^{2+} ions, factor V is first activated to V_a by thrombin (cf. [58–61] and Ch. 2A). However, on prolonged incubation the factor V_a is degraded in a way that implies that activated protein C is involved. Salem et al. [62] have recently demonstrated that this is due to factor V_a participating as a cofactor in the thrombin-catalysed activation of protein C. Salem et al. subsequently demonstrated that the isolated light chain of factor V_a retained full cofactor activity [63]. Thrombomodulin was estimated to be at least 20 times more effective as cofactor in protein C activation, than was the light chain of factor V_a. An important difference between the two cofactors is that factor V_a does not inhibit the procoagulant activity of thrombin [63]. In contrast to human factor V_a, bovine factor V_a has no cofactor activity [64] and it is also well established that in bovine serum the factor V activity is much more stable than it is in human serum.

The light and heavy chains of human factor V_a are linked non-covalently in the presence of Ca^{2+} ions [58,60,65]. If the Ca^{2+} is complexed by EDTA, the two chains dissociate and the factor V_a procoagulant activity is lost. Protein C has several Gla-dependent Ca^{2+}-binding sites and one with higher affinity that is not Gla-dependent. Thus, it is not surprising that the interactions between protein C and thrombin are considerably affected by Ca^{2+} ions. In the thrombin–thrombomodulin system the non-Gla-dependent Ca^{2+}-binding site in protein C must be saturated for rapid activation [37]. In the thrombin–factor V_a system the role of Ca^{2+} ions is complex [64,66]. Thus, Ca^{2+} ions inhibit the protein C activation when factor V_a is used as the thrombin cofactor, whereas it has virtually no effect when the isolated factor V_a light chain is used. In contrast to the thrombin–thrombomodulin system, activation of protein C by thrombin, with the light chain of factor V_a as cofactor, progressed more slowly if the protein C lacked the Gla region [64]. Another observation that may be of physiological importance is that, under certain conditions, thrombomodulin and factor V_a act synergistically on the surface of endothelial cells [66]. In this context it should be borne in mind that factor V is synthesized in endothelial cells [67].

(5) Function of protein C as an anticoagulant

Of utmost importance for the rapid advance of our knowledge on the function of protein C was the discovery that the activated protein C is identical to auto-prothrombin IIA [44], which is known to be a strong anticoagulant [44–50].

In 1977, Kisiel et al. [68] reported of the anticoagulant effect of activated protein C and demonstrated that it was obviated by prior incubation of the enzyme with diisopropylphosphorofluoridate (DFP) or phenylmethanesulphonyl fluoride (PMSF). They also found that activated protein C inactivated bovine factor V by limited proteolysis, and that the reaction depended on the presence of phospholipid and calcium ions. Two years later, Walker et al. [14] demonstrated that activated protein C selectively inactivated the thrombin-activated form of bovine factor V, whereas intact factor V was relatively resistant to degradation.

Factor V_a is an important non-enzymatic cofactor in the activation of prothrombin by factor X_a, which occurs on the surface of negatively charged phospholipids in the presence of Ca^{2+} (cf. [25,69–72] and Ch. 3). The factor V_a molecule and the surrounding negatively charged phospholipid serve as a receptor for factor X_a, e.g., on the surface of platelets (cf. [73–77] and Ch. 6). The selective degradation of factor V_a on the platelets by activated protein C destroys the receptor function of factor V_a, and consequently inhibits prothrombin activation [43,78,79]. When factor X_a is bound to factor V_a the latter is protected from degradation by activated protein C, suggesting that factor X_a sterically protects the peptide bonds in factor V_a that are susceptible to activated protein C [14,15,43,78,80].

Factor V circulates as a 330-kDa single-chain precursor molecule which has little cofactor activity [58,60,72,81–83]. Limited proteolysis of factor V by catalytic amounts of thrombin (Fig. 4) activates the pro-cofactor to a biologically active cofactor (cf. [58,60,61,72,81–83] and Ch. 2A). Presumably the factor V activity measured prior to activation is the result of partial activation of factor V in the

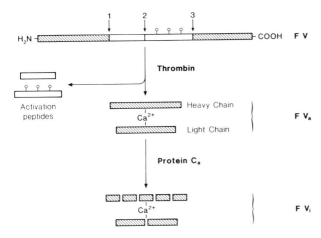

Fig. 4. Activation of factor V by thrombin and inactivation by protein C. Numbered vertical arrows above factor V denote peptide bonds cleaved by thrombin on activation of factor V to factor V_a. The shaded parts form the heavy ($M_r = 105\,000$) and the light chain ($M_r = 71\,000$–$74\,000$) of factor V_a, held
Fig. 3. Blood clotting cascade and the protein C anticoagulant system.
two activation peptides formed. Protein C_a inactivates factor V_a to factor V_i by several proteolytic cleavages in both chains of factor V_a. The number and the exact positions of the cleavages have not been determined, although the heavy-chain cleavages are probably the most important ones for the inactivation.

assay. Factor V_a consists of two polypeptide chains, a heavy chain (M_r 105 000) and a light chain (M_r 74 000). In the presence of Ca^{2+} ions the two chains associate non-covalently. The light chain bears the phospholipid-binding site of factor V_a [15,76,86,87]. In bovine factor V_a both the heavy and the light chains were found to be degraded by activated protein C [14,79,88], whereas in the human system the heavy chain is degraded much more rapidly [15]. In both species the loss of factor V_a activity is the result of the heavy-chain cleavage [15,88]. The cleaved light chain of bovine factor V_a retains full biological activity [88]. In both human and bovine factor V_a the heavy chain is degraded to several fragments ranging in molecular weight from 20 to 70 kDa, whereas the light chain is cleaved to two fragments with apparent M_r of 50 and 25–30 kDa. The only notable difference in the two species seems to be the higher sensitivity of the bovine factor V_a light chain for proteolysis by activated protein C.

Factor VIII:c is a cofactor to factor IX_a in the activation of factor X on the phospholipid surface (cf. [69–71] and Ch. 3). Factors V and VIII:c thus seem to have analogous functions in the activation of prothrombin and factor X, respectively. It is therefore interesting that the two proteins have sequence similarities indicating that they are homologous (cf. [89] and Ch. 2A and 2B). In 1980, Vehar and Davie [90] reported that bovine activated protein C inactivated bovine factor VIII:c by limited proteolysis in a reaction that required phospholipid and Ca^{2+}. By analogy with factor V, the thrombin-activated bovine factor VIII:c was more susceptible to degradation by activated protein C than was unactivated factor VIII:c. The same results have also been obtained with human factor VIII:c [16,91]. In recent years, factor VIII:c has been highly purified both from bovine [90], porcine [92], and human [91,93–98] plasma but most preparations are apparently partially proteolytically degraded and the structural organisation of the factor VIII:c molecule is still preliminary (see Ch. 2B for more details). Thrombin-activated human factor VIII:c, when analysed by SDS–polyacrylamide gel electrophoresis, showed fragments similar to those obtained by thrombin activation of factor V (cf. Ch. 2A and 2B). The generation of a 92-kDa polypeptide correlated with the increase in factor VIII:c activity [94,98], by analogy with the formation of the heavy chain of factor V_a. Factor VIII:c polypeptides with M_r of 79000–80000 and 71000–72000 were suggested to be the structural analogues to the light phospholipid-binding chain of factor V_a [94]. Human activated protein C selectively cleaved the 92-kDa factor VIII:c species, cleavage correlated with the loss of activity [91]. Similar findings were also reported by Vehar and Davie for the degradation of bovine factor VIII:c by activated protein C [90]. These results, together with the reported sequence homology between factor V and factor VIII:c [89], point to a strong structural and functional analogy between these two cofactors, and activated protein C apparently degrades both in a similar way.

A very important property of activated protein C is its high selectivity favouring the degradation of phospholipid-bound, thrombin-activated, forms of both factor V and factor VIII:c [14–16,90,91]. Thus, activated protein C when infused into experimental animals or endogenously formed by infused thrombin, does not affect the concentrations of the circulating procofactors, i.e., factor V and factor VIII:c [99,100]. In this context it is also important to note that in vitro and in vivo activated protein C is inactivated very slowly by its physiological inhibitor [99,101–103] (see below). This suggests that activated protein C not only has a local regulatory function on blood coagulation but that it also has a systemic anticoagulant effect. Under physiological conditions a delicate balance exists between the rate of formation of activated cofactors (V and VIII:c) in vivo, and the concentration of local or circulating activated protein C. Disturbance of this balance will result either in an increased tendency to thrombus formation or in an enhanced anticoagulant effect. In this context it should be mentioned that Emekli and Ulutin [104] have found that activated protein C has a protective effect on experimental disseminated coagulation in animals.

The vitamin K-dependent part of activated protein C is essential for its function and binds the protein to the phospholipid surface. Recently, Esmon et al. [37] demonstrated that Gla-domainless protein C (formed by limited proteolysis using chymotrypsin) has no anticoagulant effect.

6. Protein S, a cofactor to activated protein C

Walker [105–107] has presented evidence that the function of activated protein C is regulated by another vitamin K-dependent plasma protein called protein S.

Protein S is a single-chain 70–80-kDa protein [108–111] with a plasma concentration of approximately 25 mg/l [111]. About 60% of protein S in human plasma circulates in a 1:1 non-covalently linked complex with C4b-binding protein [112–115], which is an important regulator of the rate of activation of the classical complement pathway [116]. The functional significance of this interaction for the regulation of the complement and coagulation systems is still largely unknown [111–115]. In contrast to the other vitamin K-dependent coagulation proteins, protein S does not seem to be a serine protease since it cannot be activated by e.g. trypsin [109–111]. Bovine protein S seems to have a higher affinity for Ca^{2+} and for negatively charged phospholipids than protein C [117]. When studying the degradation of bovine factor V by activated protein C [105], Walker found that plasma contained a cofactor to activated protein C. He identified the cofactor as protein S which had just been purified to homogeneity. The cofactor function of protein S is most pronounced in experiments using low concentrations of phospholipid [6,105–107,118], or when platelets are used instead of the phospholipid [119]. The effect of protein S in the inactivation of factor V_a by activated protein C has been attributed to an enhancement by protein S of the binding of activated protein C to phospholipid vesicles [6,105–107]. It has been suggested that protein S and activated protein C form a 1:1 complex on the phospholipid surface [6,107]. In this context it is interesting to note that a single peptide bond close to the NH_2-terminal of protein S is very susceptible to cleavage by thrombin [111]. The Gla-containing peptide is linked to the large COOH-terminal fragment by a disulphide bridge [111]. Thrombin-modified protein S has lost much of its calcium-binding capacity [111,120] and has no activated protein C cofactor activity in the degradation of phospholipid-bound factor V_a [6,118,120]. Both human and bovine activated protein C has been observed to be species specific, e.g. when assayed by an activated partial thromboplastin (APT) time [12,49,50,68]. Thus, bovine activated protein C did not influence the APT time when added to human plasma. However, when bovine protein S was added together with bovine activated protein C, the species specificity was lost [106]. Furthermore, bovine activated protein C, added to bovine plasma from which protein S had been removed by immunoadsorption, exhibited very little anticoagulant activity [6]. These results show that protein S is an important cofactor to activated protein C.

7. A protease inhibitor for activated protein C

An inhibitor for activated protein C was identified in human plasma by Marlar and Griffin [101]. On addition of activated protein C to plasma, its activity was reduced to less than 25% of the preincubation activity in approximately 30 min. Thus the inhibitor inhibited activated protein C very slowly in vitro, in comparison with the previously studied protease inhibitors in human plasma. Comp et al. [99] have also found that active protein C is cleared very slowly from the circulation in dogs.

The inhibitor for activated protein C was recently purified from human plasma and characterized by Suzuki et al. [102,103,121]. The starting material for the purification was plasma from which the vitamin K-dependent plasma proteins had been removed by barium citrate adsorption. The subsequent purification steps were polyethylene glycol fractionation, followed by chromatographies on DEAE–Sepharose, dextran sulphate agarose, gel filtration on Ultrogel AcA 44 and DEAE–Sephacel. The purification steps, up to the dextran sulphate agarose chromatography, are the same as used for the purification of human factor V [60]. Generous use of DFP and benzamidine seems to be required as in factor V purification procedures. The overall recovery of protein C inhibitor was 9%, and 0.4 mg of purified inhibitor was obtained per litre plasma.

The purified protein C inhibitor was separated into two biologically active fractions by chromatography on DEAE–Sephacel [102]. It did not react with antisera against α_1-antitrypsin, α_1-antichymotrypsin, antithrombin III, inter-α-trypsin inhibitor, α_2-plasmin inhibitor, α_2-macroglobulin or C_1-esterase inhibitor. A monospecific antiserum against protein C inhibitor completely precipitated the protein C inhibitor activity in plasma, suggesting that protein C inhibitor is the functionally important protein C inhibitor in vivo. The inhibitor is non-competitive and forms a 1:1 complex with activated protein C. The inhibitor constant is 58 nM [102].

The rate of complex formation between activated protein C and protein C inhibitor increases in the presence of heparin. However, the optimum heparin concentration is higher than required for rapid inhibition of thrombin by antithrombin III [103,121]. The complex between activated protein C and protein C inhibitor is stable during SDS–polyacrylamide gel electrophoresis and has an apparent M_r of 102 000. It is slowly cleaved at neutral pH, and a degraded, inactive inhibitor ($M_r = 54 000$) is formed, while the protease regains activity. Nucleophilic agents such as hydroxylamine rapidly cleave the enzyme–inhibitor complex. The inhibitor thus seems to be functionally similar to α_1-antitrypsin and antithrombin III. The NH_2-terminal acid sequence does not show any homology to antithrombin III, heparin cofactor II or APC-binding protein [121].

8. Protein C and fibrinolysis

An involvement of protein C in fibrinolysis was first found by Zolton and Seegers, who demonstrated that it stimulated fibrinolysis in dogs, and suggested that the activated protein C depressed the function of plasmin inhibitors [122]. More recently Comp and Esmon [123] found that infusion of physiological concentrations of activated bovine protein C into dogs increased the lysis rate of clots formed from postinfusion blood. This effect was primarily caused by increased concentrations of tissue plasminogen activator in the blood [7,123]. Treatment of dog blood in vitro with activated bovine protein C, and infusion of the treated blood after the protein C had been neutralized by antibodies, also resulted in increased plasminogen activator concentrations, suggesting that the involvement of activated protein C in the release of the plasminogen activator is indirect [123]. Fibrinolysis is also stimulated when protein C is activated in vivo. Thus, infusion of small doses of thrombin into dogs is followed by an increased concentration of circulating plasminogen activator [99]. The role of protein C in fibrinolysis is unclear, and may differ from one species to another. Thus, recent experiments on squirrel monkeys [100] have failed to demonstrate an effect on fibrinolysis by activated protein C (cf. Ch. 8).

9. Determination of the plasma concentration of protein C

Several immunological methods have been used to measure the concentration of protein C in plasma. In 1981, Griffin et al. [124] successfully used the Laurell rocket technique, supplemented with ^{125}I-labelled antiprotein C antibodies, to make the first identification of protein C deficiency in a patient. They later reported that the protein C concentration is approximately 4 mg/l plasma [125], a value since confirmed in studies from other laboratories [126–129]. Stenflo et al. [126] used a modification of the Laurell rocket technique, in which the immunoprecipitates were enhanced by a second peroxidase-conjugated goat antirabbit IgG antiserum. Although other laboratories have since successfully used ordinary protein-stained Laurell rocket techniques [127,129–131], enhancement of the immunoprecipitates makes the assays more sensitive. Protein C in plasma has also been measured by radioimmunoassay [128]. More sensitive and specific assays using well-defined monoclonal antibodies and peptide-specific antisera are currently under development in several laboratories, but have so far not been published.

Several functional assays have recently been developed for protein C [127,128,132,133] and have proved useful in the identification of patients with functionally abnormal protein molecules, but with a normal protein C concentration as determined by immunological methods [127,128,133,134]. In the assay described by Francis and Patch [132], protein C is separated from its inhibitor by barium citrate adsorption. After elution it is activated by thrombin. The thrombin is then inhibited by antithrombin III and the amount of activated protein C is estimated by its anticoagulant activity in a partial thromboplastin time assay. Bertina et al. [133] used a similar approach, but measured the activated protein C with a chromogenic substrate (S2266). In an assay described by Sala et al. [128], the protein C in the barium eluate is activated by a thrombin–thrombomodulin mixture. After inhibition of the thrombin, the amidolytic activity of activated protein C is measured using a chromogenic substrate (S2266). In the approach used by Comp et al. [127], protein C is activated directly in plasma by the thrombin–thrombomodulin complex. The activated protein C is then immunoadsorbed with a solid-phase polyclonal antiprotein C antibody and measured using a chromogenic substrate (S2238). The assay of Comp et al. [12] measures both acarboxy protein C (formed under dicoumarol treatment), and carboxylated protein C, whereas, owing to the barium or $Al(OH)_3$ adsorption, the other 3 assays are capable of measuring carboxylated protein C only. The measurement of the activated protein C by its inhibitory activity in a partial thromboplastin time assay, distinguishes the method of Francis and Patch [132] from the other 3 methods [127,128,133] and may prove useful in the identification of protein C species that are functionally defect in, for instance, factor V or factor VIII:c binding, but have full amidolytic activity.

(a) Protein C deficiency

The mean plasma concentration of protein C in healthy adults is approximately 4 mg/l, with 95% of the values encountered lying between 70% and 150% of the mean value [124–129]. No differences relating to age, sex, or normal pregnancy have been found [131]. Concentrations around 30% of the adult value (with a 95% range of 18–57%) have been found in normal full-term infants [131].

During oral anticoagulant therapy with vitamin K-antagonistic drugs such as Warfarin and dicoumarol, the concentration of protein C antigen in plasma decreases to approximately 40% of its pretreatment value [124–133]. Abnormal, acarboxy protein C, with poor Ca^{2+}-binding properties is found in plasma during treatment with, for instance, Warfarin [135], and the concentration of functionally active protein C is thus lower than that indicated by the immunological assays [127,128,132,133]. Upon initiation of anticoagulant therapy, the fall in protein C concentration (both antigen and functional activity) is more rapid than that of factors II, IX and X and similar to that of factor VII [135,136]. From experience with infusion of protein C into an infant with homozygous protein C deficiency, it appears that the half-life of protein C is approximately 8 h [136]. The more rapid decrease in protein C concentrations than in those of the other vitamin K-dependent clotting factors (II, IX and X) has been suggested as the cause of the severe skin necroses that may develop in heterozygous protein C-deficient patients after the initiation of oral anticoagulant therapy with vitamin K-antagonistic drugs [137–139]. The current hypothesis is that the temporary imbalance between procoagulant and anticoagulant vitamin K-dependent proteins results in the progressive local venular thrombosis that is characteristic of coumarin necrosis.

Low concentrations of protein C antigen have also been demonstrated in patients with disseminated intravascular coagulation, adult respiratory distress syndrome, or chronic liver disease [125,131,132,140]. In hepatocellular disorders and vitamin K deficiency (e.g. coumarin therapy) the concentrations of all of the vitamin K-dependent plasma proteins are decreased. Low concentrations of protein C resulting from any of these conditions may be distinguished from hereditary specific protein C deficiency (see below) by relating the protein C antigen concentration to the concentration of one of the other vitamin K-dependent proteins [124,130].

Griffin et al. [124] were the first to find a family with recurrent venous thromboembolism during early adulthood in conjunction with a low protein C concentration. The proband had 40% of the normal protein C antigen concentration.

Several similar patients and families have since been identified in various laboratories, both in the U.S.A. and in Europe [127–131,133,134,137–152]. Among individuals with heterozygous protein C deficiency, there is a very high incidence of venous thrombosis and pulmonary embolism during early adulthood. Broekmans et al. [143] studied 18 heterozygous patients from 3 families, and reported that by the age of 30 more than half of the protein C-deficient patients had suffered from venous thromboembolism. However, in another family with a homozygous newborn infant (see below) and with 14 heterozygous for protein C deficiency, there was no history of thrombosis among the heterozygotes [129]. The pattern of inheritance is consistent with an autosomal dominant trait with variable expression. As previously discussed, the heterozygotes for protein C deficiency have an increased incidence of skin necrosis after initiation of oral anticoagulant therapy [137–139]. Recently, patients with venous thromboembolism and functionally abnormal protein C but with normal protein C antigen concentrations, have been identified [127,128,133,134]. Often, patients with venous thromboembolism are treated with oral anticoagulants when referred to a coagulant laboratory. The heterozygotes for protein C deficiency can be identified in this group, for instance, by estimating the ratios of protein C to factor X or of protein C to prothrombin [124,130]. Altogether the identification of protein C deficiency in patients on anticoagulant therapy is less reliable than in untreated patients.

Homozygous protein C deficiency (unmeasurable protein C concentration, i.e., below 5% of normal) has recently been described in a newborn infant with massive venous thrombosis [129]. The proband died shortly after birth and the autopsy showed extensive venous thrombosis, although no thrombi were found in the arteries. Two siblings of the proband had died in the neonatal period. The parents were first cousins and both had heterozygous protein C deficiency. Other infants manifesting homozygous protein C deficiency have been reported [129, 136,142,151,152], one of whom was succesfully treated with protein C-rich factor IX concentrates [151] and another one with fresh plasma [152]. Another newborn with a coumarin-responsive chronic relapsing purpura fulminans and inherited protein C deficiency (protein C concentration of 6%) was described by Branson et al. [142]. Such cases as these demonstrate that severe isolated protein C deficiency is incompatible with life.

Approximately 50% of heterozygous protein C-deficient individuals develop thrombosis, which suggests that additional factors may be involved. In a recent report Scully et al. [146] indicate that in the unstimulated platelets from a protein C-deficient patient there was an increase in the number of prothrombinase-binding sites, although whether this is a general phenomenon in protein C deficiency remains to be established. Other factors such as the protein S concentration or the amount of protein S complexed to C4b-binding protein [111–113], may also exacerbate any tendency to thrombosis in protein C-deficient individuals. Comp et al. [153] recently identified two related youths, who both had thrombosis and protein S deficiency; they had reduced protein S antigen concentrations and apparently no free protein S in plasma. The small amount of protein S antigen detected in their plasma was complexed with the C4b-binding protein. To elucidate in detail the clinical significance of protein S and its complex with C4BP, independent measurements of free and complexed protein S are required as well as a functional assay for protein S.

10. Concluding remarks

During the last couple of years a rapid increase in the understanding of the regulation of blood coagulation has been witnessed. Much of this development has centred around protein C, which is now recognized as a most important regulator of blood coagulation. The role of protein C was definitely established when certain families with hereditary tendency to develop venous thrombosis in young adulthood were found to have protein C deficiency. The most dramatic illustration of the role of protein C has been obtained in the few children, who apparently have been homozygous for protein C deficiency and who developed fatal thrombosis during the first week of life.

The activation of protein C by thrombin bound to the endothelial cell cofactor thrombomodulin illustrated the importance in the regulation of haemostasis of the large endothelial cell surface to blood volume in the capillary bed. It has also given us an example of how the substrate specificity of a serine protease can be altered by another macromolecule i.e. the conversion of thrombin from a coagulant protein into an anticoagulant (protein C activator) by complex formation with thrombomodulin.

The anticoagulant activity of activated protein C is due to degradation of factors V_a and VIII_a by limited proteolysis. It now seems to be established that another vitamin K-dependent plasma protein, protein S, is required as a cofactor to protein C in vivo. Unlike the other vitamin K-dependent plasma proteins protein S is not a serine protease. Little is known about its mode of action. Recently the term 'the protein C anticoagulant system' has been used to emphasize that several components are involved together with protein C. We are now only in the beginning of the elucidation of this pathway and it seems safe to predict that hitherto unrecognized proteins will ultimately prove important as modulators of protein C activity. The rapid development in this field of research holds promise for an improvement in our ability to find out the causes of thrombosis in affected individuals and may ultimately enable successful intervention by the clinician, based on rational appreciation of cause and effect.

References

1 Kisiel, W. and Davie, E.W. (1981) Methods Enzymol. 80, 320–332.
2 Seegers, W. (1981) Semin. Thromb. Hemostas. 7, 257–262.
3 Esmon, C.T. (1983) Blood 62, 1155–1158.
4 Stenflo, J. (1984) Semin. Thromb. Hemostas. 10, 109–121.

5 Esmon, C.T. and Esmon, N.L. (1984) Semin. Thromb. Hemostas. 10, 122–130.

6 Walker, F.J. (1984) Semin. Thromb. Hemostas. 10, 131–138.

7 Comp, P.C. (1984) Semin. Thromb. Hemostas. 10, 149–153.

8 Griffin, J.H. (1984) Semin. Thromb. Hemostas. 10, 162–166.

9 Gardiner, J.E. and Griffin, J.H. (1983) in: Progress in Hematology (Brown , E.B., Ed.) Vol. 13, pp. 265–278, Grune and Stratton, New York.

10 Comp, P.C. (1984) Surv. Synth. Pathol. Res. 3, 31–37.

11 Stenflo, J. (1976) J. Biol. Chem. 251, 355–363.

12 Kisiel, W. (1979) J. Clin. Invest. 64, 761–769.

13 Sugo, T., Björk, I., Holmgren, A. and Stenflo, J. (1984) J. Biol. Chem. 259, 5705–5710.

14 Walker, F.J., Sexton, P.W. and Esmon, C.T. (1979) Biochim. Biophys. Acta 571, 333–342.

15 Suzuki, K., Stenflo, J., Dahlbäck, B. and Teodorsson, B. (1983) J. Biol. Chem. 258, 1914–1920.

16 Marlar, R.A., Kleiss, A.J. and Griffin, J.H. (1982) Blood 59, 1067–1072.

17 Bajaj, S.P., Rapaport, S.I., Maki, S.L. and Brown, S.F. (1983) Prep. Biochem. 13, 191–214.

18 Comp, P.C., Nixon, R.R. and Esmon, C.T. (1984) Blood 63, 15–21.

19 Kisiel, W., Ericsson, L.H. and Davie, E.W. (1976) Biochemistry 15, 4893–4900.

20 Miletich, J.P., Leykam, J.F. and Broze, G.J. (1983) Blood 62, Suppl. 1, 306a.

21 Foster, D. and Davie, E.W. (1984) Proc. Natl. Acad. Sci. (U.S.A.) 81, 4766–4770.

22 Long, G.L., BeLagaje, R.M., MacGillivray, R.T.A. (1984) Proc. Natl. Acad. Sci. (U.S.A.) 81, 5653–5656.

23 Fernlund, P. and Stenflo, J. (1982) J. Biol. Chem. 257, 12170–12179.

24 Stenflo, J. and Fernlund, P. (1982) J. Biol. Chem. 257, 12180–12190.

25 Jackson, C.M. and Nemerson, Y. (1980) Annu. Rev. Biochem. 49, 765–811.

26 Huschka, P.V., Lian, J.B. and Gallop, P.M. (1975) Proc. Natl. Acad. Sci. (U.S.A.) 72, 3925–3929.

27 Price, P.A., Otsuka, A.S., Poser, J.W., Kristaponis, J.K. and Raman, N. (1976) Proc. Natl. Acad. Sci. (U.S.A.) 73, 1447–1451.

28 Drakenberg, T., Fernlund, P., Roepstorff, P. and Stenflo, J. (1983) Proc. Natl. Acad. Sci. (U.S.A.) 80, 1802–1806.

29 Fernlund, P. and Stenflo, J. (1983) J. Biol. Chem. 258, 12509–12512.

30 McMullen, B.A., Fujikawa, K. and Kisiel, W. (1983) Biochem. Biophys. Res. Commun. 115, 8–14.

31 McMullen, B.A., Fujikawa, K., Kisiel, W., Sasagawa, T., Howald, W.N., Kwa, E.Y. and Weinstein, B. (1983) Biochemistry 22, 2875–2884.

32 Sugo, T., Fernlund, P. and Stenflo, J. (1984) FEBS Lett. 165, 102–106.

33 Kurachi, K. and Davie, E.W. (1982) Proc. Natl. Acad. Sci. (U.S.A.) 79, 6461–6464.

34 Choo, K.H., Gould, K.G., Rees, D.J.G. and Brownlee, G.G. (1982) Nature (London) 299, 178–180.

35 Leytus, S.P., Chung, D.W., Kisiel, W., Kurachi, K. and Davie, E.W. (1984) Proc. Natl. Acad. Sci. (U.S.A.) 81, 3699–3702.

36 Blow, D.M. (1971) Enzymes 3, 185–212.

37 Esmon, N.L., DeBault, L.E. and Esmon, C.T. (1983) J. Biol. Chem. 258, 5548–5553.

38 Esmon, C.T. and Owen, W.G. (1981) Proc. Natl. Acad. Sci. (U.S.A.) 78, 2249–2252.

39 Lewis, J.H. and Szeto, I.L.F. (1962) J. Lab. Clin. Med. 60, 261–273.

40 Izak, G. and Galewsky, K. (1966) Thromb. Diath. Haemorrh. 16, 228–242.

41 Esmon, C.T., Stenflo, J., Suttie, J.W. and Jackson, C.M. (1976) J. Biol. Chem. 251, 3052–3056.

42 Amphlett, G.W., Kisiel, W. and Castellino, F.J. (1981) Biochemistry 20, 2156–2161.

43 Dahlbäck, B. and Stenflo, J. (1980) Eur. J. Biochem. 107, 331–335.

44 Seegers, W.H., Novoa, E., Henry, R.L. and Hassouna, H.I. (1976) Thromb. Res. 8, 543–552.

45 Mammen, E.F., Thomas, W.R. and Seegers, W.H. (1960) Thromb. Diath. Haemorrh. 5, 218–250.

46 Seegers, W.H., McCoy, L.E., Groben, H.D., Sakuragawa, N. and Agrawal, B.L. (1972) Thromb. Res. 1, 443–460.

47 Seegers, W.H., Marlar, R.A. and Walz, D.A. (1978) Thromb. Res. 13, 233–243.

48 Herman, G.E., Seegers, W.H. and Henry, R.L. (1978) Thromb. Haemostas. 40, 61–65.

49 Marciniak, E. (1970) Science 170, 452–453.

50 Marciniak, E. (1972) J. Lab. Clin. Med. 79, 924–934.

304

51 Owen, W.G. and Esmon, C.T. (1981) J. Biol. Chem. 256, 5532–5535.
52 Busch, P.C. and Owen, W.G. (1982) in: Pathology of the Endothelial Cell (Possel, H.L. and Vogel, H.J., Eds.) pp. 97–101, Academic Press, New York.
53 Esmon, N.L., Owen, W.G. and Esmon, C.T. (1982) J. Biol. Chem. 257, 859–864.
54 Johnson, A.E., Esmon, N.L., Lane, T.M. and Esmon, C.T. (1983) J. Biol. Chem. 258, 5554–5560.
55 Morita, T., Isaacs, B.S., Esmon, C.T. and Johnson, A.E. (1984) J. Biol. Chem. 259, 5694–5704.
56 Esmon, C.T., Esmon, N.L. and Harris, K.W. (1982) J. Biol. Chem. 257, 7944–7947.
57 Esmon, N.L., Carrol, R.E. and Esmon, C.T. (1983) J. Biol. Chem. 258, 12238–12242.
58 Esmon, C.T. (1979) J. Biol. Chem. 254, 964–973.
59 Nesheim, M.E. and Mann, K.G. (1979) J. Biol. Chem. 254, 1326–1334.
60 Dahlbäck, B. (1980) J. Clin. Invest. 66, 583–591.
61 Suzuki, K., Dahlbäck, B. and Stenflo, J. (1982) J. Biol. Chem. 257, 6556–6564.
62 Salem, H.H., Broze, G.J., Miletich, J.P. and Majerus, P.W. (1983) Proc. Natl. Acad. Sci. (U.S.A.) 80, 1584–1588.
63 Salem, H.H., Broze, G.J., Miletich, J.P. and Majerus, P.W. (1983) J. Biol. Chem. 258, 8531–8534.
64 Salem, H.H., Esmon, N.L., Esmon, C.T. and Majerus, P.W. (1984) J. Clin. Invest. 73, 968–972.
65 Guinto, E.R. and Esmon, C.T. (1982) J. Biol. Chem. 257, 10038–10043.
66 Maruyama, J., Salem, H.H. and Majerus, P.W. (1984) J. Clin. Invest. 74, 224–230.
67 Cerveny, T.J., Fass, D.N. and Mann, K.G. (1984) Blood 63, 1467–1474.
68 Kisiel, W., Canfield, W.M., Ericsson, L.H. and Davie, E.W. (1977) Biochemistry 16, 5824–5831.
69 Davie, E.W., Fujikawa, K., Kurachi, K. and Kisiel, W. (1979) Adv. Enzymol. 48, 277–318.
70 Stenflo, J. and Suttie, J.W. (1977) Annu. Rev. Biochem. 46, 157–172.
71 Nemerson, Y. and Furie, B. (1980) CRC Crit. Rev. Biochem. 9, 45–85.
72 Nesheim, M.E., Katzmann, J.A., Tracy, P.B. and Mann, K.G. (1981) Methods Enzymol. 80, 249–274.
73 Dahlbäck, B. and Stenflo, J. (1978) Biochemistry 17, 4938–4945.
74 Kane, W.H. and Majerus, P.W. (1982) J. Biol. Chem. 257, 3963–3969.
75 Tracy, P.B., Nesheim, M.E. and Mann, K.G. (1981) J. Biol. Chem. 256, 743–751.
76 Miletich, J.P., Jackson, C.M. and Majerus, P.W. (1977) Proc. Natl. Acad. Sci. (U.S.A.) 74, 4033–4036.
77 Tracy, P.B. and Mann, K.G. (1983) Proc. Natl. Acad. Sci. (U.S.A.) 80, 2380–2384.
78 Comp, P.C. and Esmon, C.T. (1979) Blood 54, 1272–1281.
79 Tracy, P.B., Nesheim, M.E. and Mann, K.G. (1983) J. Biol. Chem. 258, 662–669.
80 Nesheim, M.E., Canfield, W.M., Kisiel, W. and Mann, K.G. (1982) J. Biol. Chem. 257, 1443–1447.
81 Kane, W.H. and Majerus, P.W. (1981) J. Biol. Chem. 256, 1002–1007.
82 Nesheim, M.E., Myrmel, K.H., Hibbard, L. and Mann, K.G. (1979) J. Biol. Chem. 254, 508–517.
83 Katzmann, J.A., Nesheim, M.E., Hibbard, L.S. and Mann, K.G. (1981) Proc. Natl. Acad. Sci. (U.S.A.) 78, 162–166.
84 Foster, B.W., Tucker, M.M., Katzmann, J.A. and Mann, K.G. (1983) J. Biol. Chem. 258, 5608–5613.
85 Nesheim, M.E., Foster, W.B., Hewick, R. and Mann, K.G. (1984) J. Biol. Chem. 259, 3187–3196.
86 Higgins, D.L. and Mann, K.G. (1983) J. Biol. Chem. 258, 6503–6508.
87 van de Waart, P., Bruls, H., Hemker, C. and Lindhout, T. (1983) Biochemistry 22, 2427–2432.
88 van de Waart, P., Bruls, H., Hemker, H.C. and Lindhout, T. (1984) Biochim. Biophys. Acta 799, 38–44.
89 Fass, D., Hewick, R., Knutson, G., Nesheim, M. and Mann, K. (1983) Thromb. Haemostas. 50, 255.
90 Vehar, G.A. and Davie, E.W. (1980) Biochemistry 19, 401–410.
91 Fulcher, C.A., Gardiner, J.E., Griffin, J.H. and Zimmermann, T.S. (1984) Blood 63, 486–489.
92 Fass, D.N., Knutson, G.J. and Katzmann, J.A. (1982) Blood 59, 594–600.
93 Fulcher, C.A. and Zimmerman, T.S. (1982) Proc. Natl. Acad. Sci. (U.S.A.) 79, 1648–1652.
94 Fulcher, C.A., Roberts, J.R. and Zimmerman, T.S. (1983) Blood 61, 807–811.
95 Fay, P.J., Chavin, S.I., Schroeder, D., Young, F.E. and Marder, V.J. (1982) Proc. Natl. Acad. Sci. (U.S.A.) 79, 7200–7204.

96 Hamer, R.J., Besser-Visser, N.H. and Sixma, J.J. (1983) Thromb. Haemostas. 50, 108.
97 Rotblat, F., O'Brien, D.P., Middleton, S.M. and Tuddenham, E.G.D. (1983) Thromb. Haemostas. 50, 108.
98 Kuo, G., Craine, B., Masiarz, F., Rall, L., Truett, M., Valenzuela, P., Nordfang, O. and Ezban, M. (1983) Thromb. Haemostas. 50, 262.
99 Comp. P.C., Jacocks, R.M., Ferrell, G.L. and Esmon, C.T. (1982) J. Clin. Invest. 70, 127–134.
100 Colucci, M., Stassen, J.M. and Collen, D. (1984) J. Clin. Invest. 74, 200–204.
101 Marlar, R.A. and Griffin, J.H. (1980) J. Clin. Invest. 66, 1186–1189.
102 Suzuki, K., Nishioka, J. and Hashimoto, S. (1983) J. Biol. Chem. 258, 163–168.
103 Suzuki, K., Nishioka, J., Kusumoto, H. and Hashimoto, S. (1984) J. Biochem. 95, 187–195.
104 Emekli, N.B. and Ulutin, O.N. (1980) Haematologica 65, 644–651.
105 Walker, F.J. (1980) J. Biol. Chem. 255, 5521–5524.
106 Walker, F.J. (1981) Thromb. Res. 22, 321–327.
107 Walker, F.J. (1981) J. Biol. Chem. 256, 11128–11131.
108 DiScipio, R.G., Hermodson, M.A., Yates, S.G. and Davie, E.W. (1977) Biochemistry 16, 698–706.
109 DiScipio, R.G. and Davie, E.W. (1979) Biochemistry 18, 899–904.
110 Stenflo, J. and Jönsson, M. (1979) FEBS Lett. 101, 377–381.
111 Dahlbäck, B. (1983) Biochem. J. 209, 837–846.
112 Dahlbäck, B. and Stenflo, J. (1981) Proc. Natl. Acad. Sci. (U.S.A.) 78, 2512–2516.
113 Dahlbäck, B. (1983) Biochem. J. 209, 847–856.
114 Dahlbäck, B. and Hildebrand, B. (1983) Biochem. J. 209, 857–863.
115 Dahlbäck, B., Smith, C.A. and Müller-Eberhard, H.J. (1983) Proc. Natl. Acad. Sci. (U.S.A.) 80, 3461–3465.
116 Nussenzweig, V. and Melton, R. (1981) Methods Enzymol. 80, 124–133.
117 Nelsestuen, G.L., Kisiel, W. and DiScipio, R.G. (1978) Biochemistry 17, 2134–2138.
118 Suzuki, K., Nishioka, J. and Hashimoto, S. (1983) J. Biochem. 94, 699–705.
119 Suzuki, K., Nishioka, J., Matsuda, M., Murayama, H. and Hashimoto, S. (1984) Biochem. J. 96, 455–460.
120 Walker, F.J. (1984) J. Biol. Chem. 259, 10335–10339.
121 Suzuki, K. (1984) Semin. Thromb. Hemostas. 10, 154–161.
122 Zolton, R.P. and Seegers, W.H. (1973) Thromb. Res. 3, 23–33.
123 Comp, P.C. and Esmon, C.T. (1981) J. Clin. Invest. 68, 1221–1228.
124 Griffin, J.H., Evatt, B., Zimmerman, T.S., Kleiss, A.J. and Wideman, C. (1981) J. Clin. Invest. 68, 1370–1373.
125 Griffin, J.H., Mosher, D.F., Zimmerman, T.S. and Kleiss, A.J. (1982) Blood 60, 261–264.
126 Stenflo, J., Dahlbäck, B., Fernlund, P. and Suzuki, K. (1982) in: Pathobiology of the Endothelial Cell (Nossel, H.L. and Vogel, H.J., Eds.) pp. 103–119, Academic Press, New York.
127 Comp, P.C., Nixon, R.R. and Esmon, C.T. (1984) Blood 63, 15–21.
128 Sala, N., Owen, W.G. and Collen, D. (1984) Blood 63, 671–675.
129 Seligsohn, U., Berger, A., Abend, M., Rubin, L., Attias, D., Zivelin, A. and Rapaport, S.I. (1984) New Engl. J. Med. 310, 559–562.
130 Bertina, R.M., Broekmans, A.W., Van der Linden, I.K. and Mertens, K. (1982) Thromb. Haemostas. 48, 1–5.
131 Mannucci, P.M. and Vigano, S. (1982) Lancet 2, 463–464.
132 Francis, R.B. and Patch, M.J. (1983) Thromb. Res. 32, 605–613.
133 Bertina, R.M., Broekmans, A.W., Krommenhoek-van Es, C. and van Wijngaarden, A. (1984) Thromb. Haemostas. 51, 1–5.
134 Barbui, T., Finazzi, G., Mussoni, L., Riganti, M., Donati, M.B., Colucci, M. and Collen, D. (1984) Lancet 6, 819.
135 Vigano, S., Mannucci, P.M., Solinas, S., Bottasso, B. and Mariani, G. (1984) Br. J. Haematol. 57, 213–220.
136 Epstein, D.J., Bergum, P.W. and Rapaport, S.I. (1983) Circulation 68, 316.
137 Broeckmans, A.W., Bertina, M.R., Loelinger, E.A., Hofmann, V. and Klingemann, H.G. (1983) Thromb. Haemostas. 49, 251.

138 McGehee, W.G., Klotz, T.A., Epstein, D.J. and Rapaport, S.I. (1984) Ann. Intern. Med. 100, 59–60.

139 Samama, M., Horellou, M.H., Soria, J., Conard, J. and Nicolas, G. (1984) Thromb. Haemostas. 51, 132–133.

140 Rodeghiero, F., Mannucci, P.M., Vigano, S., Barbui, T., Gugliotta, L., Cortellaro, M. and Dini, E. (1984) Blood 63, 965–969.

141 Pabinger-Fasching, I., Bertina, R.M., Lechner, K., Niessner, H. and Korninger, Ch. (1983) Thromb. Haemostas. 50, 810–813.

142 Branson, H., Katz, J., Marble, R. and Griffin, J.H. (1983) Lancet 2, 1165–1168.

143 Broekmans, A.W., Veltkamp, J.J. and Bertina, R. (1983) New Engl. J. Med. 309, 340–344.

144 Horellou, M.-H., Conard, J., Bertina, R.-M. and Samama, M. (1983) Presse Méd. 12, 2259.

145 Bercoff, E., Morcamp, D., Bourreille, J., Borg, J.Y., Piquet, H., Sovia, J., Soria, C. and Dorner, M. (1984) Presse Méd. 13, 49.

146 Scully, M.F., Ellis, V., Melissari, E. and Kakkar, V.V. (1984) Thromb. Haemostas. 51, 407.

147 Broekmans, A.W., van der Linden, I.K., Veltkamp, J.J. and Bertina, R.M. (1983) Thromb. Haemostas. 50, 350.

148 Griffin, J.H., Bezeaud, A., Evatt, B. and Mosher, D. (1983) Blood 62, 301a.

149 Marciniak, E., Wilson, H.D. and Marlar, R.A. (1983) Blood 62, 303a.

150 Marlar, R.A. and Endres-Brooks, J. (1983) Thromb. Haemostas. 50, 351.

151 Marlar, R.A., Sills, R.H. and Montgomery, R.R. (1983) Blood 62, 303a.

152 Estellés, A., Garcia-Plaza, I., Dasi, A., Aznar, J., Duart, M., Sanz, G., Pérez-Requejo, J.L., Espana, F., Jimenez, C. and Abeledo, G. (1984) Thromb. Haemostas. 52, 53–56.

153 Comp, P.C., Nixon, R.R., Copper, M.R. and Esmon, C.T. (1984) J. Clin. Invest. 74, 2082–2088.

R.F.A. Zwaal and H.C. Hemker (Eds.), *Blood Coagulation*
© 1986 Elsevier Science Publishers B.V. (Biomedical Division)

CHAPTER 10

Interplay between medicine and biochemistry

H. COENRAAD HEMKER

University of Limburg, Biomedical Centre, Maastricht (The Netherlands)

Medical science, not surprisingly, flowers at the interface of medicine and science. Its bloom thus results from the confrontation of two different cultures. Although it is good custom to emphasize the warm relations between the two, it is of no use to dissimulate the distance that separates doctors and scientists. Indeed the gap is large enough to use the expression 'two cultures' not exclusively as a description of the situation between the sciences and the humanities. There is sufficient reason to maintain that it applies as well to the sciences confronting medicine. A good doctor is primarily interested in the well-being of his patients and uses scientific insight only as one of the tools of his trade. It is rare to find him develop an expert knowledge in a branch of natural science. On the other hand a scientist opts for insight, no matter how delighted he may be to find his results of use in the diagnosis and treatment of the sick. The fundamental difference in attitude between the two makes that the exploration of the interface between science and medicine often is difficult. In fact every symposium or congress in one field or another of human pathobiology teaches us that although doctors and scientists meet frequently, their views only amalgamate with difficulty.

There is good reason to stress this point if one is to discuss the interplay between medicine and science in the field of blood coagulation. There is hardly another subject of study in human biology where the clinics have remained the most important source of information for so long. Whereas e.g. endocrinology or immunology had their science components developed already during the first half of this century, haemostasis research remained the playground of the doctors. There probably are multiple reasons for this, such as the rareness of congenital bleeding disorders, that are the most natural first object of study or the complexity of the problem that presents itself already after the first few experiments, to defy any simplifying hypothesis etc. I would not maintain that blood coagulation per se is more complicated than immunology or endocrinology or any other subject of human pathophysiology. It only presents its complexity right at the beginning of the most simple experiments. This makes people tend to shy away from an attempt at a formal scientific approach. Even in 1962, when I planned to enter the field, my colleague biochemists were shocked to see that I would consider that kettle of fish worthy of my attention. My medical colleagues did not share these objections although they failed to see why I should stop medical practice, while playing around with tubes. At that time the lab carrying most weight in the field of blood coagulation was that in Oxford where R.G. Macfarlane, M.D. and clinical pathologist, together with Rosemary Biggs, Ph.D. and originally a botanist, formed a nucleus around which many medical doctors and several scientists gathered and formed a group that was responsible for many fine contributions. Yet, even there, the application of modern biochemical techniques was less fruitful than the typical coagulation approach, that in essence exists of measuring clotting times in endless permutations and combinations of mixtures. 'After all' Rosemary Biggs used to say 'After all it is more like cooking than like anything else'. In Detroit, Walter Seegers, M.D. and professor of physiology, devoted his life to attempts at purifying prothrombin and other clotting factors. Rereading the articles from this group one is struck by the tremendous amount of work, by the many observations done that can only be explained in the light of our newest knowledge (cf. Ch. 9B). Also by the fact that the results did not even allow the construction of a refutable set of hypotheses.

It must be said that, with all their cooking and curing the doctors had done a good job. By 1960 most of the coagulation 'factors' had been defined as functions lacking in haemophilic disorders. The role of blood platelets had been discerned and the pathology of thrombosis had been described in great detail. A good start had been made with anticoagulant treatment and with the treatment of haemophilia by the use of plasma fractions.

Mentioning the pathology of thrombosis automatically evokes Virchow and the scientists of the 19th and early 20th centuries. What about the interactions between medicine and science in those days? Buchanan (M.D.) was the first to report (1836) that catalytic amounts of clotted blood could coagulate a fibrinogen solution. His fibrinogen solution was prepared involuntarily in the scrotum of patients suffering from a hydrocele. These experiments can – a posteriori – hardly be thought to be conclusive but they did introduce the concept of coagulation by enzymatic conversion that we now know to be correct. In the second half of the 19th century this concept was heavily opposed a.o. by Alexander Schmidt who favoured the idea that fibrin arises from a stoichiometric interaction between blood proteins. Others, like e.g. Hammersten sustained Buchanan's view, often with experimental evidence that up to this moment seems convincing. Nevertheless, even with all the old literature on one's desk it is hard to find out what was really meant. Some workers like Hammersten describe experiments with meticulous precision; others, like Schmidt prefer general considerations but in any case our observation of their results is tinged with our present knowledge. The controversy that dominates the blood coagulation literature in the latter half of the last century is that between those who see fibrin as the product of the catalytic action of thrombin on fibrinogen and those who think fibrin to arise from the stoichiometric action of fibrinogen and a second substance. The gist of this controversy seems to be that at that time no distinction could be made between the functions of thrombin and that of thromboplastin. In trying to repeat the old experiments it often up to this day cannot be made clear in what modern terms they should be explained. The same confusion repeats itself about half a century later when the two functions of thromboplastin are recognised: tissue thromboplastin as we know it and 'blood-thromboplastin' now known to be prothrombinase. With combinations of crude blood fractions and thromboplastin-containing preparations (cells, serum etc.) observations can be made that indeed suggest stoichiometric interactions but others suggestive of enzymatic interaction are possible as well. Join to this that nomenclature in those days was confused to the degree of complete incomprehensibility and that communications often hardly crossed the national borders then one will be hardly surprised by the fact that a communis opinio was not reached until around the turn of the century. After 1876 Schmidt began to accept reluctantly that thrombin might play a role in the generation of fibrin and he postulated that it circulates in the blood in an inactive precursor state.

The type of argument used in the 19th century discussions switched from medical observations to chemical experiments and back with an astonishing ease, especially where, as in the case of Schmidt, the borderline between discussion and speculation faded. Schmidt was a medical doctor and professor of physiology. Hammersten was a chemist. It would in my opinion be unjustified to attribute the difference in style between these two scientist to a difference in discipline. I would rather see it as a question of temper. Temper anyhow spices these discussions, even to a degree that we nowadays would think unpalatable. From the literature of the 19th century the impression remains that doctors and chemists did not work in different worlds but rather cooperated and penetrated each others fields freely. Outside coagulation one might think of the chemist Pasteur who cured rabies or, conversely, of the first generation of biochemists who were almost exclusively medical doctors. Perhaps in those times the new ground to cover was so enormous that one did not bother about subdivisions. Perhaps, on the other hand, we tend to stick too much to our disciplines these days.

In the field of blood coagulation there is a very interesting personality that up to this moment did hardly get the attention he deserves: Cornelis A. Pekelharing (Fig. 1), a medical doctor who became professor of general pathology at the University of Utrecht, The Netherlands, in 1881. In 1894 he described experiments that up to this day can be easily repeated and that demonstrate the existence of prothrombin. By repeated precipitations with NaCl and/or $MgSO_4$ he obtained two fractions from normal plasma, neither of which clotted upon addition of $CaCl_2$ and/or tissue thromboplastin. One of the preparations, however, after these additions acquired the capacity to make the other one clot. Pekelharing drew the correct conclusion: A proenzyme, prothrombin, is converted, under the influence of tissue thromboplastin and $CaCl_2$, into an enzyme, thrombin that can make fibrinogen clot.

To my knowledge this does not only mark the discovery of prothrombin but also is the first demonstration of a proenzyme–enzyme conversion. It thus shows that the work of an M.D. on a medical problem often can yield results that are of seminal importance to biological sciences, to biochemistry in this case. It thus is a per-

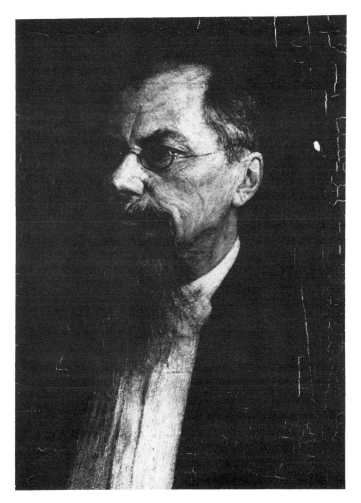

Fig. 1. Cornelis A. Pekelharing (1848–1922).

fect example of one of the main features of the interaction of medicine and chemistry: medical problems are a treasure trove for the biochemist who takes the pain to understand them correctly. Talking with a clinician and trying to understand his problems may be more difficult than running an ultracentrifuge or interpreting kinetic data but it may be at least as fruitful. The traffic between biochemists and medical doctors is often hampered by the failure of either one to try and understand the other's language. Now this can indeed be difficult. I have had the pleasure to work as a clinical assistant in the paediatric clinics of a pioneer of blood coagulation research: Prof. S. van Creveld. The astonishing ease with which he could suggest the most complicated biochemical research on the spur of a patient seen ('After this vacation we will attack von Willebrand's disease') was only rivalled by the astonishing answers that the scientists did indeed find under such guidance. I remind you of the discovery of platelet factor 3 (Paulssen) or the purification of factor VIII (van Mourik). On the other hand scientists tend to impose their way of thinking on their medical colleagues, more often focussing on problems that are likely to be solved than on those that will help to gain insight in pathophysiological mechanisms. Yet, up to this day, the liaisons and cross-fertilisations between scientists and practitioners remain many and varied. We see Prof. Magnusson, M.D., solve the primary structure of prothrombin and Prof. Duckert, Ph. D., solve many problems directly related to patient care. We see the medical doctors continuously improve on the quality of their clinical trials under the continuous criticism of the statisticians and we continue to find patients that help us pose problems of fundamental interest and solve them. It is only relatively recently that the Fletcher and Fleaujac deficiencies led to the discovery of the details of contact activation, that a study of the membrane proteins in congenital thrombopathies gave important clues to the receptor functions in platelets or that the problems of the control of oral anticoagulation inspired the experiments that led to the discovery of carboxyglutamic acid and the mechanism of action of vitamin K.

A 'more than life size' example plays just at this moment (October 1984) in our laboratory while Mrs. Scott is visiting us. Mrs. Scott is an American lady who was treated by Dr. Weiss in New York for a mild thrombopathy that he could define to be a lack of platelet procoagulant activity. Later the group of Dr. Majerus in St. Louis also did experiments with her platelets and they concluded that a membrane protein receptor for the formation of prothrombinase was lacking. On the basis of quite different experiments our group arrived at the conclusion that it is rather the transbilayer lipid movement in platelets that causes platelet procoagulant activity. It makes phosphatidyl serine available at the outside of the membrane, which is crucial to the procoagulant activity of any phospholipid preparation. Now indeed if the platelets of Mrs. Scott can be shown to lack a protein receptor the 'American' view must be deemed right. On the other hand, if Mrs. Scott's platelets do not show phospholipid flip-flop, our concept of PF 3 is the more likely one. So at this moment we are determining whether only prothrombinase-forming capacity is lacking in her platelets or whether the capacity to support the formation of the factor X-converting enzyme is lacking as well. If this is the case, either the receptor is aspecific *or* two receptors are lacking at the same time. We will also see whether or not phosphatidyl serine will show up at the outside of her triggered platelets. In this way we hope to settle a difference in opinion in a way that will convince our American colleagues (cf. Rosing et al. (1985) Blood 65, 1557–1561).

This case is a perfect modern example of the continuous need, also in modern biochemistry, of 'the experiment of nature' that is to be found in the clinics. Also of the continuous need for biochemists alert for rare cases presented by clinicians and of the need for continuous attention from the side of the doctors, in order to find those cases that may help solve scientific problems. Alas it must be said that only a small part of the doctors burdened by an everyday practice have the talent and/or interest to pay attention to this part of medical science. And also that those

312

who do, will often not find a scientist competent and willing to listen to their story and grasp its possible meaning. The fact that such contacts are rare makes one think that much valuable material slips constantly through the hands of the clinicians. This is readily illustrated by the fact that a relatively common disorder like congenital fibrinogen abnormality seems to cluster around places where good coagulation labs are to be found. One wonders how this can be remedied. Making clinical doctors responsible for the research lab, as it used to be done in the past and still is often seen nowadays is, in my opinion, not a good solution. Both tasks are so formidable that one of them – usually the fundamental research – tends to be neglected. Our solution has been to engage people with a clinical training in our research group. These doctors have a part-time function in the hospital and thus help establishing the bridge between the 'two cultures'. It may seem strange that we did not in the first place attempt a link via the routine coagulation lab. This however, was on purpose. More often than not the routine lab shields the clinics from the research department. Only in those cases where the latter is an integral part of the routine laboratory this can be avoided. If the head of the routine lab is not a research scientist with primary interest in the type of problems discussed in this article, the routine lab will not make the necessary 'traits d'union'. The clinician thinks that he has done his duty in sending his samples to 'the lab'. The clinical lab has its duty done if it applies routine tests to these samples and discusses the results with the clinicians and the research interests are nowhere to be seen. If on the contrary the routine lab joins in an existing dialogue between researchers and clinicians their contribution as 'case hunters' may be of great use. I conclude that the interplay between clinics and basic science up to this day is of paramount importance in haemostasis and thrombosis research. We must confess that the difficulties that arise in establishing the necessary links are often of an organisational and psychological nature. Recognising this may be a first step to a solution.

In view of the special subject of this article it is hardly useful to publish a list of references. To the reader interested in the history of blood coagulation research an extensive bibliography of the literature up to around 1900 is available upon request.

Subject index